Medicinal Cannabis

Medicinal Cannabis
Pearls for Clinical Practice

Deborah Malka MD, PhD

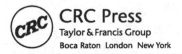

CRC Press
Taylor & Francis Group
Boca Raton London New York

CRC Press is an imprint of the
Taylor & Francis Group, an **informa** business

First edition published 2022
by CRC Press
6000 Broken Sound Parkway NW, Suite 300, Boca Raton, FL 33487–2742

and by CRC Press
2 Park Square, Milton Park, Abingdon, Oxon, OX14 4RN

© 2022 Deborah Malka MD, PhD

CRC Press is an imprint of Taylor & Francis Group, LLC

Library of Congress Cataloging-in-Publication Data
Names: Malka, Deborah, author.
Title: Medicinal cannabis : pearls for clinical practice / Deborah Malka.
Description: First edition. | Boca Raton : CRC Press, 2022. | Includes
    bibliographical references and index.
Identifiers: LCCN 2021030302 | ISBN 9780367565299 (hardback) |
    ISBN 9780367565275 (paperback) | ISBN 9781003098201 (ebook)
Subjects: LCSH: Cannabis—Therapeutic use. | Marijuana—Therapeutic use.
Classification: LCC RM666.C266 M35 2022 | DDC 615.7/827—dc23
LC record available at https://lccn.loc.gov/2021030302

ISBN: 978-0-367-56529-9 (hbk)
ISBN: 978-0-367-56527-5 (pbk)
ISBN: 978-1-003-09820-1 (ebk)

DOI: 10.1201/9781003098201

Typeset in Times
by Apex CoVantage, LLC

Contents

Part I   Introduction and Scientific Background

Part II   Patient Practice Management

Part III Clinical Case Examples for Medical Conditions

Foreword

I am a family physician with over 30 years of practice experience in Northern California. Early in my career I knew I needed to be non-judgmental about my patients' use of cannabis because it is a part of the culture here in my community. I knew people wanted to know about cannabis from a medical perspective and I wanted to be able to provide that information when possible. Thus began my scientific inquiries into the use of cannabis as real medicine, treating real medical problems.

Early on in my work with clinical cannabis, I was lucky enough to meet and collaborate with Deborah Malka. For many years, Dr. Malka and I have had a long-standing relationship regarding the use of cannabis as medicine, both of us enthusiastically learning about using the herb for our patients' best benefit. Over the years, we have continued to share a passion for educating patients and medical professionals on the clinical use of cannabis. Many hours have been spent jointly comparing notes on individual patients with all the science we could discover, and together we have built vast libraries of scientific articles on the subject.

A few years ago, Dr. Malka and I collaborated to create the first online course for professionals covering the clinical use of cannabis. We included a variety of medical conditions and were able to provide continuing education credits to physicians who were willing to take the time to learn. It was a labor of love to put together useful information for physicians interested in this herb, based on good science and our combined clinical experience.

I will never forget the first time I saw a suffering patient use cannabis. Suzanne was being treated for small cell lung carcinoma and bravely going through brutal chemotherapy sessions. She was drained of all energy and had absolutely no appetite, but she continued to do her best to stay upbeat. It was a big day when she agreed to use cannabis for the first time in her life, but she figured she didn't have anything to lose. Her experienced friend fixed her up with a water pipe fashioned from a glass teapot in her kitchen and had her inhale just two short inhalations without asking her to hold her breath. After all, she did have lung cancer.

It took about 5 minutes to take effect. The first change was in her color – she went from sickly gray to alive pink. She began to notice the beautiful view off her deck where we were sitting on that early summer day, and pretty soon was laughing and holding up her end of the conversation just like the old days before chemo. When her husband came home, he looked at her with initial confusion and then, at the sight of the herb on the table, a bit of disapproval. But when she asked him to make her a smoothie – the first food she'd asked for in several days – he dropped his disapproval and headed for the blender. Her response was truly miraculous on many levels, and while cannabis did not cure her cancer, it made those difficult days much easier and more enjoyable. I, as her primary care physician, was sold. A tiny dose of a non-lethal medicine that could make that big a difference? I wanted to know more.

Dr. Malka and I are both well aware that many patients use cannabis, but most do not discuss their use with physicians. Some patients are fearful of judgement. Many assume that their doctor will disagree with the use of the herb and will therefore refuse to treat them when they realize they are "abusing" an illicit substance. In our experience, this unfortunate situation has occurred many times, and stems from many providers' lack of knowledge or understanding.

Cannabis is medicine. But cannabis is not a pharmaceutical with specific limited indications or dosages, and that makes it confusing and strange to medical professionals. The combination of social stigmas and the challenges of recommending and managing herbal medicine are too great for many providers to overcome. While there is science to support the use of cannabis, a majority of scientific articles end their conclusions with "more studies are needed." This does not inspire confidence.

Many physicians are waiting for pharmaceutical companies to extract, synthesize and produce a pill that delivers the "medical aspects" of cannabis. But there is no one part of cannabis that can be considered the medical part. Cannabis is an herb that requires all its parts to be effective, a phenomenon we know as the *entourage effect*. A little more of one part or a little less of another may deliver the desired effects, but we know that synergy is necessary. Cannabis is firmly in the herbal medicine arena and that requires a bit of unfamiliar knowledge on the part of the provider.

Every patient has a unique endocannabinoid system and therefore a unique need and response to cannabis. Each patient is an individual and dosing the herb is truly patient-controlled, adjusted according to need and response. The provider is an essential partner in helping patients discover and manage appropriate use.

Why should medical providers educate themselves on an herbal medicine when their specialty really only requires pharmaceuticals? One clear compelling reason is that cannabis interacts with other medications. Seizure medications may need to be decreased if cannabis is being used, and opioids may need to be decreased if co-treating pain with cannabis. Working with patients who are using cannabis can provide safer treatment plans based on full disclosure. Knowing the potential benefits of appropriate use can more effectively treat many difficult medical problems, providing relief to patients without significant risk. Cannabis used correctly is safe; we simply need more physicians who know how to integrate it into their practice. Patients are willing to learn, but are their providers?

With a dearth of definitive scientific chemistry to rely upon, and countless individual responses, clinical experience is truly the gold standard for the safe and effective use of medical cannabis. And clinical experience is what Dr. Malka brings to the table. Over her years of working with patients with a wide variety of medical problems, she has seen more than most. She has kept track of risks, benefits and the use of cannabis in a variety of different situations. This book is her generous share with you, the reader, of the science she has learned and the clinical pearls she has gathered from constantly studying and from working with her patients. Here, Dr. Malka provides a strong foundation for any provider who is willing to acknowledge their patients' use of cannabis. I honor Dr. Malka for being in the forefront of those recognizing and filling the need to include cannabis as safe and effective medicine, and I commend you, the reader, for finding this reliable guide to the use of cannabis for our patients' best health. May we all benefit!

Stacey Marie Kerr, MD
Santa Rosa, CA

Preface

I make no apology for my orientation toward cannabis as a useful clinical medicinal therapy. I have been immersed in recommending its use for tens of thousands of patients for the past 13 years. When I first started working with patients who wanted a medical marijuana approval in California in 2006, I didn't know much about its medicinal effects. I knew something about herbal medicine and routinely prescribed herbal remedies in my holistic medical practice. Right then, my approach to learning about the utility of cannabis was skewed in a different direction than many physicians who were my colleagues at the time. They were trying to view it as a "medicine" along the lines of a "drug" rather than a botanical therapy: to write a "prescription," recommendation on a piece of paper and their job was done. It was the custom to spend little time with patients, maybe 10 minutes, just long enough to fill out some basic information on the chart and sign a recommendation. Physicians who did this, for the most part, in California, were not only not required to learn anything about cannabis, but they also practiced superficial medicine. Too often the practice was that of a "paper mill," with dollar signs motivating how many patients could be crammed into a clinic day. Sadly, many medical cannabis patient visits involve too little physician–patient interaction, with too sparse physician knowledge on this specialty topic.

As a new cannabis specialist, I was a staff physician for a group of clinics whose founder wanted to add depth to this model. The lead physician wanted to teach his staff about the science and utility of cannabis as a medicine, although we called it marijuana at the time. He was so overloaded from expanding his clinic base to over 30 clinics throughout California serving over 300,000 patients at its apex that he needed someone else to teach the doctors. Fortunately for me, that became my job as Assistant Medical Director, in addition to seeing 100 patients/week. I loved learning! I was trained in research, having gotten a PhD years earlier in Molecular Biology and Human Genetics. I soon began to scour the internet for educational articles about the medicinal effects of cannabis. There was a considerable amount on the chemistry of cannabinoids, many on the (negative) effects of "recreational marijuana," less on the effects of cannabis medicinal use in vitro or in vivo and, finally, a dearth of articles regarding clinical use in humans. I actually went to the stacks of a medical library to look up articles from a now defunct journal – *The Journal of Cannabis Therapeutics*. I was sponsored to go to cannabis educational conferences, national and international, and learned from many knowledgeable speakers. The one thing that the speakers almost all had in common was that their knowledge was derived from basic science, was primarily theoretical in regard to human subjects and clinical knowledge was mostly anecdotal.

I remember attending an international cannabis conference in 2008, where it was queried as to whether cannabis was helpful for attention deficit disorder (ADHD). Many participants had opinions, and some had seen a few cases. I recall sitting there dumbfounded. Did they really have such a paucity of real patient data on a global scale? I asked myself if I should stand up and talk about the approximately three to four cases per month of patients with ADHD who were using medicinal cannabis that I was seeing in the Central Coast of California, which I ultimately did. I didn't have any proof that cannabis was helpful, all I knew was what the patients were telling me. And to this day, that is where I have encountered the greatest learning environment, in working with over 30,000 medical cannabis patients. Each patient story has at least one learning "pearl," shared in this book along with their case reports found in the clinical case examples chapters. I have found that being a student of my patients, combined with my enforced task of having to teach a staff of 40 cannabis physician specialists, resulted in my becoming somewhat of an expert in clinical cannabis. This led me to develop the first comprehensive online CME-approved course for cannabis health professionals – the Clinical Cannabinoid Medicine Curriculum approved by the Postgraduate Institute of Medicine for 12 credits, offered by The Medical Cannabis Institute from 2015 to 2017. We had stellar faculty contributing to the course, yet I feel my greatest contribution was not merely getting it out there for public consumption, but to hold us to a clinical orientation. How to use cannabis for real patients, its pitfalls and challenges, as well as rewards, is still an undercovered topic. Now that some form of medical cannabis is approved in almost all states, doctors and patients throughout the country *Need to Know*. This book is offered in an attempt to fill that void.

Acknowledgments

There are several people who have inspired me to make the effort to put this book out to health care professionals. The first was my medical school mentor, Scott Obenshain, MD, who was then the Dean of Medical Education. When I wanted to bring an Integrative Medicine program to our school, he supported my effort to write a grant for this purpose, opening the resources of his office and helping me to get submission of the grant accomplished. While it was not ultimately funded, I will never forget his belief in me as I have neither truly let go of my desire to broaden medical education. When I wanted to initiate a postgraduate CME program in cannabis medical education, there was one person at the Society of Cannabis Clinicians, a society in which I was then the education director, who cheered this project on. This was David Bearman, MD, a cannabis clinician specialist and activist of long-standing. Fortunately, this was more successful, and our program became the first of its kind to educate thousands of participants. My friend and coeditor of this CME project, Stacey Marie Kerr, MD, spent many long hours with me to achieve the success of this enterprise. I thank her also for writing the Foreword to this book. I am indebted to my colleague and friend, Connie McLaughlin-Miley, Pharm D, for reviewing and editing several of the more challenging scientific chapters in this book. And most of all, I want to acknowledge all the thousands of patients who have been my partners, if not guinea pigs, in discovering the multitude of ways that cannabis can be therapeutic in restoring and maintaining homeostasis in human health.

Author

Deborah Malka, MD, PhD, is a holistic physician with certification in Integrative Holistic Medicine. Prior to clinical practice, Dr. Malka completed her PhD in Human Genetics from Columbia University, and studied both natural and traditional medicine, with degrees from the University of New Mexico School of Medicine and the Santa Fe College of Natural Medicine. She has been supportive of patient empowerment and alternative medicine throughout her career. She practiced as a primary care physician, directing a holistic medical clinic in Aptos, California, for 15 years. Following this, she specialized in cannabis medical consulting serving over 30,000 patients to date. Her private practice, "Cannabis Plus," provided medical cannabis evaluations and natural health consulting with offices in Monterey and Santa Cruz, California. She has been committed to educating the public and professionals about medicinal cannabis, teaching at conferences nationally and internationally. She developed and served as faculty director for the first online CME accredited course in Clinical Cannabinoid Medicine sponsored by the Society of Cannabis Clinicians. She currently provides private cannabis medical consultations and natural health guidance for clients from her home office in New Mexico.

Abbreviations

2-AG – 2-Arachidonoylglycerol
5-HT – 5-Hydroxytryptamine (serotonin)
11-OH-THC – 11-Hydroxy-tetrahydrocannabinol
AE – Adverse effect
AEA – Anandamide (*N*-arachidonoylethanolamide)
ATP – Adenosine triphosphate
CAM – Complementary and alternative medicine
CB – Cannabinoid
CB1 – Cannabinoid receptor type 1
CB2 – Cannabinoid receptor type 2
CBD – Cannabidiol
CBDA – Cannabidiolic acid
CBC – Cannabichromene
CBCA – Cannabichromenic acid
CBDV – Cannabidivarin
CBG – Cannabigerol
CBGA – Cannabigerolic acid
CBN – Cannabinol
CBNA – Cannabinolic acid
CBr – Cannabinoid receptor
COX – Cyclooxygenase
CNS – Central nervous system
CUD – Cannabis use disorder
CYP – Cytochrome P
DA – Dopamine
DDI – Drug–drug interaction
eCB – Endocannabinoid (such as AEA and 2-AG)
EC – Endocannabinoid
ECS – Endocannabinoid system
FAAH – Fatty acid amide hydrolase
FABP – Fatty acid-binding protein
FDA – Food and Drug Administration
GABA – Gamma(γ)-aminobutyric acid
GPCR – G-protein coupled receptor
IL – Interleukin
LOX – Lipoxygenase
MAGL – Monoacylglycerol lipase
MRSA – Methicillin-resistant *Staphylococcus aureus*
NASEM – National Academies of Sciences, Engineering, and Medicine
NSAID – Non-steroidal anti-inflammatory drug
n-AChR – Nicotinic acetylcholine receptor
NF-κ – Nuclear factor kappa

PK – Pharmacokinetic

PPAR – Peroxisome proliferator-activated receptor

REM – Rapid eye movement

ROS – Reactive oxygen species

THC – Tetrahydrocannabinol

THCA – Tetrahydrocannabinolic acid (a THC precursor)

THC-COOH – Tetrahydrocannabinol carboxylic acid (a THC metabolite)

THCV – Tetrahydrocannabivarin

TRPA – Transient receptor potential subfamily A (ion channel)

TRPV – Transient receptor potential vanilloid (ion channel)

TRPM – Transient receptor potential melastin (ion channel)

TNF – Tumor necrosis factor

VA – US Department of Veterans Affairs

Part I

Introduction and Scientific Background

1 The Evolution of Cannabis in Medical Practice

PHYSICIANS' LEGAL STATUS

We begin with recounting the shift that has taken place over the past 20 years; this offered from my vantage point as a physician practicing in California from 2006 to 2018. California was the first state to decriminalize the use of cannabis for patients for whom a medical "recommendation" was written as of 1996. There is a 20+ year history of achievements, challenges and pitfalls that we progressed through in the medical cannabis arena here, culminating in decriminalization for all adult use for those 21 and older, which took effect in 2018 in this state. At first, there were rare few physicians, medical doctors (MDs) or doctors of osteopathic medicine (DOs) who, as required by law, took the risk of signing their name to a recommendation certificate, or even a note written on a prescription pad. Until 2004, the Medical Board of California penalized some physicians who did so by either suspending their license or more often placing them under probation for a period of 3–5 years. Cited infractions included poor documentation, lack of appropriate demonstration that other more traditional approaches had not worked or not reviewing a patient's medical history. This changed in 2004.

On May 7, 2004, the Medical Board of California adopted an informational statement to give further guidance to physicians who may recommend the use of medicinal cannabis to their patients. The statement stressed that physicians would not be subject to investigation or disciplinary action if they arrive at the decision to recommend medicinal cannabis in accordance with accepted standards of medical responsibility that "any reasonable and prudent physician would follow when recommending or approving any other medication or prescription drug treatment."[1] As of 2014, the Board amended the original guidelines to include telehealth visits for the initial visit. Prior to this, an in-person visit was required to meet the standard. Also, most importantly, they began to use the word cannabis instead of marijuana, where previously *Cannabis sativa* consultations were referred to exclusively as medical marijuana. These standards include a history and examination of the patient, development of a treatment plan, informed consent, periodic review (at least annually), consultation as needed and elaboration of the decision to recommend medical cannabis.[1]

In California, for the most part, the mere adoption of these standards was successful at reducing license suspensions. Unfortunately, most physicians doing recommendations during this time, from 2004 up until the present, did not follow these standards, resulting in poor outcomes for the patients and poor reputations

DOI: 10.1201/9781003098201-2

for physicians approving medicinal cannabis. They have been referred to as "pot-docs." Some of us followed these standards and may have gone beyond, incorporating additional medical advice into the visit. Most often, for myself, this included holistically guided basic advice concerning nutrition, exercise, lifestyle and/or mood management. Little did I understand in these early years that these questions are central in determining how a patient will respond to cannabis therapy, reflecting the "endocannabinoid tone" of the patient (discussed in Chapters 2 and 7). One aspect of these standards provided for follow-up and a treatment plan. I incorporated this into a treatment plan including referrals to the appropriate clinician, physician, therapist, chiropractor, etc. It soon became apparent that the standard of practice requiring annual follow-up visits with the cannabis physician was woefully inadequate. This policy has been the greatest detriment to the successful practice of cannabis medicine to date, in my opinion. As the typical cannabis consulting visit was neither billed to nor covered by insurance, especially in these early years, follow-up visits were an out-of-pocket optional expense. In my practice I invited all patients to see me before the year was up, or at least to call with questions or feedback, especially for ongoing management. Maybe 10% of my patients took advantage of this invitation. The lack of support existing in their current medical paradigm or in what was typically advised medically resulted in the patients' undervaluing the benefit of ongoing cannabis care. Often, they would go back to their primary care clinician who knew nothing about what we were trying to achieve with cannabis, and who was frankly suspicious of this quasi-illegal, totally unconventional practice, so these patients were deterred from continuing. Other challenging areas were dosing advice and ensuring the procurement of legitimate, safe cannabis medicine. To understand the evolution of this potential dilemma, we must revisit the dichotomy of cannabis still being a Schedule I drug, while yet giving professional advice about its use. How can this be done legally?

Physicians sought protection under federal law, even though they might be acting in accordance with legislation from their state. The evolution of this protection took several years, put forth in a series of rulings known as "the Conant decisions." The Ninth Circuit US District Court has affirmed that the First Amendment protects physicians' right to recommend or advise that their patients use medicinal cannabis so long as the physicians do not aid and abet or conspire with their patients to violate the federal drug laws. Regarding discussion of marijuana, *Conant v. McCaffrey* (N.D. Cal. 1997) 172 F.R.D. 681) ruled that physicians would be protected from federal penalties if advising patients with cancer, glaucoma, HIV disease and/or seizures or muscle spasms associated with a chronic, debilitating condition, and that physicians would be breaking the law if they were directly involved in helping a patient to acquire marijuana. The judge defined this limit as "criminal conduct" under federal law, meaning "aiding and abetting or conspiracy" to violate federal drug laws.[2] In *Conant v. McCaffrey* (N.D. Cal. 2000) 2000 WL 1281174), it was extended that doctors may recommend marijuana to patients who may benefit from it (i.e., no diagnosis restriction) without fear that federal authorities may revoke their medical license or impose other sanctions. The opinion stated, "[I]t will be the professional opinion of doctors that marijuana is the best therapy or at least should be tried. If such recommendations could not be communicated, then the physician-patient relationship would be seriously impaired."[2] In *Conant v. Walters* (9th Cir. 2002) 309 F.3d 629), the Ninth US Circuit Court of Appeals unanimously ruled that the federal government may not sanction doctors who recommend marijuana therapy to their patients.[3] A review of the legal evolution of medical cannabis written in 2010 explaining federal and state positions provides a more thorough legal history of this paradoxical issue.[4] Cannabis' utility as a medicine was becoming more well known. More states have approved its medical use, growing from one state in 1996 to 36 states plus Washington, DC, by 2020. An additional 11 states have approved the use of CBD extracted from cannabis or hemp as well. Figure 1.1 illustrates the current regulatory status of the United States, by state as of 2021. Please note that there are only three states in which cannabis in any form is still illegal. These are Idaho, Kansas and Nebraska.[5]

Direction given by the California Medical Association (CMA) attempted to further provide guidelines that have also evolved. Originally these instituted a standard whereby dosing was strongly advised to be absent from communication, a hugely untenable position! Guidance taken from the 2009–2011 directive, regarding dispensing advice on what medical cannabis to use tells physicians that their advice may not be too specific, and especially to avoid writing anything may appear as a prescription, or be construed as a type of aiding and abetting. The CMA directive advises that physicians must avoid

> a) Providing cannabis to a patient; b) Describing to a patient how the patient may obtain cannabis . . .; c) Communicating with a cannabis distributor, such as a cannabis dispensary, to confirm a recommendation made to a patient in an office dialogue; d) Offering a specific patient individualized advice concerning appropriate dosage timing, amount, and route of administration.[6]

And so began the irrational practice of recommending the use of cannabis as a medicine, yet being cautioned against giving dosing advice or direction to reputable sources for product. In fact, cannabis dispensaries routinely contacted the physician's office to confirm that a recommendation is valid, a process called verification. Patients were left to do their own research online or learn from friends about how much to take and where to get it. And even worse, they relied on the non-medical "expertise" of the sales agents at dispensaries, so-called "budtenders." For many years there was no formal training, not even available for physicians, patients or budtenders to provide knowledgeable information. Fortunately, that is not the case any longer.

At this time, several states actually require a prescription type of recommendation, with exact determination of delivery method, some with dose suggested, and some counseled not by physicians but by pharmacists. Some states as well require specific medical cannabis continuing medical education (CME) training in order to provide cannabis recommendations. As more states began to decriminalize medical cannabis use, the recommended standards varied between states. To ensure uniformity, in April 2016, the Federation of State Medical Boards (FSMB) adopted guidelines that incorporated most of the aforementioned standards set out by California.[7] The group reviewed marijuana statutes, rules, state medical board

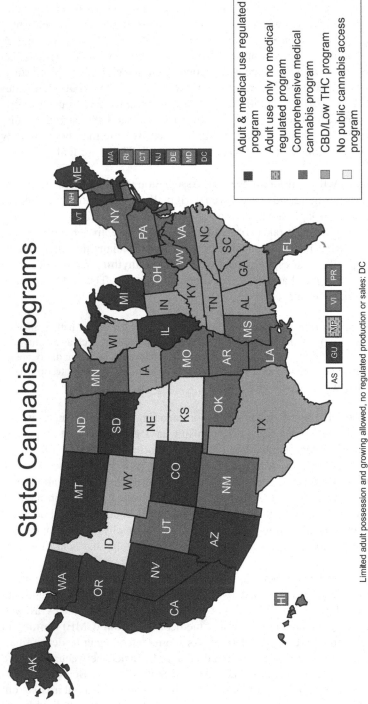

State Cannabis Programs

Adult & medical use regulated program

Adult use only no medical regulated program

Comprehensive medical cannabis program

CBD/Low THC program

No public cannabis access program

November 2020

Limited adult possession and growing allowed, no regulated production or sales: DC

FIGURE 1.1   Current cannabis laws by state.

Source: National Conference of State Legislatures. State Medical Marijuana Laws. As of February 5, 2021. www.ncsl.org/research/health/state-medical-marijuana-laws.aspx.

policies, peer-reviewed articles and policy statements regarding the recommendation of cannabis. A survey of FSMB member boards indicated that the most important issues included guidance on recreational cannabis use by physicians (31.4%), guidance on medical cannabis use by physicians (47.1%) and guidelines for recommending medical cannabis to patients (49%).[7]

As of my opening of a private practice in cannabis consulting, rather than as a staff physician working under a larger umbrella, I was able to slowly change the nature of provider support for my patients. This happened during 2012–2018. This period of time included my presentations at Grand Rounds of several local hospitals. Slowly I began to build a referral base of local practitioners. Nevertheless, the time was ripe for embracing cannabis as a prevalent, viable alternative to pharmaceuticals, and many physicians were interested. The stigma of cannabis medicinal use was decreasing. More and more physicians need and want an educational framework they could trust to help them navigate through the pros and cons of cannabis use in their patients. Then came the opiate crisis. All of a sudden there was an emergent, urgent need for a pain therapy that not only could replace opiates but also could help patients wean off of it. I started getting referrals from pain specialists, primary care physicians, emergency room physicians and psychiatrists. Finally, my cannabis medicine practice was part of a cohesive strategy that my patients' other providers not only knew about but also supported. We were then able to have improved outcomes. Patients did not disappear as often and were not discouraged by their primary health care team from seeking benefit from cannabis. I wish I could say this was the positive end of the story, but there is one more chapter that brings us up to the current situation in California among other states.

This was the advent of adult use decriminalization, now approved in 11 US states. This legalized expansion of access has been much to the detriment of medical cannabis programs. Yet again, patients are left to their own, uninformed, unregulated, often poorly advised status. Now that adults can walk into a dispensary and ask the person behind the counter (far from a medically trained provider), what to get to treat their complaint, we are back to the dark ages of recreational marijuana. Most of my medical cannabis patients have chosen not to renew their medical status with me, erroneously believing that because they are no longer required to do so by law, there's not enough benefit. Yet again, many are using the wrong products, in the wrong amounts, to treat superficial symptoms, while not addressing underlying problems. For instance, in the case of neuropathy with neuropathic pain, if patients find a way to lessen the pain, they no longer feel the need to treat the neuropathy. Cannabis is one of the few products that patients can take that actually is neuroprotective, antioxidant and anti-inflammatory. Thus, over a long-enough period of time, their neuropathy can reverse, or at least slow its trajectory of progression. But who is going to reiterate this approach? Not the budtender, not their primary care provider who doesn't realize what cannabis can do and, sadly, the patient, if they ever understood this nuance will likely have forgotten.

So, as other states in the United States go through this progression of overcoming bias and stigma of cannabis use and recommendation, building up a trust base between patients and their providers, I hope they can learn from California's mistakes. No medicine can be used correctly unless instructions are repeatedly given and understood. If the providers don't yet understand these instructions, how can we expect patients to be more knowledgeable on their own behalf?

CANNABIS MEDICINE IS AN ALTERNATIVE THERAPY

My exposure to herbal medicine during holistic medical training has led me to take a more integrative approach to cannabis as a medicine than most physicians are oriented toward it. There are many terms used somewhat interchangeably to define medicine that incorporates alternative concepts – including holistic, alternative, complementary and integrative. The National Center for Complementary and Alternative Medicine, established in 1998 as a branch of the National Institutes of Health, promoted the term "complementary and alternative medicine" known as CAM. The agency has now evolved into the National Center for Complementary and Integrative Health (NCCIH), which defines these terms as follows; "If a non-mainstream practice is used together with conventional medicine, it's considered 'complementary.' If a non-mainstream practice is used in place of conventional medicine, it's considered 'alternative.'"[8] They specify that complementary health approaches may include biologically based therapies (herbs, foods, vitamins and other dietary supplements, including natural products). Cannabis falls into the category of "natural products" as it is an herbal medicine. The NCCIH now lists cannabis as a therapy for cancer and pain and is sponsoring new research into the medical benefits of cannabinoids. The interest in cannabis and cannabinoids for therapeutic use is growing rapidly. Cannabis is one of the fastest growing natural products for sale in the United States. Currently, consumers spend more money on cannabis than any other CAM product. The sale of cannabidiol (CBD) alone in the United States is in billions of dollars.[9] It is estimated that one in five patients is asking their primary care provider for information about cannabinoids and/or cannabis. With cannabis medicine, not only are we dealing with a natural product but also with an alternative practice with a philosophy that is considered to be outside the scope of traditional medicine – one for which classically trained practitioners lack the expertise to give informed guidance. For a long time, cannabis medicine has not only lived on the fringe of medical therapies, but it also remains today an alternative therapy.

The experience of integrating CAM therapies into traditional practice ensuing over the past 40 years has followed a trajectory similar to what cannabis medicine is now facing. We may be able to learn from the challenges faced by CAM proponents. In a survey of general practice physicians regarding their opinions about CAM in 2010, 76% said they were poorly informed about herbal medicines, 47% said their own knowledge on this topic was very poor or quite poor and 77% feared patients would take herbal medicines without telling them.[10] The consensus of the survey was that physicians lack the resources and training to respond to patients' inquiries about many CAM therapies. Similarly, surveys about physician's attitudes about cannabis medicine have shown like sentiments, reviewed later in this chapter. So, what have we learned from the incorporation of CAM into a traditional medicine practice over the past 40 years? During this time, integrative medicine, which integrates conventional, complementary and alternative medicine and reemphasizes the relationship between health care practitioners and patients, has gained in popularity. This is a newly recognized subspecialty with Board-certified fellows in Integrative and Holistic Medicine approved as of 2014. One can envision that the evolution of cannabis medical expertise may take a similar course, with incorporation of its use into a more comprehensive primary or subspecialty practice.

In questioning why CAM therapies are still on the sidelines, we recall that conventional medicine is structured upon therapies that are evidence based. While scientific evidence exists for some CAM therapies, there are key questions that are yet to be answered. Why has there been so little researched evidence about CAM? One reason for the lack of research in alternative treatments is that large, carefully controlled medical studies are costly and most commonly funded by pharmaceutical companies. This is a case we see all too often in herbal medicine in general, and especially for cannabis research. Research in cannabis medicine, especially for human trials, is additionally hampered by the fact that it is a Schedule I drug – approvals to do research in the United States are hard to come by, the approval process can take many years to achieve and research materials are difficult to obtain. Support for research into cannabis and cannabinoids has been espoused by several significant medical groups, yet human trials have been few, most likely due to the constraints herein outlined. As far back as 1999, the Institute of Medicine (IOM) prepared a report for the White House Office of National Drug Control Policy about health benefits and risks of marijuana and its constituent cannabinoids. They concluded in part as follows:

> Recommendation 1: Research should continue into the physiological effects of synthetic and plant-derived cannabinoids and the natural function of cannabinoids found in the body. Recommendation 2: Clinical trials of cannabinoid drugs for symptom management should be conducted with the goal of developing rapid-onset, reliable, and safe delivery systems. Recommendation 3: Psychological effects of cannabinoids such as anxiety reduction and sedation, which can influence medical benefits, should be evaluated in clinical trials. Recommendation 4: Studies to define the individual health risks of smoking marijuana should be conducted, particularly among populations in which marijuana use is prevalent.[11]

The American College of Physicians produced a position statement in 2008, which said that evidence supports medical use of cannabis, and further

> suggests numerous indications for [use of] cannabinoids. Additional research is needed to further clarify the therapeutic value of cannabinoids and determine optimal routes of administration. The science on medical marijuana should not be obscured or hindered by the debate surrounding the legalization of marijuana for general use.[12]

In 2019, the American Medical Association (AMA) opined:

> We also applaud the Surgeon General's commitment to furthering research on cannabis. . . . Due to legal and regulatory barriers to cannabis and cannabinoid research, physicians and patients do not currently have the evidence needed to understand the health effects of these products and make sound clinical decisions regarding their use.[13]

Now over 20 years later, research results into some of these areas is beginning to emerge. Much of the basic scientific as well as clinical research on cannabis therapeutics has come from outside the United States. Almost all reviews, government-funded workshops and, indeed, scientific consensus suggest that more research needs to be done using cannabis in human trials.

Hard lessons learned from the CAM movement can serve as a roadmap in the growth of cannabis as a medicine. Considering cannabis as a type of CAM therapy may help both patients and health care providers make the paradigm shift from viewing it as a drug of abuse to an alternative medicine. One author's comments on the subject are applicable to the challenge we now face in cannabis practice as clinicians.

> Raw plant-based products such as marijuana often fall under the classification of complementary and alternative medication, partly due to the imprecise estimates of the potentially useful substances. . . . However, traditional medical school pharmacology is focused on a prescriptive pill containing one precisely quantitated chemical element or possibly two, with well-studied efficacy and risks.[14]

PHYSICIAN ATTITUDES ABOUT CANNABIS

Physician attitudes toward patient use of cannabis cover a wide range of evolving responses. An early 1999 article from a family practice journal typifies the primarily negative advice that has prevailed.

> Prolonged use of cannabis leads to a dependence syndrome similar to that of alcohol, affecting approximately one in 10 users. In adolescents, heavy cannabis use is associated with academic underachievement, job instability, problems in family relationships, involvement in crime and use of other illicit substances.[15]

This cautious attitude has continued, mixed with a more informed, practical opinion that has evolved as evidenced by the following opinion.

> Regardless of personal views and perceptions, to deny or disregard the implications of use of this substance on patient health and the infrastructure of the health care system is irresponsible; clinicians must be aware of these implications and informed about how this therapy may influence practice in a variety of health care settings.[16]

In a survey of 1,544 doctors in 2014, 67% thought cannabis should be a medical option. However, they were reluctant to recommend a drug whose form, contents, dosage and type cannot be specified, had concern about adverse effects and possibility for addiction and there was a lack of hard clinical data regarding its efficacy in treating certain conditions.[17] Regarding physician apprehensions about medical cannabis, a poll revealed:

> Several studies over the past decade have ascertained that physicians are apprehensive about adult use of MM [medical marijuana]. This reluctance appears to be driven by the potential for side effects, scant high-quality scientific data, unclear dosage guidelines, and a lack of regulatory oversight by the FDA, unlike other therapeutic and supportive care drugs.[18]

In a comprehensive review of health professionals' beliefs, knowledge and concerns surrounding medicinal cannabis, 15,775 studies were retrieved and a final 26 were included. It was found,

> The general impression was that health professionals supported the use of medicinal cannabis in practice; however, there was a unanimous lack of self-perceived knowledge surrounding all aspects of medicinal cannabis. Health professionals also voiced concern regarding direct patient harms and indirect societal harms.[19]

Several common themes have emerged in studies of physicians' beliefs in surveys of clinicians in multiple settings, especially in states that have adopted medical cannabis programs. Familiarity with it and ability to provide guidance remains a challenge. Almost all reflected a need for more education. Specific feedback are as follows:

1. Little familiarity with the state program and a modest knowledge of the endocannabinoid system (New York).[20]
2. Lack of training opportunities. Low knowledge and comfort level related to recommending medical cannabis (Washington).[21]
3. Not convinced of marijuana's health benefits and believe its use carries risks. Few are comfortable with the topic. Need for more education (Colorado).[22]
4. Provider knowledge gaps about the effectiveness of medical cannabis for qualifying conditions need to be addressed. Concern about addiction, safety, legality (Minnesota).[23]
5. Most were not likely to recommend marijuana to their patients. Concern about legality and addiction (Ohio).[24]
6. Lack of guidance, concern about dosing, risks. Need for more education (Canada).[25]

There are now some more progressive attitudes.

> [P]rimary care physicians (PCPs) are faced with more patients seeking information on medical cannabis. Even if the PCP is not prescribing medical cannabis, their patients may be using it and providers should be able to discuss the pros and cons of cannabis use and help to monitor for improvements and for potential adverse outcomes.[26]

And regarding those physicians who take a "don't ask, don't tell" stance about cannabis, one author opined:

> I have come to see willful ignorance about cannabinoids as a form of patient abandonment. The message to the patient seems to be figure it out yourself and do not tell me about it. Such a stance is not consistent with the highest values and aspirations of medicine.[27]

Recommendations of how to be informed about cannabis medical therapeutics may be summarized in the following conclusions:

1. Patients/consumers need to be educated about medical efficacy and appropriate use.

12

2. Physicians need more (ANY) education about medical cannabis, herbal medicine in general and the endocannabinoid system.
3. Evidence-based research goes a long way toward acceptance in the conventional medical community.
4. Research restrictions are in transition, slowly lifting.
5. More communication is needed between patients and their providers about their health care choices.

CANNABIS MEDICAL EDUCATION

There is broad agreement that more education about cannabis, cannabinoids and the endocannabinoid system is needed. In a study of how US physicians who actually practice cannabis medicine are educated, self assess their knowledge and describe their practice, it was found that physicians gained knowledge through conferences (71%), the medical literature (64%) and websites (62%). As much as 56% felt that there was sufficient information available to practice cannabis medicine. The authors conclude:

> Findings of this study suggest the need for more formal education and training of physicians in medical school and residency, more opportunities for cannabis-related continuing medical education for practicing physicians, and clinical and basic science research that will inform best practices in cannabis medicine.[28]

The Cannabis and Cannabinoids Knowledge Assessment Survey (CCKAS) of 55 physicians, of whom half were in clinical practice, found that 64% reported self-education via the internet, literature and other means, 33% said that they rely on online CME resources and 22% take live CME. Only 21% received such training in an academic setting and said they are not using any form of training to better understand cannabis/cannabinoids. The survey revealed physicians exhibit significant knowledge gaps regarding safety, pharmacological activity of cannabinoids and FDA regulations.[29]

The push for cannabis medical education has received much attention in Canada, where medical cannabis has been nationally decriminalized. A physician survey reported 79% had been approached by a patient and/or his/her family to discuss the use of cannabis medicine, and 66% had medical cannabis patients. Physicians showed a preference for online education and peer-reviewed summaries on specific medical cannabis subtopics. The authors conclude, "Our results support the need for further medical education and training on CTP [cannabis for therapeutic purposes]."[25] A leading proponent of cannabis medical education in Canada and globally comments:

> The global regulatory landscape regarding the medical use of cannabis and cannabinoids is changing rapidly. . . . We propose a "cannabis curriculum" that covers the spectrum of historical, botanical, physiological, clinical and legal issues to allow health care professionals to engage in meaningful discussions with their patients and colleagues around this stigmatized and controversial subject.[30]

The situation in US medical education is stark, there is little to no academic instruction for physicians. A reviewer of this topic – regarding physicians' cannabis and/or cannabinoid education states:

They didn't learn about it in medical school, and, because it is not a US Food and Drug Administration – approved drug backed by randomized controlled trials, they can't turn to the Physicians' Desk Reference for information about dosage, indications, and contraindications.[31]

The opinion goes on to point out that physicians lack the basic knowledge to even distinguish among cannabinoids, and the fact that while THC "makes marijuana users high," CBD does not.[31] A survey of physicians in Washington State revealed that 77% thought MC (medical cannabis) should be included in undergraduate medical curricula, 87% thought MC should be included in graduate medical curricula and 96% thought continuing medical education on MC should be available. The authors comment: "Currently, MC and the endocannabinoid system are rarely if ever part of health care providers' graduate or postgraduate training, and Continuing Medical Education (CME) opportunities exist but are scarce."[21] As aforementioned, CME is available, but what about medical school training? An inquiry into the 2015–2016 AAMC (Association of American Medical Colleges) curriculum revealed that only 9% had any content on medical cannabis, while two-thirds reported that their graduates were not prepared to prescribe it.[32] As of 2017, the directors of the curriculum of the 157 accredited American medical schools were asked if they teach about the endocannabinoid system (ECS) or had education in cannabis. None taught endocannabinoid science as an organized course, and only 21 of the 157 schools surveyed had the ECS mentioned in any course.[33] The relevance of the ECS in understanding human health and disease cannot be underestimated! This important topic is presented in Chapter 3. It is imperative that this topic be included in all health professionals' training, minimally as a component of a comprehensive Human Physiology course. In addition, as patients are encouraged to discuss their interest in medical cannabis with their providers, the need for informed decision-making requires the incorporation of this topic into medical and pharmaceutical training. Hopefully, it will be without the bias of old that presents cannabis as a drug of abuse without therapeutic benefit.

REFERENCES

1. Medical Board of California. Guidelines for the recommendation of cannabis for medical purposes. April 2018. www.mbc.ca.gov/Download/Publications/guidelines-cannabis-recommendation.pdf Accessed July 15, 2020.
2. Conant v. McCaffrey. Opinion. Case Text website. https://casetext.com/case/conant-v-mccaffrey-1 Accessed December 5, 2020.
3. Conant v. Walters. Opinion. Case Text website. https://casetext.com/case/conant-v-walters Accessed December 5, 2020.
4. Eddy M. CRS Report for Congress. Medical marijuana: review and analysis of federal and state policies. April 2, 2010. https://fas.org/sgp/crs/misc/RL33211.pdf Accessed July 15, 2020.

5. National Conference of State Legislatures. State medical marijuana laws. 2021. www. ncsl.org/research/health/state-medical-marijuana-laws.aspx Accessed February 5, 2021.

6. CMA On-call: The California Medical Association's Information-on-Demand Service. Document #1315 CMA Legal Counsel. The Compassionate Use Act of 1996: the medical marijuana initiative. January 2009. www.cmanet.org Accessed June 10, 2011.

7. Federation of State Medical Boards. Report of the FSMB Workgroup on Marijuana and Medical Regulation. Model guidelines for the recommendation of marijuana in patient care. Adopted as policy by the Federation of State Medical Boards April 2016. www. fsmb.org/siteassets/advocacy/policies/model-guidelines-for-the-recommendation-of-marijuana-in-patient-care.pdf Accessed July 15, 2020.

8. NCCIH National Center for Complementary and Integrative Health. Complementary, alternative, or integrative health: what's in a name? www.nccih.nih.gov/health/complementary-alternative-or-integrative-health-whats-in-a-name Accessed July 15, 2020.

9. Mikulic M. Total U.S. cannabidiol (CBD) product sales 2014–2022. Statista website. November 5, 2020. www.statista.com/statistics/760498/total-us-cbd-sales/ Accessed December 5, 2020.

10. Ventola CL. Current issues regarding complementary and alternative medicine (CAM) in the United States part 1: the widespread use of CAM and the need for better-informed health care professionals to provide patient counseling. *PT*. 2010;35(8):461–468.

11. Joy JE, Watson SJ Jr, Benson JA Jr, eds. Institute of Medicine. *Marijuana and Medicine: Assessing the Science Base*. Washington, DC: National Academies Press (US); 1999.

12. American College of Physicians. Supporting research into the therapeutic role of marijuana. Philadelphia: American College of Physicians; 2008: Position Paper. www.acponline. org/acp_policy/policies/supporting_research_therapeutic_role_of_marijuana_ 2016.pdf Accessed December 5, 2020.

13. Harris PA. President, American Medical Association. AMA applauds surgeon general's advisory on cannabis. August 29, 2019. www.ama-assn.org/press-center/ama-statements/ ama-applauds-surgeon-general-s-advisory-cannabis Accessed December 5, 2020.

14. Schrot RJ, Hubbard JR. Cannabinoids: medical implications. *Ann Med*. 2016;48(3): 128–141.

15. Walling AD. How should physicians counsel patients about cannabis use? *Am Fam Physician*. 1999;59(7):1985.

16. Bridgeman MB, Abazia DT. Medicinal cannabis: history, pharmacology, and implications for the acute care setting. *PT*. 2017;42(3):180–188.

17. Rappold S. Legalize medical marijuana, doctors say in survey. April 2, 2014. Webmd website. www.webmd.com/pain-management/news/20140225/webmd-marijuana-survey-web#1 Accessed December 5, 2020.

18. Adler JN, Colbert JA. Clinical decisions. Medicinal use of marijuana: polling results. *New Engl J Med*. 2013;368(22):e30.

19. Gardiner KM, Singleton JA, Sheridan J, Kyle GJ, Nissen LM. Health professional beliefs, knowledge, and concerns surrounding medicinal cannabis: a systematic review. *PLoS ONE*. 2019;14(5):e0216556.

20. Sideris A, Khan F, Boltunova A, et al. New York physicians' perspectives and knowledge of the state medical marijuana program. *Cannabis Cannabinoid Res*. 2018;3:74–84.

21. Carlini BH, Garrett SB, Carter GT. Medicinal cannabis: a survey among health care providers in Washington state. *Am J Hosp Palliat Care*. 2017;34(1):85–91.

22. Kondrad E, Reid A. Colorado family physicians' attitudes toward medical marijuana. *J Am Board Fam Med*. 2013;26(1):52–60.

23. Philpot LM, Ebbert JO, Hurt RT. A survey of the attitudes, beliefs and knowledge about medical cannabis among primary care providers. *BMC Fam Pract*. 2019;20(1):17.

24. Lombardi E, Gunter J, Tanner E. Ohio physician attitudes toward medical cannabis and Ohio's medical marijuana program. *J Cannabis Res.* 2020;2:16.
25. Ziemianski D, Capler R, Tekanoff R, et al. Cannabis in medicine: a national educational needs assessment among Canadian physicians. *BMC Med Educ.* 2019;15:52.
26. Slawek D, Meenrajan SR, Alois MR, et al. Medical cannabis for the primary care physician. *J Prim Care Community Health.* 2019;10:1–7.
27. Strouse TS. Cannabinoids in medical practice. *Cannabis Cannabinoid Res.* 2016;1(1): 38–43.
28. Takakuwa KM, Mistretta A, Pazdernik VK, Sulak. Education, knowledge, and practice characteristics of cannabis physicians: a survey of the Society of Cannabis Clinicians. *Cannabis Cannabinoid Res.* 2021;6(1):58–65.
29. Neurology Reviews. Survey identifies gaps in physician knowledge about cannabis and cannabinoids. www.neurologyreviewsdigital.com/neurologyreviews/nord_march_2020/MobilePagedArticle.action?articleId=1566841#articleId1566841 Accessed July 15, 2020.
30. Ware MA, Ziemianski D. Medical education on cannabis and cannabinoids: perspectives, challenges, and opportunities. *Clin Pharmacol Ther.* 2015;97(6):548–550.
31. Rubin R. Medical marijuana is legal in most states, but physicians have little evidence to guide them. *JAMA.* 2017;317(16):1611–1613.
32. Evanoff AB, Quan T, Dufault C, Awad M, Bierut LJ. Physicians-in-training are not prepared to prescribe medical marijuana. *Drug Alcohol Depend.* 2017;180:151–155.
33. Allen DB. Survey shows low acceptance of the science of the ECS (endocannabinoid system) at American medical schools. www.outwordmagazine.com/inside-outword/glbt-news/1266-survey-shows-low-acceptance-of-the-science-of-the-ecs-endocannabinoid-system Accessed July 15, 2020.

2 Cannabis as a Botanical Medicine

HISTORY OF CANNABIS AS A MEDICINAL PLANT

The history of cannabis use as a medicine documents its source as a botanical medicine in many early cultures. Its first recorded medical use was around 2300 BC in China. The Chinese called cannabis "tai-ma" (great hemp) or "chu-ma" (meaning female hemp) possibly indicating that they knew that the female variety had medicinal properties. Cannabis was listed in the Ayurvedic Materia Medica, and Egyptian medical texts as far back as 1000 BC. Many other ancient cultures such as the Persians, Greeks, East Indians, Romans and the Assyrians documented cannabis medicinal application for the control of muscle spasms, reduction of pain and for indigestion, among other uses. Cannabis as a name for this plant likely came later, with Cana – Sanskrit for hemp, Bis – bosma, Aramaic for fragrant and cannabis – kannabis, Greek for hemp.[1] The cultivation of this plant has been spread worldwide as a source of food, energy, fiber and medicinal preparations. Cannabis as a medicine was common throughout most of the modern world in the 1800s. It was used as the primary pain reliever until the invention of aspirin. In 1890, England's *Lancet* journal said cannabis extract was good for neuralgia, fits, migraine and psychosomatic disorders. Extracts, tinctures and herbal packages of cannabis manufactured by many drug companies were available in any pharmacy from about 1850 until 1942 when the US pharmacopeia eliminated cannabis from its listing.[2] The 1918 United States Dispensatory described cannabis as such:

> Cannabis is used in medicine to relieve pain, to encourage sleep, and to soothe restlessness. Its action upon the nerve centers resembles opium, although much less certain, but it does not have the deleterious effect on the secretions. As a somnifacient it is rarely sufficient by itself, but may at times aid the hypnotic effect of other drugs. For its analgesic action it is used especially in pains of neuralgic origin, such as migraine, but is occasionally of service in other types. As a general nerve sedative it is used in hysteria, mental depression, neurasthenia, and the like. It has also been used in a number of other conditions, such as tetanus and uterine hemorrhage, but with less evidence of benefit. One of the great hindrances to the wider use of this drug is its extreme variability.[3]

As far as dosing is concerned, it said:

> The only way of determining the dose of an individual preparation is to give it in ascending quantities until some effect is produced. The fluid extract is perhaps as useful a preparation as any; one may start with two or three minims of this three times a day, increasing one minim every dose until some effect is produced.[3]

DOI: 10.1201/9781003098201-3

Today, this guidance holds true, in that dosage is determined in each individual user by slowly titrating up, by the drop if using a tincture, until the most effective level is achieved. We have a better understanding of the therapeutic range now, the active components (multiple active components have been identified) and something about their therapeutic interactions, known as the entourage effect.

Since the beginning of the 20th century, most countries have enacted laws against the cultivation, possession, or transfer of cannabis. Strong public reaction led to a federal anti-marijuana law in 1937, the Marijuana Tax Act. This act placed a tax of $1 for medical use and $100 for recreational use. This was a large factor in why doctors stopped using it as a medicine. After 1937, it became virtually impossible for physicians to obtain or prescribe cannabis preparations for their patients.[4] Thus, the medical profession, as well as patients were denied access to a versatile herbal medicine with a history of therapeutic utility going back thousands of years. It actually did not become federally illegal to prescribe until 1970, when cannabis was placed in a Schedule I category, defining it as having a high potential for abuse, no currently accepted medical use in treatment in the United States and lack of accepted safety for use under medical supervision. Under federal law, Congress defined marijuana to focus on those parts of the cannabis plant that are the source of tetrahydrocannabinol (THC). The US federal code states:

> The term "marihuana" means all parts of the plant *Cannabis sativa* L., whether growing or not; the seeds thereof; the resin extracted from any part of such plant; and every compound, manufacture, salt, derivative, mixture, or preparation of such plant, its seeds or resin. Such term does not include the mature stalks of such plant, fiber produced from such stalks, oil or cake made from the seeds of such plant, any other compound, manufacture, salt, derivative, mixture, or preparation of such mature stalks (except the resin extracted therefrom), fiber, oil, or cake, or the sterilized seed of such plant which is incapable of germination.[5]

Even though the raw plant is devoid of THC, rather its non-psychoactive precursor, tetrahydrocannabinolic acid (THCA) is found in "marijuana" plants; both of these compounds are in a Schedule I class. With industrial hemp characterized by being low in THC, the current legal level for cultivation are plants containing <0.3% THC. This has created confusion in the status of cannabidiol (CBD), which has been available for sale over the counter for many years. The Farm Bill of 2018 has clarified that hemp cultivation and products made from hemp are now federally approved. This does not technically remove all sources of CBD from federal prohibition. If CBD is extracted from a plant with >0.3% THC, the CBD is still considered to be a form of marijuana.[6]

After cannabis was placed into Schedule I, a synthetic version of THC was produced and was approved by the US Food and Drug Administration (FDA) in the 1970s. This drug, Marinol® (dronabinol), contains only synthetic THC and is devoid of the array of cannabinoids, terpenes and flavonoids and other constituents that the whole plant offers. Sativex® (nabiximols) is a full plant extract and was introduced in Europe in 2003 as a legal substance, containing approximately equivalent amounts of THC and CBD. It is more accurately described as an herbal compound than a drug. It wasn't until 1996, when California became the first state to decriminalize the use of cannabis medically that much interest resurfaced in producing cannabis for medicinal purposes. Cannabidiol oral solution/Epidiolex® (liquid), which is highly purified CBD originating from cannabis, has been FDA approved in 2018 for use in certain pediatric seizure disorders.

Now in several countries and states with passage of legalization of cannabis as medicine, we are faced with reintroducing herbal products into an industry that is regulated by single drug, allopathic standards. Currently, 37 states and the District of Columbia have passed medical marijuana laws (see Figure 1.1). The use of cannabis as an herbal medicine is undergoing a resurgence at a grassroots level.

WHAT IS AN HERBAL/BOTANICAL MEDICINE?

One of the most relevant distinguishing features in understanding how to use cannabis therapeutically is to be mindful that it is a botanical or herbal medicine in contrast to a pharmaceutical medicine. Often the terms botanical and herbal are used interchangeably. The distinction is that a botanical is a substance obtained from a plant, while an herbal refers to a specific use of the botanical – as it is used for food, medicine, flavoring or perfume. So medicinal plants fall more specifically under the herbal category. Physicians and other practitioners of conventional medicine are not only more familiar with the use of pharmaceuticals but also entrained in the paradigm of one drug-one outcome conditioning, with accompanying dosing expectations. These concepts simply do not apply here. Physicians are in a position of acting as gatekeepers to approve the use of cannabis as a medicine, yet few are trained in herbal prescribing. In fact, the allopathic approach, not considering the array of effects of herbals on human physiology, does not embrace the full complexity of this plant medicine. There are significant differences between an herbal medicine and a drug. Cannabis has paradoxically been termed a "drug" of abuse; however, it is not a drug! Most simply, a drug is made from purified chemical(s) and is most often composed of a single substance. In fact, it is estimated that many drugs (up to 70%) have been derived from botanical progenitors. Active ingredients in drugs are generally more concentrated than in plants. This is in contrast to herbal medicines that may contain dozens of therapeutic ingredients at lower doses. In general, herbs have a greater safety profile than drugs, causing less adverse effects and are less likely to cause adverse interactions with other pharmaceuticals. Most herbal compounds can be used as an adjunct to concurrent pharmaceutical use, and/or may reduce the dosage of some medications.

Herbalists believe that all the elements are in balance within a plant and it's important to keep them together. Remedies are extracted from roots, stalks, leaves and flowers of plants. An herbal formulation can include the fresh or dried herb or herb part, whole, chopped or powdered, or a concentrated form of the herb usually made via extraction by a solvent such as water, ethanol, glycerin or an organic solvent. Herbs often have nutritional value and are assimilated as food for the body. Herbs can balance the metabolism in a general way in addition to having specific therapeutic properties. Herbs may be matched to a person's constitution, thus making an herbal therapy individualized. The use of plants may promote the linkage of

patients to their environment, facilitating a healing process encompassing a therapeutic ecology.[7]

Herbal medicine has been used for over 5,000 years and was the only documented
medicine in use during that time. Until about 150 years ago, all medicines were
derived from natural materials. As late as the 1890s, 59% of the products in the
US Pharmacopoeia were based on herbs or herbal combinations.[8] Herbal medicine
remains the most widely practiced form of medicine across the world still today.
It is estimated that 80% of the world's population in the developing world rely on
herbal medicinal products as a primary source of health care.[9] Throughout much of
the 20th century, the focus of medicine in the developed world changed, and herbal
remedies were being replaced with new pharmaceutical formulations, albeit many
of which were derived from plant components. After a 100-year decline in use in
the Western world, herbal medicine has been undergoing a revival in the modern
consumer market. In 2013, herbal products sales in the United States reached a total
of $6 billion, with a global market at least ten times that.[9] Now in the United States,
cannabis alone is outselling herbals (their sale estimated to be $8 billion in 2018),
while cannabis sales reached $10 billion in 2018, with an additional $2 billion for
CBD products.[10] Cannabis is now recognized as the most popular herbal medicine
in the United States.

Cannabis as a botanical medicine may be understood by applying established
herbal medicine concepts. Much is known about how to work with herbal products,
supported by scientific research. Phytotherapy, the practice of modern Western
herbal medicine, applies scientific research and high professional standards to
its practice. In phytotherapy, plant medicines are selected mainly to stimulate or
strengthen the body's normal functions, and so help the body heal itself.[11] Basic
science research bridging the gap between botany, phytochemistry and drugs is
provided by a discipline called pharmacognosy. This is the branch of knowledge
concerned with medicinal drugs obtained from plants or other natural sources.
"It is historically true that pharmacognosy, the study of medicinal plants, has
frequently pointed us in the proper direction to better understand our own body
chemistry."[12] As far back as 1969, in an article on the pharmacognosy of cannabis,
including an in-depth description of its botany and cannabinoid content, the author
opines:

> In order to fully understand those problems associated with the control of marihuana,
> both legal and moral, one must have some knowledge of the plant itself, the chemi-
> cal constituents in the plant, methods for identifying marihuana samples, the inherent
> variability in the plant and the type of biological test systems that are used to detect
> marihuana activity in laboratory animals.[13]

For an in-depth reference, an excellent monograph describing the botanical aspects
of cannabis including a pharmacognosy view has recently been published.[14]

There are, of course, many challenges to the standardized use of an herbal medicine that do not translate into a pharmaceutical medicine structure, the most frequently cited regarding dosing parameters. Single substance drugs are easier to
research, standardize and regulate the dosage versus herbal medicines. "The lack of

standardized procedures for herbal preparations and the absence of posology [dosing] protocols complicate the role of physicians in prescribing targeted therapies."[15]

> Researchers increasingly agree that it is important to establish a rational basis for dosing and standardization of biologically active compounds before conducting large-scale treatment trials. These efforts can improve investigators' ability to assess the risks and benefits of participation in large-scale herbal medicine trials.[9]

The situation with cannabis is no different:

> Besides obvious legal implications, Cannabis as an herbal medicine poses serious challenges to modern medicine, which operates according to the "single compound, single target" paradigm of pharmacology. An obvious question therefore is how the chemical constituents found in Cannabis reflect different medicinal properties.[16]

BOTANICAL AND TAXONOMICAL ASPECTS OF *CANNABIS SATIVA* L.

It is instructive to understand the basic botanical aspects of cannabis regarding its growth as a plant and how this affects potential therapeutic applications. *Cannabis sativa* L. is an annual plant, which belongs to the family Cannabaceae. The members of this family include cannabis (hemp, marijuana), humulus (hops) and celtis (hackberries). Cannabis is a somewhat weedy plant and may grow as high as 18 ft. It is a dioecious plant, that is, it bears male and female flowers, developing on separate plants. It is illustrated in Figure 2.1.

It is only the female plant that produces the medicinal components in any significant amount (i.e., cannabinoids, terpenoids), and such are selected for medicinal cultivation.[17–20] The secretory cavity of glandular trichomes located in the flowering tips and upper leaves occur most abundantly in female plants. These flowering tips secrete a sticky resin containing cannabinoids, flavonoids, terpenes, alkaloids and calcium.[18] A flowering tip ("bud") is shown in Figure 2.2.

The phytochemistry of cannabis is very complex with more than 500 compounds identified thus far, representing different chemical classes. Some belong to the primary metabolism of the plant, for example, amino acids, fatty acids and steroids, while cannabinoids, flavonoids, stilbenoids, terpenes, lignans and alkaloids represent secondary metabolites.[17] About 200 compounds have now been identified as cannabinoids, with over 200 terpenes isolated.

Historically and continuing through the present, cannabis cultivators (growers) and recreational users have distinguished among the hundreds of cultivar (strain) varieties by referring to these according to their strain names, often associated with distinguishing characteristics. This has resulted in the loose classification of three types of categories of plants: indica, sativa and hybrid. In the past, indica cultivars were recognized as shorter plants with wide leaflets. Generally, the effects of indica cultivars have been described as predominantly physical and sedative. Terms such as couch-lock or sleepy, dreamlike or melancholic were attributed to these strains, containing primarily THC or including some CBD and THC

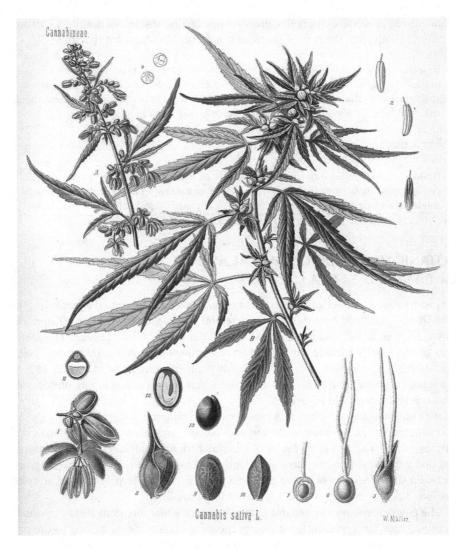

FIGURE 2.1   Drawing of the parts of *Cannabis sativa* L.

Source: Hermann Adolph Köhler (1834–1879) – http://caliban.mpiz-koeln.mpg.de/koehler (index) http://
caliban.mpiz-koeln.mpg.de/koehler/CANNABIS.jpg (image).

combinations. Indicas have been sought more for nighttime use due to their sup-
posedly sedating qualities. Sativa cultivars were recognized as taller plants with
more slender leaflets. The primary properties of the sativa cultivars have been
described as having greater effect on the mind and emotions, giving users an
increased sense of energy, well-being or euphoria. They were thought to be better
for daytime use due to their stimulating nature, having mostly THC as the primary cannabinoid. The third general category, the hybrid cultivar, has been created through selective cross-pollination of different cannabis varieties. In crossed

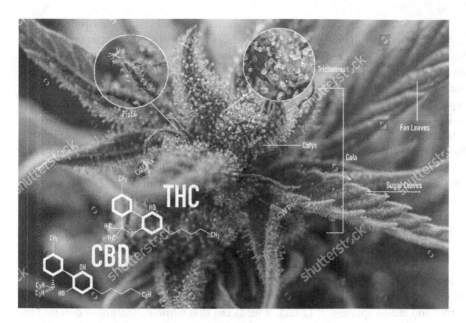

FIGURE 2.2 Cannabis flowering tip (bud).

varieties, the characteristics and effects of one cultivar will usually be dominant. There has been a huge effort to create hybrid strains (cultivars) with a range of new attributes, especially in the years of black-market cannabis cultivation. Due to selective enrichment in the United States during the 1960s until recently, all readily available cultivars were selected to contain high levels of THC and minimal levels of CBD. In fact, cultivar selection has led to a dearth of true indica or sativa phenotypes, almost all cultivars now are of a hybrid type. This legacy system has not proven to be useful for the scientific or medicinal classification of cannabis, as has been pointed out by several cannabis researchers.

> There are biochemically distinct strains of Cannabis, but the sativa/indica distinction as commonly applied in the lay literature is total nonsense and an exercise in futility. One cannot in any way currently guess the biochemical content of a given Cannabis plant based on its height, branching, or leaf morphology.[21]

"Categorizing Cannabis as either 'Sativa' and 'Indica' has become an exercise in futility. Ubiquitous interbreeding and hybridization renders their distinction meaningless."[22] The taxonomic classification of the multitude of varieties of *Cannabis sativa* L. remains an ongoing endeavor. Although patients as well as dispensaries will likely continue to talk about the properties of indicas and sativas, there is no valid scientific basis for such inaccurate categorization. Additionally, dispensaries, patients and public marketing refer to cannabis varieties as strains, not as cultivars. In speaking with patients, the "strain" terminology is still most useful, while researchers may refer to cultivars or chemovars.

Since the early 1970s, a classification system was advanced that reflected the importance of identifying the cannabinoid content of the plant, a categorization based upon the chemical phenotype or "chemotype" assessing the amount of THC and CBD produced, and on the ratio of THC to CBD. There have been three primary types of plants categorized based upon their chemotype; these are chemotype I or "drug"-type plants, commonly referred to as marijuana, that have a high THC/CBD ratio (much >1), chemotype II or intermediate-type plants that have an intermediate THC/CBD ratio (close to 1) and chemotype III or fiber-type plants that have a low THC/CBD ratio (much <1), also called hemp and used for textile or seed oil purposes.[23] More recently, other proposals have included the incorporation of chemotype IV and V to reflect 5% propyl cannabinoids, cannabigerol (CBG) derivatives and fiber types mostly devoid of cannabinoids.[24]

The chemotyping system originated prior to appreciating the medicinal importance of the terpene content of the cultivar. Historically, plants were considered to have either THC or CBD as the main cannabinoid, as little was understood about the effects of other cannabinoids, or even the progenitor cannabinoid acids. "More recently, PCA (principal component analysis) seemed to point to terpenoid content as the most convincing distinguishing chemotaxonomic markers between putative sativa and indica species."[25] In fact, it turns out that while cannabinoid content certainly determines many of the therapeutic properties of a cannabis cultivar, the terpene content is more indicative of whether a plant will be stimulating or sedating (see Chapter 5).

> Research suggests these effects are not likely due purely to CBD:THC ratios, as there are no significant differences in CBD:THC ratios between Sativa and Indica strains. Rather these different subjective effects are likely due to varying ratios of major cannabinoids as well as minor cannabinoids, terpenes and probably additional phytochemicals.[26]

For example, many researchers believe that sedation in most common cannabis cultivars is attributable to the β-myrcene (a monoterpene) content, thought to impart a narcotic-like effect with sedating properties. Furthermore, it is thought that a high limonene content lends an uplifting mood and highly energetic effect to some cultivars. Currently, cultivar names are applied to domesticated plants that have undergone years of breeding and genetic stabilization to express desired traits. It turns out, that chemical content, rather than appearance determines cultivar characteristics. The resulting mix of cannabinoids, terpenes and flavonoids are dictated by the genetic profile of the particular cultivar. *Thus, it is the plant's genetics that drives the characteristics of a specific cultivar of cannabis.*

CANNABIS SYNERGY

It is becoming apparent that the multifold components of cannabis work synergistically with each other to produce entourage effects.[27] The entourage effect may be defined as the interaction of the plant's individual constituents in producing synergy, thereby increasing its therapeutic potential. It was first suggested in 1998 that the endocannabinoid system demonstrated an "entourage effect," in which a multitude of metabolites modified the activity of the endocannabinoids anandamide and 2-arachidonoylglycerol.[28] Of course, this is to be expected in a botanical preparation, where the whole is often more efficacious than the sum of the individual components. The authors who coined the entourage effect hypothesis also postulated that this helped to explain how botanical drugs were often more efficacious than their isolated components.[29] Understanding herbal synergy is a cornerstone of herbal medicine practice. In fact, the concept of the entourage effect ascribed to endocannabinoid and cannabis interactions is but one example of herbal synergy. Synergy has been proven to occur between cannabis, endocannabinoids, cannabinoids and terpenes as they act on human physiology. Understanding these interactions is integral to assessing efficacy and choice of cultivar.

It has been proposed that the basis for entourage in cannabis or in any plant extract occurs through mechanisms that include pharmacokinetic effects (e.g., improved bioavailability or solubility), action of synergistic partners in the same cascade (multitarget effects), modulation of cellular transport and binding to target proteins, activation or deactivation of active compounds, inhibition of adverse effects and improved bacterial resistance.[30,31] Synergy provides for additive effects to occur in a potentiated way when single or multiple constituents bind to multiple targets.[31] As one author commenting on this complex issue says, that single cannabinoid preparations may be less effective than whole plant formulations due to

> the possibility of unique therapeutic benefit from a dynamic interaction between the myriad chemicals found in the cannabis plant. Referred to as the "entourage effect," unique therapeutic effects of cannabis are hypothesized to be achieved through a complex synergy between phytocannabinoids and the many other secondary constituents of the plant.[32]

Importantly, the authors further point out that *effects generated from one chemovar cannot be generalized to other varieties*, sadly, a fact that is not yet well recognized in cannabis marketing and consumer advice.

Some examples of synergy between cannabinoids might include the effect of CBD on THC pharmacology and physiological effects (see Chapter 4). CBD is now routinely being suggested as a complement to THC preparations due to its anxiolytic, antipsychotic effects. "In support of this view, CBD may potentiate the beneficial effects associated with ΔTHC (analgesia, antiemesis, and anti-inflammation) and reduce the negative psychoactive effects of Δ9-THC (impaired working memory, sedation, tachycardia, and paranoia)."[31] Other less prevalent cannabinoids are of consequence as well. For example, a cannabis extract was more efficacious than pure THC in treating breast cancer in vitro, possibly due to the presence of small concentrations of cannabigerol (CBG) and tetrahydrocannabinolic acid (THCA).[25] Synergy between cannabinoids and terpenes in cannabis has also been documented (see Chapter 5). It has been proposed that terpenes may modulate the affinity of THC for the CB1 receptor and interact with neurotransmitter receptors, affecting mood, analgesia and/or cognitive function among other effects.[27,33] With the exception of β-caryophyllene and potentially others, it has been determined that cannabis terpenes do not directly activate cannabinoid receptors.[34,35] Terpenes may also alter the pharmacokinetics of cannabinoids by increasing the blood–brain barrier permeability allowing greater cannabinoid access to target receptors. "In view of the potential of phytocannabinoid-terpene synergy, it has been suggested to tailor novel therapeutic treatments such as CBD-terpene extracts to be used against acne, MRSA, depression, anxiety, insomnia, dementia and addiction."[27]

Testing for and listing the complete cannabinoid and terpene profile is not yet common practice, even in cultivars used in clinical research. As the significance of the entourage effect becomes more widely appreciated, more studies need to be done to characterize the medicinal effects of full plant flower or extracts.

CONCLUSION

We are not yet at a place where the significance and diversity of cannabis is being recognized due to its nature as a plant, rather than a single purified drug. The trend in modern research has been to attempt to isolate its active components, study them, categorize them, standardize them and regulate and package them. Examples of this include purified cannabinoids such as THC or CBD as isolates. Nabiximols, such as Sativex, and a purified CBD oil such as Epidiolex have attempted to standardize and purify a full plant extract. In most therapeutic assessments using cannabis as a medicine, the full plant extract has proven to be more efficacious at a lower dose than the purified cannabinoid counterpart(s). The safety profile of this herbal medicine is superior to many pharmaceuticals that it may substitute for effectively. The versatility and value of this botanical medicine often surpasses any other substance, or multiple substances that cannabis may serve to replace. As one author comments, "*C. sativa* and cannabinoids constitute one of the most paradigmatic examples of the deep impact that natural products can have on biochemistry, pharmacology, and toxicology."[18] We will see that dosing remains a challenge and much work needs to be done to analyze, standardize and regulate this botanical, as has been accomplished for a multitude of herbal medicines thus far. A Harvard psychiatry professor who became a forerunner in the medical cannabis field after his research found it was less toxic or addictive than alcohol or tobacco, Dr. Lester Grinspoon said of cannabis:

> Countless clinicians and patients the world around ... have observed that it often provides better relief with fewer serious side effects than conventionally prescribed medicines. Presently we are beginning to see two powerful forces collide: the growing acceptance of medical cannabis and the proscription against any use of herbal marijuana, medical or non-medical.[36]

REFERENCES

1. Russo EB. The pharmacological history of cannabis. In: Pertwee R, ed. *Handbook of Cannabis*. Oxford, UK: Oxford University Press; 2014:23–43. www.researchgate.net/publication/312414874_The_pharmacological_history_of_cannabis Accessed July 13, 2020.

2. Bridgeman MB, Abazia DT. Medicinal cannabis: history, pharmacology, and implications for the acute care setting. *PT.* 2017;42(3):180–188.

3. Remington JP, Wood HC Jr, et al. *The Dispensatory of the United States of America.* Reprinted from *Dispensary of the United States of America.* 20th ed. Philadelphia, PA: Lippincott; 1918:276–281. www.onlinepot.org/medical/Dr_Tods_PDFs/s5_3.pdf Accessed July 13, 2020.

4. Lee MA. *Smoke Signals: A Social History of Marijuana: Medical, Recreational, and Scientific.* New York, NY: Scribner; 2012.

5. US Department of Justice, DEA, Diversion Control Division. Controlled Substance Schedules, Marijuana. Clarification of the New Drug Code 7350 for marijuana extract. www.deadiversion.usdoj.gov/schedules/marijuana/m_extract_7350.html Accessed November 20, 2020.

6. US Food and Drug Administration. FDA regulation of cannabis and cannabis-derived products, including cannabidiol (CBD). www.fda.gov/news-events/public-health-focus/ fda-regulation-cannabis-and-cannabis-derived-products-including-cannabidiol-cbd Accessed July 13, 2020.

7. Hoffmann D. *Medical Herbalism: The Science and Practice of Herbal Medicine.* Rochester, VT: Healing Arts Press; 2003.

8. Rashrash M, Schommer JC, Brown LM. Prevalence and predictors of herbal medicine use among adults in the United States. *J Patient Exp.* 2017;4(3):108–113.

9. Tilburt JC, Kaptchuk TJ. Herbal medicine research and global health: an ethical analysis. *Bull World Health Organ.* 2008;86(8):577–656.

10. Ponieman N. 5 drivers of the correlated growth of cannabis, herbal medicine. Benzinga website. January 06, 2020. www.benzinga.com/markets/cannabis/20/01/15047483/5-drivers-of-the-correlated-growth-of-cannabis-herbal-medicine Accessed July 13, 2020.

11. What is phytotherapy? The College of Practitioners of Phytotherapy website. http://phytotherapists.org/about.php Accessed July 13, 2020.

12. Russo E. Introduction to the endocannabinoid system. Phytecs website. www.phytecs.com/wp-content/uploads/2015/02/IntroductionECS.pdf Accessed July 20, 2020.

13. Farnsworth NR. Pharmacognosy and chemistry of "cannabis sativa". *J Am Pharm Assoc.* 1969;9(8):410–414.

14. Upton R, Craker L, ElSohly M, Romm A, Russo E, Sexton M, eds. *Cannabis Inflorescence (cannabis spp.): Standards of Identity, Analysis, and Quality Control.* Scotts Valley, CA: American Herbal Pharmacopoeia; 2014.

15. Brunetti P, Pichini S, Pacifici R, Busardò FP, Del Rio A. Herbal preparations of medical cannabis: a vademecum for prescribing doctors. *Medicina (Kaunas).* 2020;56(5):237.

16. Hazekamp A, Tejkalova K, Papadimitriou S. Cannabis: from cultivar to chemovar ii: a metabolomics approach to cannabis classification. *Cannabis Cannabinoid Res.* 2016;1(1):202–215.

17. Flores-Sanchez IJ, Verpoorte R. Secondary metabolism in cannabis. *Phytochem Rev.* 2008;7:615–639.

18. Appendino G, Taglialatela-Scafati O. Cannabinoids: chemistry and medicine. In: Ramawat K, Mérillon JM, eds. *Natural Products.* Berlin, Heidelberg: Springer; 2013: 3417–3435. www.researchgate.net/publication/300516737_Cannabinoids_Chemistry_ and_Medicine Accessed July 20, 2020.

19. Hanus LO. Pharmacological and therapeutic secrets of plant and brain (endo)cannabinoids. *Med Res Rev.* 2009;29(2):213–271.

20. Lynch RC, Vergara D, Tittes S, et al. Genomic and chemical diversity in Cannabis. *Crit Rev Plant Sci.* 2015;35(5–6):349–363.

21. Piomelli D, Russo EB. The Cannabis sativa Cannabis indica debate: an interview with Ethan Russo, MD. *Cannabis Cannabinoid Res.* 2016;1(1):44–46.
22. McPartland JM. Cannabis systematics at the levels of family, genus and species. *Cannabis Cannabinoid Res.* 2018;3:203–212.
23. Elzinga S, Fischedick J, Podkolinski R, Raber JC. Cannabinoids and terpenes as chemotaxonomic markers in cannabis. *Nat Prod Chem Res.* 2015;3(4):181.
24. Aizpurua-Olaizola O, Soydaner U, Öztürk E, et al. Evolution of the cannabinoid and terpene content during the growth of cannabis sativa plants from different chemotypes. *J Nat Prod.* 2016;79(2):324–331.
25. Russo EB. 2019. The case for the entourage effect and conventional breeding of clinical cannabis: no "strain," no gain. *Front Plant Sci.* 2019;9:1969.
26. Baron EP, Lucas P, Eades J, et al. Patterns of medicinal cannabis use, strain analysis, and substitution effect among patients with migraine, headache, arthritis, and chronic pain in a medicinal cannabis cohort. *J Headache Pain.* 2018;19:37.
27. Russo EB. Taming THC: potential cannabis synergy and phytocannabinoid-terpenoid entourage effects. *Br J Pharmacol.* 2011;163:1344–1364.
28. BenShabat S, et al. An entourage effect: inactive endogenous fatty acid glycerol esters enhance 2-arachidonoyl-glycerol cannabinoid activity. *Eur J Pharmacol.* 1998;353:23–31.
29. Mechoulam R, BenShabat S. From gan-zi-gun-nu to anandamide and 2-arachidonoylglycerol: the ongoing story of cannabis. *Nat Prod Rep.* 1999;16(2):131–143.
30. Andre CM, Hausman JF, Guerriero G. Cannabis sativa: the plant of the thousand and one molecules. *Front Plant Sci.* 2016;7:19.
31. Wagner H, Ulrich-Merzenich G. Synergy research: approaching a new generation of phytopharmaceuticals. *Phytomedicine.* 2009;16:97–110.
32. Bonn-Miller MO, ElSohly MA, Loflin MJE, Chandra S, Vandrey R. Cannabis and cannabinoid drug development: evaluating botanical versus single molecule approaches. *Int Rev Psychiatry.* 2018;30(3):277–284.
33. McPartland J, Russo E. Cannabis and cannabis extracts: greater than the sum of their parts? *J Cannabis Ther.* 2001;1;103–132.
34. Santiago M, Sachdev S, Arnold JC, McGregor IS, Connor M. Absence of entourage: terpenoids commonly found in Cannabis sativa do not modulate the functional activity of δ9-thc at human CB1 and CB2 receptors. *Cannabis Cannabinoid Res.* 2019;4(3):165–176.
35. Finlay DB, Sircombe KJ, Nimick M, Jones C, Glass M. Terpenoids from cannabis do not mediate an entourage effect by acting at cannabinoid receptors. *Front Pharmacol.* 2020;11:359.
36. Grinspoon L. On the future of cannabis as medicine. *Cannabinoids.* 2007;2(2):13–15.

3 The Endocannabinoid System

ENDOCANNABINOID SYSTEM – AN OVERVIEW

This is likely the most relevant chapter in this book for all medical professionals. As one author puts it,

> The discovery of the endocannabinoid system (ECS) is the single most important scientific medical discovery since the recognition of sterile surgical technique. As our knowledge expands, we are coming to realize that the ECS is a master control system of virtually all physiology.[1]

Due to the significant impact of the ECS on health and disease, and the lack of education about this in medical curriculums, this chapter will provide an in-depth review.

The endocannabinoid system was first proposed in the early 1990s when cannabinoid receptors (CBrs), the first internal receptor that binds to phytocannabinoids, was defined. The discovery of a specific cell membrane receptor for THC was followed by the isolation and identification of endogenous (animal) ligands termed endocannabinoids (eCBs). The ECS carries the cannabinoid name because study of cannabis chemistry led to the system's discovery. It has been found in all animals, vertebrates and even invertebrates, the oldest identified being the sea squirt, a creature thought to have developed nearly 600 million years ago. CBrs are present in every vertebrate investigated to date being absent in non-chordate invertebrates (insects, nematodes, Hydra), fungi, and plants. Of note, CBrs existed long before cannabis evolved. This begs the question, why do animals have receptors that apparently have an origin apart from the plant cannabinoids that bind to them? That is because animals synthesize endogenous molecules, eCBs, that bind to these receptors, which turn out to be crucial in maintenance of the organism's homeostasis. The components of the ECS are expressed in nearly all parts of the human body throughout every stage of life. The complexity of the ECS is still being elucidated, but currently is thought to include CB type 1 (CB1) and type 2 (CB2) receptors (at minimum), multiple endocannabinoids, the most well-known being *N*-arachidonoylethanolamide (AEA) most commonly referred to as anandamide, 2-arachidonoylglycerol (2-AG), and the enzymes involved in the synthesis and degradation of eCBs. New information is being discovered, as yet poorly identified, about cellular uptake mechanisms and potential storage mechanisms involving fatty acid-binding proteins (FABPs).[2]

> After 50 years since the discovery of THC, and nearly 20 years since that of AEA (1992) and 2-AG (1995), only recently it is emerging that the correct interaction between the different components of ECS is essential for a proper function of eCB [endocannabinoid] as signaling molecules.[3]

DOI: 10.1201/9781003098201-4

And further,

> Thus, in order to understand the many-faceted actions elicited by eCBs (and hence by
> eCB-related drugs) it appears now crucial to understand how after getting to the right
> place eCBs can be concentrated to suitable amounts for receptor activation at the right
> time.[3]

The function of the ECS is vast, and vastly underrated as of yet. The ECS is
involved in regulating homeostatic physiological and cognitive processes, controlling an array of physiological functions, such as energy storage, immune
regulation, appetite regulation, pain, mood, memory, learning, stress response,
autonomic response, endocrine responses, temperature regulation and sleep.
Modulation of the ECS has been documented during disease or injury. The ECS
is ubiquitously found in the brain, skin, digestive tract, liver, cardiovascular system, immune system, endocrine tissues, genitourinary tissues, reproductive system and bone. It plays an important role in migration of hematopoietic stem and
progenitor cells as well. Recent evidence points to its involvement in the control
of cellular metabolism, differentiation, proliferation, aging and death. Several
comprehensive reviews have been published about the ECS.[4–8] "An overwhelming body of scientific evidence now indicates the existence of this elaborate and
previously unknown but ubiquitous EPCS [endocannabinoid physiological control
system] whose fundamental role in human development, health, and disease is
unfolding."[4] The author goes on to say that the presence of endocannabinoids in
all animals at all stages of development indicates a "fundamental role in human
biology." Lifestyle factors such as diet, exercise and stress management also affect
ECS function.[9] The functions of the ECS can be summed up by an acronym which
is to *Protect, Relax, Eat, Forget and Sleep.*[10] Table 3.1 provides a list of the main
functions of the ECS.

TABLE 3.1
Functions of the ECS

Primary function is cellular homeostasis
Embryological development
Regulation of cellular differentiation and aging
Modulation of growth and development
Autonomic regulation
Neuroprotection and neuroplasticity
Immune regulation and inflammation
Modulation of hunger, feeding and glucose metabolism
Antinociception and pain regulation
Regulation of apoptosis and carcinogenesis

Unfortunately, almost 30 years after its discovery, the ECS is still not taught in medical training curricula. The result of this omission is aptly summarized with the following observation, "Although the biology of cannabinoids and the variety of their central and peripheral actions have been studied for over half a century, these early findings have gone largely unnoticed by the overwhelming majority of physicians and scientists."[5]

STRUCTURE OF ENDOCANNABINOIDS

Endocannabinoids are derivatives of polyunsaturated fatty acids, differing in chemical structure from the phytocannabinoids of the cannabis plant. The first to be discovered was AEA in 1992 – named from the Sanskrit word *ananda*, which means bliss. Multiple endocannabinoids other than AEA and 2-AG have been identified, including, 2-arachidonylglyceryl ether (noladin ether), *O*-arachidonoyl-ethanolamine (virodhamine), *N*-arachidonoyl-dopamine (NADA), *N*-dihomo-γ-linolenoylethanolamine and *N*-docosatetraenoylethanolamine. More recently, both *N*-docosahexaenoylethanolamine (DHEA), *N*-eicosapentaenoylethanolamine (EPEA) and oleamide have been shown to activate CBrs as well.[11] Figure 3.1 shows the structure of the two main endocannabinoids, AEA and 2-AG.

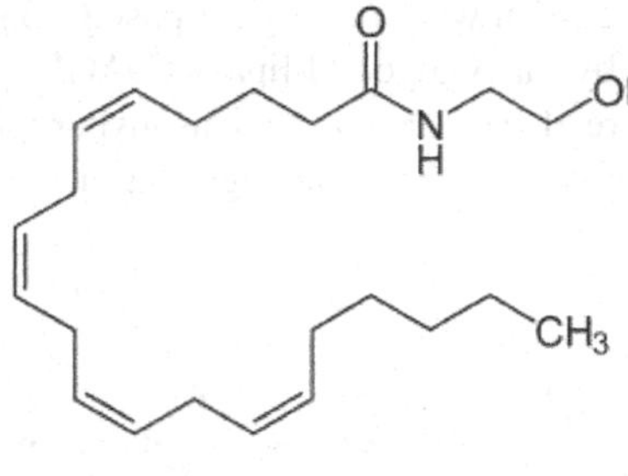

Anandamide

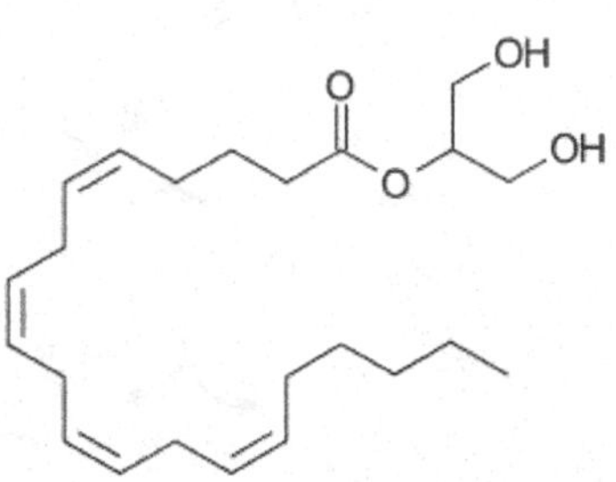

2-Arachidonylglycerol

FIGURE 3.1 Structure of endocannabinoids.

ENDOCANNABINOID SYNTHESIS AND METABOLISM

Prior to understanding how the ECS acts on human health and disease, we must first delve deeper into its component actions. How are endocannabinoids synthesized and degraded, what constitutes a cannabinoid receptor, what is the mechanism of receptor–ligand interaction and what overlap exists with components of cannabis? The eCBs AEA and 2-AG are lipophilic compounds produced from membrane phosphoglycerides via Ca^{2+} sensitive biosynthetic pathways.

> Since the biosynthetic precursors for endocannabinoids seem to be ubiquitous in membranes, it is the reciprocal pattern of expression of endocannabinoid biosynthesizing enzymes and cannabinoid receptors that determines the specificity of endocannabinoid action, whereas the localization of the degrading enzymes sets its duration.[12]

The synthesis and degradation of the two primary eCBs have been reviewed in detail.[2,3,11]

Endocannabinoids are generated on demand from cell membrane phospholipid precursors. Anandamide is synthesized and degraded at postsynaptic neurons. The synthesis of AEA from arachidonic acid has been proposed as a one- or two-step process, involving first the action of N-acyltransferase (NAT) and then N-acylphosphatidylethanolamine-hydrolyzing phospholipase D (NAPE-PLD), or directly in one step by NAPE-PLD. The biosynthesis of 2-AG occurs at postsynaptic neurons, while degradation is localized to presynaptic neurons. 2-AG is synthesized in a two-step process in which phospholipase C-β generates diacylglycerol, which is then hydrolyzed by diacylglycerol lipase (DAGLα and β) to yield 2-AG. Other synthetic enzymes are also emerging, such as glycerophosphodiesterases. See Figure 3.2 for endocannabinoid synthesis and degradation.

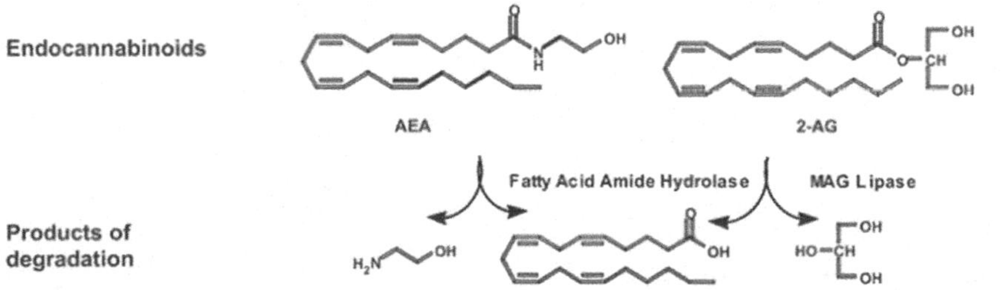

FIGURE 3.2   Endocannabinoid synthesis and degradation.

Source: Gatta-Cherifi B, Cota D. 2016. New Insights on the Role of the Endocannabinoid System in the Regulation of Energy Balance. *Int J Obes*. 40: 210–219.

Endocannabinoid lipid mediators are largely insoluble in an aqueous environment; thus they are likely carried by intracellular transporters such as FABPs. The effect of FABPs on endocannabinoid regulation is just starting to be understood. These proteins have been implicated in the intracellular transport of AEA to its catabolic enzyme fatty acid amide hydrolase (FAAH). FABPs also bind to phytocannabinoids. In fact, THC and CBD have been shown to inhibit the cellular uptake and catabolism of AEA by targeting FABPs. It has been proposed that, "Competition for FABPs may in part or wholly explain the increased circulating levels of endocannabinoids reported after consumption of cannabinoids."[13] After cellular uptake, AEA is hydrolyzed by FAAH into arachidonic acid and ethanolamine. FAAH appears postsynaptically and is thought to be primarily localized to intracellular organelles that serve as Ca^{2+} storage sites. Degradation of 2-AG occurs by a membrane-associated, soluble enzyme, monoacylglycerol lipase (MAGL), that appears presynaptically at axon terminals. Alternatively, AEA and 2-AG may be oxidized by cyclooxygenase-2 (COX-2), distinct lipoxygenases (LOXs) or cytochrome P (CYP) 450 enzymes.[3]

The action of AEA and 2-AG may be enhanced by "entourage compounds" that inhibit their hydrolysis via substrate competition, thereby increasing their concentration and prolonging their activity. Entourage compounds include N-palmitoylethanolamide (PEA), N-oleoylethanolamide (SEA) and cis-9-octadecenoamide (OEA, oleamide).[9] Both OEA and PEA share the catabolic routes of AEA, thereby potentiating the activity of eCBs by inhibiting their degradation, resulting in an entourage effect.[11] The phytocannabinoid, CBD, is also thought to impede the degradation of AEA by FAAH.

CANNABINOID RECEPTORS

Cells recognize endogenous cannabinoids by their membrane protein cannabinoid receptors. As discussed previously, these are the binding sites that previously had been determined to bind to the phytocannabinoid, THC.

> The discovery of specific genes coding for cannabinoid receptors (CBrs) that are activated by smoking marijuana and the finding of endogenous cannabinoids that also activate CBrs have transformed marijuana-cannabinoid research into mainstream science with significant implications in human health and disease.[4]

Cannabinoid receptors belong to the family of G protein-coupled receptors (GPCRs). Their activation causes inhibition of adenylate cyclase, thus inhibiting the conversion of adenosine triphosphate (ATP) to cyclic AMP (cAMP) and stimulating different members of the mitogen-activated protein kinase (MAPK) family, which is a mechanism by which cannabinoids affect synaptic plasticity.[8,14] Anandamide shows preferential affinity for CB1 compared to CB2 receptors, while 2-AG is considered a full agonist at both CB1 and CB2 receptors. A number of other receptors for both phytocannabinoids and endocannabinoids outside of the CBr system have been found, but the CB1 and CB2 mechanism is still thought to be primary for eCBs. Cannabinoid receptors are ubiquitous throughout the nervous system, being 12 times more prevalent than mu-opiate receptors.

The most important physiological effects triggered by stimulation of CBrs can be identified as the (a) psychotropic effects, (b) analgesic effects, (c) immunomodulatory effects and (d) cardiovascular effects.[15] The ECS plays a critical role in managing pain, inflammation and hyperalgesia through both CB1 and CB2 mechanisms. By limiting glutamate release when stimulated at the presynaptic nerve terminals, eCBs decrease glutamate cytotoxicity, limiting neuronal cell death and decreasing reactive oxygen species (ROS). Endocannabinoids in the central nervous system (CNS) affect both short-term and long-term forms of synaptic plasticity, including depolarization-induced suppression of both excitatory and inhibitory neurotransmission, long-term potentiation and depression and long-term depression of inhibition, and decrease glutamate excitotoxicity. The ECS regulates metabolic functions not only in the CNS but also by affecting a multitude of other cells, including adipocytes, hepatocytes, and multiple other non-neuronal systems.

> While initially it was believed that this endocannabinoid signaling system would only facilitate energy intake, we now know that perhaps even more important functions of endocannabinoids and CB(1) receptors in this context are to enhance energy storage into the adipose tissue and reduce energy expenditure by influencing both lipid and glucose metabolism.[16]

CANNABINOID RECEPTOR TYPE 1

Cannabinoid receptor type 1 was discovered in 1988 and has major homeostatic influence in the central nervous system where it is the most abundant and widely distributed GPCR. These receptors are found on nerve cells in the brain, with particularly dense expression in (ranked in order) the substantia nigra, globus pallidus, hippocampus, cerebral cortex, putamen, caudate, cerebellum and amygdala, and the spinal cord as well as some in the peripheral nervous system. They are present and active from the earliest phases of ontogenetic development, including during the embryonal stages, which has proved to be of importance in neuronal development and newborn suckling. One of the few places where cannabinoid receptors are not found is within the portion of the brain stem devoted to respiration. This helps explain cannabis' lethal dose safety profile, with no Lethal Dose 50 (LD50) determined at maximum doses. Frequently, CB1 receptors are found at the terminals of central and peripheral nerves and modulate the release of other neurotransmitters. Thus, CB1 receptor activation protects the nervous system from overactivation or overinhibition by neurotransmitters.[8] Although the activation of presynaptic CB1 receptors can lead to inhibition of the release of a number of different excitatory or inhibitory neurotransmitters both in the brain and in the peripheral nervous system, there is also evidence that CB1 receptor agonists can stimulate dopamine (DA) release in the nucleus accumbens.[14] A particularly well-researched topic is the role of CB1 activation, by endocannabinoids or otherwise (i.e., phytocannabinoids or synthetic cannabinoids) in neural modulation. Type 1 receptors are involved in γ-aminobutyric acid (GABA) and glutamate neurotransmission, as they are found on GABAergic and glutamatergic neurons. Type 1 receptors are found primarily on central and peripheral neurons in the presynapse. These locations facilitate the modulation of neurotransmitter release, which is one of the major functions of the endocannabinoid system. The high CB1 levels in sensory and motor regions are consistent with the important role of CB1 receptors in motivation and cognition. "The neuromodulatory actions of endocannabinoids in the sensory and autonomic nervous systems also result, mostly through CB1 receptors, in the regulation of pain perception and of cardiovascular, gastrointestinal and respiratory functions."[17]

Type 1 receptors are also expressed in non-neuronal cells, such as adipocytes and hepatocytes, connective and musculoskeletal tissues of the endocrine glands, salivary glands, leukocytes, spleen, heart and parts of the reproductive, urinary and gastrointestinal tracts.

[T]heir effects on the release of hypothalamic hormones and peptides, and the regulation of their levels by steroid hormones, lead to modulation of food intake and of the pituitary – hypothalamus – adrenal axis, as well as of both female and male reproduction.[17]

The physiological and pathological roles of CB1 receptors have been comprehensively reviewed.[18]

CANNABINOID RECEPTOR TYPE 2

Cannabinoid receptor type 2 is expressed principally in immune cells, among them leukocytes, in blood, spleen and tonsils. Originally, it was assumed that CB2 receptors were present only in cells of the immune system, but they have now also been identified throughout the central nervous system particularly in microglial cells.[14] CB2 receptor activation results in inhibition of neuroinflammatory signaling pathways, reducing inflammation in microglial cells potentially through modulation of extracellular signal-regulated protein kinases 1 and 2 (ERK1/2) activation.[19] As previously mentioned, 2-AG is a full agonist at CB2 receptors, while anandamide has less binding affinity for CB2. The ECS is intimately involved in the regulation of mature immune cell tracking, effector cell functions and in the regulation of adaptive immunity. Taken together, these examples indicate that the ECS is a key regulator of the immune system; therefore, any treatment that modulates its function will have immunological effects.[20] One of the actions of CB receptors in the immune system is modulation of release of cytokines, which modulate inflammation and immune function. A major consequence of CB2 receptor activation is immunosuppression, which limits inflammation and associated tissue injury. Type 2 receptor density is increased during inflammation or bone injury. The physiological importance of CB2 receptors in cellular and humoral immune responses is only now starting to be revealed. Type 2 receptors are also considered to be involved in neuroinflammation, atherosclerosis and bone remodeling. Newer studies have demonstrated the presence of CB2 receptors in the CNS with properties that extend their neuro-immunological function. The function of CB2 receptors in the CNS has been shown to occur by a cellular hyperpolarization event that may be occurring postsynaptically.[21] The physiological and pathological roles of CB2 receptors have been comprehensively reviewed.[8,19] The location and summary of function of CB1 and CB2 receptors is shown in Figure 3.3.

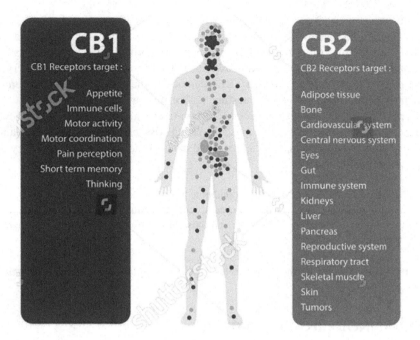

FIGURE 3.3   CB1 and CB2 distribution and function.

ADDITIONAL RECEPTORS

Additional GPCR receptors, such as GPR55, GPR18 and GPR119, have been discovered to interact with the endocannabinoids and some phytocannabinoids, contributing to the non-CB1, non-CB2-mediated effects reported for some cannabinoids. While interaction with multiple cannabinoids have been found at these GPCR receptors, the activity of the primary endocannabinoids, AEA and 2-AG, at these sites has not yet been confirmed. Another orphan GPCR receptor has been proposed, tentatively called CB3, which shares low sequence homology with CB1 and CB2, yet it activates GTPases and MAPK kinases.[11]

Non GCPR receptors that bind to cannabinoids have also been identified. Other binding sites for eCBs include the transient receptor potential vanilloid 1 (TRPV1) ion channel, highly expressed in some primary sensory neurons, both centrally and peripherally, and in various non-neuronal cells.

TRPV1 interaction (that occurs at the inner side of the plasma membrane) leads to the control of CNS functions including nociception, and of basic biological processes like the induction of apoptosis. An important consequence of its activation is the release of sensory neuropeptides that then produce effects such as pain, tachycardia, vasodilation and bronchoconstriction.[3]

Both AEA and 2-AG bind (directly or indirectly) to nuclear peroxisome proliferator-activated receptors (PPARs) α and γ, which regulate gene transcription, cell differentiation and lipid metabolism.[3,11] There is evidence for the presence of allosteric regulation of AEA and other cannabinoids on several non-cannabinoid receptors.

These are 5-HT2 receptors, 5-HT3 receptors, α1-adrenoceptors, M1 and M4 muscarinic receptors and α-amino-3-hydroxy-5-methyl-4-isoxazolepropionic acid (AMPA) GLUA1 and GLUA3 glutamate receptors. The mechanism of action of eCBs at many of these non-CB receptors is not yet well elucidated.

> As compared to the great wealth of descriptive and mechanistic information available on the function and dysfunction of CB1 in metabolism, much work is still required to fully understand the exact role of CB2, or of PPARs and TRPV1 in endocannabinoid control of metabolism.[22]

RETROGRADE MECHANISM OF ACTION

Endocannabinoids have long been thought to be triggered on demand, rather than being prestored in secretory vesicles. Endocannabinoids, therefore, do not typically function like hormones, but have been thought to act as local (autocrine or paracrine) mediators, with a retrograde inhibition effect. The retrograde mechanism of action has been primarily demonstrated for eCB action in neuronal cells at CB1 receptors. CB1 receptors are found on both excitatory and inhibitory neurons, suppressing both GABAergic and glutamatergic transmission, a process called depolarization-induced suppression of inhibition (DSI) or depolarization-induced suppression of excitation (DSE).

> The net effect from this process is determined by the ratio of DSI to DSE and represents the "fine tuning" of neurotransmission in the CNS and the peripheral nervous system; the release or uptake of other neurotransmitters such as dopamine and serotonin is influenced, too.[2]

Endocannabinoids in fact exert influence on nearly all other receptor systems' neurotransmitters, such as dopamine, serotonin, melatonin, and acetylcholine, glutamate and GABA. The ECS employs a unique retrograde feedback loop of postsynaptic and presynaptic signaling. Both AEA and 2-AG are found in the postsynaptic neuron membrane within a lipid ring encircling synapses that keep the endocannabinoids and their receptors sequestered from their aqueous surroundings and are produced on-site and on demand. The cannabinoids then travel retrograde (backward) to the presynaptic cannabinoid receptor associated with that neuron to inhibit the release of all other neurotransmitters. AEA functions as a partial receptor agonist affecting the neurons that regulate pain. By contrast, 2-AG is a total agonist, fully activating the cannabinoid receptors. The retrograde mechanism of action of eCBs at neuronal synapses is shown in Figure 3.4.

The retrograde mechanism of action may, however, be too simplistic. Recalling that eCBs are largely insoluble in an aqueous environment and may be carried by intracellular transporters FABPs, the paracrine nature of action may not provide the full picture. The transport and concentration of ECs at receptor sites is an area undergoing ongoing research. One author comments:

> A re-examination of the widely accepted "dogma" issuing that eCBs are exclusively synthesized and released on demand could be proposed, whereby intracellular trafficking, in addition to storage in specific reservoirs like adiposomes, could play a key role in determining signal transduction triggered by the same eCB in different cellular contexts.[3]

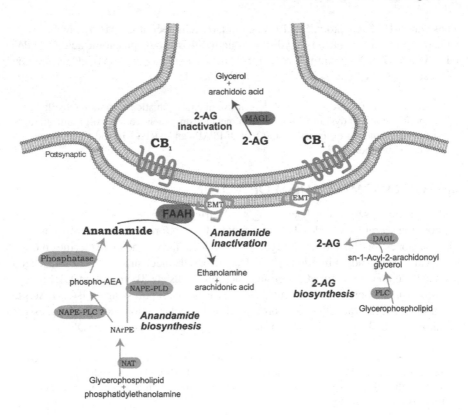

FIGURE 3.4   Retrograde synaptic transmission.

Source: Pacher P, Batkai S, Kunos G. 2006. The Endocannabinoid System as an Emerging Target of Pharmacotherapy. *Pharmacol Rev.* 58(3): 389–462.

While retrograde synaptic transmission has long been thought to be the primary mechanism of action for eCBs (Figure 3.5A), recent evidence suggests that eCBs also participate in non-retrograde autocrine signaling with CB and non-CB receptors located on neural and non-neural cells. These include binding to receptors located on or within the postsynaptic cell, including CB and TRPV1 receptors (Figure 3.5B). While AEA is a partial agonist at the CB1 receptor, it is a full agonist at TRPV1 receptor; 2-AG does not exhibit binding affinity for this receptor. The additional binding of eCBs to astrocytes is presumably by a CBr mechanism, indirectly modulating presynaptic or postsynaptic function (Figure 3.5C).[23]

In addition to neuronal mechanisms, it has been proposed:

There are three possible mode[s] of action for cannabinoids to regulate cell function independently of CB1 and CB2: 1) cannabinoids may regulate cell function independently of a protein target (e.g. by changing cell membrane fluidity), 2) cannabinoids may interact with proteins that do not directly transduce signals (e.g. by inhibiting dopamine and adenosine transport) and/or 3) cannabinoids may produce their effects through other receptors.[24]

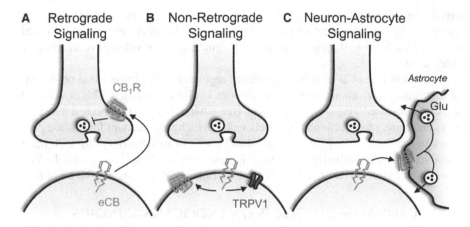

A Retrograde Signaling **B** Non-Retrograde Signaling **C** Neuron-Astrocyte Signaling

FIGURE 3.5 Alternative endocannabinoid signaling.

Source: Castillo PE, Younts TJ, Chávez AE, Hashimotodani Y. 2012. Endocannabinoid Signaling and Synaptic Function. *Neuron* 76(1): 70–81.

ENDOCANNABINOID TONE

A specific term, "endocannabinoid tone," has been coined to refer to an individual's state of endocannabinoid balance, with accompanying descriptors such as excess or deficiency. This term is a reflection of the overall ECS function – dependent upon the density of cannabinoid receptors, their functional status (upregulated or downregulated) and relative abundance or dearth of eCBs.[25] Endocannabinoid tone reflects the state of balance, excess or deficiency of the endocannabinoids, receptors and enzymes that constitute the endocannabinoid system.[26] "ECS 'tone' within a biological system is mostly the result of the regulation of endocannabinoid levels as modulated by different, often concurring, enzymatic cascades, which are nearly ubiquitously expressed."[22] In a review of the effect of components of daily living, many factors were listed as having an effect on eCB tone or expression. This includes the effect of diet, especially dietary fat, herbals, caffeine, nicotine, alcohol, drugs such as NSAIDS and glucocorticoids, stress, exercise, massage and cannabis.[9] A correlation between physical activity (PA) and eCB tone has been demonstrated. One study showed that exercise increased blood concentrations of AEA, but interestingly not of 2-AG, after 30–45 minutes and up to 5 hours of aerobic exercise.

> Indeed, eCBs are crucial in controlling locomotor activity. . . . Yet, in the majority of reports, unlike exercise, eCB tone negatively affects peripheral energy homeostasis towards fat accumulation, which better describes an obesity-directed condition or a sedentary lifestyle. It seems necessary, therefore, that eCBs are tightly regulated during PA, in order to maintain their beneficial effects.[27]

Physical activity has been presented as a significant factor that may lead to the activation of the EC signaling pathway. Positive ECS-related effects of physical activity on the attenuation of obesity and type 2 diabetes mellitus are potential outcomes. The involvement of physical activity in the treatment of neurological diseases by affecting the endocannabinoid signaling is not yet well researched or understood.[28]

It turns out that eCB tone is a significant regulator of the impact that phytocannabinoids may have upon cannabis therapeutics in clinical practice. This is a crucial factor in individualizing dosage regimens (see Chapter 7). Furthermore, a new theory is emerging of endocannabinoid deficiency, which may account for disease processes in some individuals, who would then benefit from supplementing with plant cannabinoids.[29] Additionally, some pathologies, such as chronic stress, might lead to overstimulation of the ECS, for whom cannabinoid antagonists may be helpful.

PHYTOCANNABINOID EFFECTS ON ENDOCANNABINOIDS

Phytocannabinoids, especially ones that are direct CBr agonists such as THC, affect endocannabinoid tone and function. It has been proposed that cannabis may work, in part, by "kick-starting" the ECS. Animal studies have shown that THC upregulates CB1 receptors in rodent brains, upregulates CB1 mRNA in rats and stimulates AEA biosynthesis.[11] Chronic, high dosing of THC causes desensitization and subsequent downregulation of CB1 and CB2 receptors producing tolerance and affecting endocannabinoid tone. Effects of THC upon the ECS are varied, dependent upon acute versus chronic dosing, modulating between potentiation and suppression.[9]

CBD, which is not a CB1 nor a CB2 agonist, inhibits FAAH levels, thereby slowing AEA degradation. Circulating AEA levels are increased in humans following consumption of CBD. It has been proposed that THC and CBD can inhibit the cellular uptake and degradation of AEA by targeting FABPs:

> CBD does not inhibit the enzymatic actions of human FAAH, and thus FAAH inhibition cannot account for the observed increase in circulating AEA in humans following CBD consumption. Competition for FABPs may in part or wholly explain the increased circulating levels of endocannabinoids reported after consumption of cannabinoids.[13]

CBD stimulates TRPV1 activity as well. The extent to which CBD appears to activate and potentially over time may desensitize TRPV1 through receptor downregulation may affect eCB binding at these channels representing yet another measure of endocannabinoid tone.[25] Other examples of phytocannabinoid–endocannabinoid interactions are found in Part III, within the presentations of specific conditions.

ENDOCANNABINOIDS IN HEALTH AND DISEASE

The physiological effects of endocannabinoids are vast, as has already been outlined. Their effect on human health and disease is equally widespread. One frequently quoted comment about the significance of the ECS in human physiology is as follows:

> Modulating endocannabinoid system activity may have therapeutic potential in almost all diseases affecting humans, including obesity/metabolic syndrome; diabetes and

diabetic complications; pain; neurodegenerative, inflammatory, cardiovascular, liver, gastrointestinal and skin diseases; psychiatric disorders; cachexia; cancer; and chemotherapy-induced nausea and vomiting, amongst many others.[30]

It has also been described as follows:

> An ancient lipid signaling network which in mammals modulates neuronal functions, inflammatory processes, and is involved in the etiology of certain human lifestyle diseases. . . . The system is able to downregulate stress-related signals that lead to chronic inflammation and certain types of pain, but it is also involved in causing inflammation-associated symptoms, depending on the physiological context.[31]

The multitude of effects that eCBs have on almost all neuronal signaling affects neurological function and dysfunction found in a host of conditions. The following list reviews some of the effects that eCBs have on neurotransmitter functions in pathogenesis of dysfunctional conditions[32]:

- Seizure disorders and neurotoxicity diseases – glutamate function
- Seizure disorders, motor function disorders, anxiety – GABA function
- Depression – noradrenaline function
- PTSD – adrenaline function
- Depression, anxiety, depression, migraine, vomiting – serotonin function
- ADHD, Parkinson's disease, schizophrenia – dopamine function
- Neuromuscular disorders, dementia – acetylcholine function

Endocannabinoids do not only affect neural functions, but have wide-reaching effects on metabolic, immunological and stress-regulated functions, as illustrated in Figure 3.6.

The ECS regulates appetite and food intake by modulating the activity of hypothalamic, mesolimbic and brain stem neurons with the release of neuropeptides in an eCB-dependent manner. This regulation is mediated, at least in part, through the action of feeding-regulated hormones, leptin, ghrelin or glucocorticoids, which affects eCB levels within the hypothalamus resulting in elevated hypothalamic endocannabinoid tone.[33]

Excellent in-depth reviews of the current state of knowledge of the endocannabinoid system as a target of pharmacotherapy, with reviews of relevant studies have been published, including a comprehensive listing of its effect on multiple pathophysiological conditions. These include reviews of diseases of energy metabolism, pain and inflammation, central nervous system disorders, cardiovascular and respiratory disorders, eye disorders, cancer, gastrointestinal and liver disorders, musculoskeletal disorders and reproductive functions.[30,34] These functions will be reviewed in Part III within the context of specific medical conditions. The current state of our understanding of the endocannabinoid system and how it affects human health and disease is yet in its infancy. The longer we study the complexity of the endocannabinoid system and its effects in promoting homeostasis, we realize the less we know about how it functions and what to expect from phytocannabinoid intervention, that is, cannabis therapy.

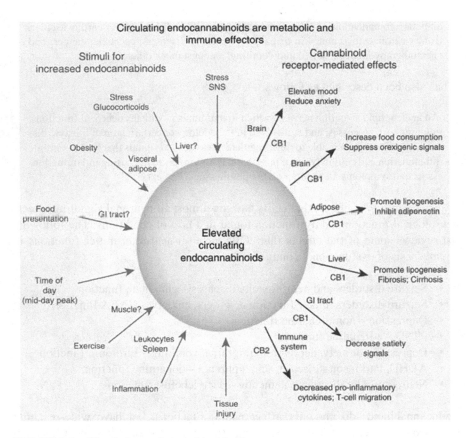

FIGURE 3.6 Circulating endocannabinoid effects.

Source: Hillard, C. 2018. Circulating Endocannabinoids: From Whence Do They Come and Where Are They Going? *Neuropsychopharmacology* 43: 155–172.

REFERENCES

1. Allen, DB. Survey shows low acceptance of the science of the ECS (endocannabinoid system). Outword Magazine website. www.outwordmagazine.com/inside-outword/glbt-news/1266-survey-shows-low-acceptance-of-the-science of the-ecs-endocannabinoid-system Accessed July 14, 2020.
2. Karst M, Wippermann S. Cannabinoids against pain. Efficacy and strategies to reduce psychoactivity: a clinical perspective. *Expert Opin Investig Drugs*. 2009;18(2):125–133.
3. Maccarrone M, Bab I, Bíró T, et al. Endocannabinoid signaling at the periphery: 50 years after THC. *Trends Pharmacol Sci*. 2015;36(5):277–296.
4. Onaivi ES, Sugiura T, Di Marzo V, eds. *Endocannabinoids: The Brain and Body's Marijuana and Beyond*. Boca Raton, FL: CRC Press Taylor & Francis Group; 2006.
5. Pagotto U, Kunos G, Marsicano G, Ghigo E (eds). The neuronal, endocrine, metabolic effects of endocannabinoid system and the potential clinical implications of the cannabinoid type 1 (CB1) blocker. *J Endocrinol Invest*. 2006;28(Supple3).

6. Pacher P, Batkai S, Kunos G. The endocannabinoid system as an emerging target of pharmacotherapy. *Pharmacol Rev.* 2006;58:389–462.

7. Pertwee RG. Pharmacological actions of cannabinoids. *Handb Exp Pharmacol.* 2005;(168): 1–51.

8. Grotenhermen F. Cannabinoids and the endocannabinoid system. *Cannabinoids.* 2006;1(1): 10–14.

9. McPartland JM, Guy GW, Di Marzo V. Care and feeding of the endocannabinoid system: a systematic review of potential clinical interventions that upregulate the endocannabinoid system. *PLoS One.* 2014;9(3):e89566.

10. Di Marzo V. 'Endocannabinoids' and other fatty acid derivatives with cannabimimetic properties: biochemistry and possible physiopathological relevance. *Biochim Biophys Acta Lipids Lipid Metab.* 1998;1392:153–175.

11. Tantimonaco M, Ceci R, Sabatini S, et al. Physical activity and the endocannabinoid system: an overview. *Cell Mol Life Sci.* 2014;71(14):2681–2698.

12. Di Marzo V, Bisogno T, De Petrocellis L. Endocannabinoids and related compounds: walking back and forth between plant natural products and animal physiology. *Chem Biol.* 2007;14(7):741–756.

13. Elmes MW, Kaczocha M, Berger WT, et al. Fatty acid-binding proteins (FABPs) are intracellular carriers for Δ9-tetrahydrocannabinol (THC) and cannabidiol (CBD). *J Biol Chem.* 2015;290(14):8711–8721.

14. Mechoulam R, Parker LA. The endocannabinoid system and the brain. *Annu Rev Psychol.* 2013;64:21–47.

15. Appendino G, Taglialatela-Scafati O. Cannabinoids: chemistry and medicine. In: Ramawat K, Mérillon JM, eds. *Natural Products.* Berlin, Heidelberg: Springer; 2013: 3417–3435. www.researchgate.net/publication/300516737_Cannabinoids_Chemistry_ and_Medicine Accessed July 13, 2020.

16. Di Marzo V, Piscitelli F, Mechoulam R. Cannabinoids and endocannabinoids in metabolic disorders with focus on diabetes. *Handb Exp Pharmacol.* 2011;(203):75–104.

17. Di Marzo V, Melck D, Bisogno T, De Petrocellis L. Endocannabinoids: endogenous cannabinoid receptor ligands with neuromodulatory action. *Trends Neurosci.* 1998;21(12):521–528.

18. Zou S, Kumar U. Cannabinoid receptors and the endocannabinoid system: signaling and function in the central nervous system. *Int J Mol Sci.* 2018;19(3):833.

19. Bie B, Wu J, Foss JF, Naguib M. An overview of the cannabinoid type 2 receptor system and its therapeutic potential. *Curr Opin Anaesthesiol.* 2018;31(4):407–414.

20. Almogi-Hazan O, Or R. Cannabis, the endocannabinoid system and immunity-the journey from the bedside to the bench and back. *Int J Mol Sci.* 2020;21(12):4448.

21. Stempel AV, Stumpf A, Zhang HY, et al. Cannabinoid type 2 receptors mediate a cell type-specific plasticity in the hippocampus. *Neuron.* 2016;90(4):795–809.

22. Silvestri C, Di Marzo V. The endocannabinoid system in energy homeostasis and the etiopathology of metabolic disorders. *Cell Metab.* 2013;17(4):475–490.

23. Castillo PE, Younts TJ, Chávez AE, Hashimotodani Y. Endocannabinoid signaling and synaptic function. *Neuron.* 2012;76(1):70–81.

24. Stella N. Cannabinoid and cannabinoid-like receptors in microglia, astrocytes, and astrocytomas. *Glia.* 2010;58(9):1017–1030.

25. Russo EB. Beyond cannabis: plants and the endocannabinoid system. *Trends Pharmacol Sci.* 2016;37(7):594–605.

26. Howlett AC, Reggio PH, Childers SR, Hampson RE, Ulloa NM, Deutsch DG. Endocannabinoid tone versus constitutive activity of cannabinoid receptors. *Br J Pharmacol.* 2011;163(7):1329–1343.

27. Sparling PB, Giuffrida A, Piomelli D, Rosskopf L, Dietrich A. Exercise activates the endocannabinoid system. *Neuroreport.* 2003;14(17):2209–2211.
28. Charytoniuk T, Zywno H, Konstantynowicz-Nowicka K, et al. Can physical activity support the endocannabinoid system in the preventive and therapeutic approach to neurological disorders? *Int J Mol Sci.* 2020;21(12):4221.
29. Russo EB. Clinical endocannabinoid deficiency reconsidered: current research supports the theory in migraine, fibromyalgia, irritable bowel, and other treatment-resistant syndromes. *Cannabis Cannabinoid Res.* 2016;1(1):154–165.
30. Pacher P, Kunos G. Modulating the endocannabinoid system in human health and disease: successes and failures. *FEBS J.* 2013;280:1918–1943.
31. Gertsch J. Anti-inflammatory cannabinoids in diet: towards a better understanding of CB(2) receptor action? *Commun Integr Biol.* 2008;1:26–28.
32. Grotenhermen F. Pharmacology of cannabinoids. *Neuro Endocrinol Lett.* 2004;25(1–2): 14–23.
33. Di Marzo V, Ligresti A, Cristino L. The endocannabinoid system as a link between homoeostatic and hedonic pathways involved in energy balance regulation. *Int J Obes (Lond).* 2009;33 Suppl 2:S18–24.
34. Di Marzo V, Bifulco M, De Petrocellis L. The endocannabinoid system and its therapeutic exploitation. *Nat Rev Drug Discov.* 2004;3(9):771–784.

4 Cannabinoid Chemistry and Physiology

The knowledge of how cannabis acts biochemically, pharmacologically and physiologically started with a dissection of its chemical components and their mechanism of action on human cells and tissues. Until recently, this investigation focused mainly on the cannabinoids in the plant and primarily on the actions of the cannabinoid associated with "marijuana," delta-9-tetrahydrocannabinol (D9-THC aka Δ9-THC). Research into the effects of cannabinoids has been ongoing for over 50 years since the discovery of THC as the active psychomimetic component in cannabis, with much of cannabinoid chemistry elucidated. Now we know that other cannabinoids in the plant also affect physiological outcomes as do the terpenes and flavonoids. It was originally postulated that the physiological actions of cannabis were mediated primarily by THC, although many cannabinoids from the plant had been identified as far back as the 1960s. A large part of this work was done by Dr. Raphael Mechoulam's group in Israel, who isolated cannabidiol (CBD) in 1963, and then Δ9-THC in 1964.[1] An understanding and appreciation of the action of the terpenes in cannabis is just beginning to be researched in detail and will be presented in the following chapter. Here we start with the cannabinoids, as the story became known. Cannabinoids may be defined as compounds that bind to a cannabinoid receptor. Generally, there are thought to be three categories of cannabinoids: endogenous – occurring within the organism (see Chapter 3), phytocannabinoids – derived from plants, and synthetic – fully or semisynthesized in a laboratory. The cannabinoids derived from cannabis are then, phytocannabinoids, a group of C21 or C22 (for the carboxylated forms) terpenophenolic compounds. Currently, over 200 phytocannabinoids are identified as derived from the cannabis plant. At one time, it was thought that they occurred naturally only in *Cannabis sativa* L., but researchers have now found cannabinoids in lower concentration in other plants as well, such as liverwort, hops and helichrysum.[2] Botanical compounds that influence cannabinoid receptors as well have a slightly different structure than classical cannabinoids called "cannabimimetic" compounds.

There are currently four FDA-approved cannabinoids available in the United States. Cannabidiol oral solution/Epidiolex® (liquid), which is highly purified CBD originating from cannabis, indicated for rare seizure disorders, dronabinol/Marinol® (capsule) and dronabinol/Syndros® (liquid) are oral forms of synthetic THC, both indicated for chemotherapy-induced nausea and vomiting (CINV) and HIV-related anorexia, and nabilone/Cesamet® (capsule) oral form of synthetic THC indicated for CINV. Countries outside of the United States have approved nabiximols/Sativex® (oromucosal liquid spray), a standardized cannabis extract containing approximately a 1:1 ratio of CBD to THC and is indicated for moderate to severe spasticity in

DOI: 10.1201/9781003098201-5

multiple sclerosis patients. Since the passage of the Farm Act in December 2018, hemp-derived CBD is no longer a federally restricted substance, but still subject to FDA regulation.[3,4]

Focusing on the phytocannabinoids in cannabis, there are relatively few that occur in significant amounts that are of interest due to their proven or potential therapeutic activity. These include Δ9- THC (commonly listed as THC), cannabidiol (CBD), cannabigerol (CBG) and cannabichromene (CBC), along with their corresponding carboxylic acids.[5] Propyl cannabinoids (cannabinoids with a C3 side chain, instead of a C5 side chain), such as tetrahydrocannabivarin (THCV) and cannabidivarin (CBDV), as well as their carboxylic acid counterparts are of therapeutic interest as well.[6] We also find cannabinol (CBN) in cannabis samples, which is a degradation product of THC. There are several excellent detailed reviews of cannabinoids.[7-12]

PHYTOCANNABINOID SYNTHESIS AND DEGRADATION

It is a little-known fact that the cannabis plant contains little to no THC, nor CBD. Rather, cannabinoids exist in the raw form as prenylated aromatic carboxylic acids. The biosynthetic pathway that occurs in the plant trichomes derives from three molecules of malonyl-CoA, (a short-chain fatty acyl-coenzyme A) and hexanoyl-CoA (a medium-chain fatty acyl-coenzyme A) combining to form olivetolic acid, a benzoic acid. This combines with geranyl diphosphate (a diphosphate of a polyprenol, geraniol) to yield the parent cannabinoid acid, cannabigerolic acid (CBGA). This is transformed into either tetrahydrocannabinolic acid (THCA), cannabidiolic acid (CBDA) or cannabichromenic acid (CBCA) according to the genetics of the plant.[13] The structure and synthesis of phytocannabinoids is depicted in Figure 4.1.

From CBGA, the following conversions occur: CBGA + THCA synthase converts CBGA to THCA, CBDA synthase yields CBDA and CBCA synthase produces CBCA. This creates three potential pathways of development: THCA dominant, CBDA dominant or CBCA dominant.[14] Production of neutral cannabinoids ultimately occurs with decarboxylation, usually by applying heat. That is likely why cannabis has historically been smoked or cooked, to introduce the heating element, but the precursor cannabinoid acids also have therapeutic benefit. Mature plants with CBCA are rare. CBCA has been reported to dominate in young plants and with levels declining upon maturation. Traditionally, the THCA-dedicated chemovars have been associated with recreational use, while the CBDA-dedicated chemovars are of the hemp variety (with hemp now defined in both federal and state regulatory structures as containing less than 0.3% THC by dry weight).

The cannabinoid content of cannabis can change upon storage. Light, heat, air and time causes THC to degrade to CBN, and THCA to degrade to cannabinolic acid (CBNA). The degradation of THC is greatest in the first year of storage with the content of CBN increasing during storage over time. The degradation rates are higher in the samples exposed to light at 22°C than in those stored in the darkness at 4°C, substantiating the heat and light sensitivity of cannabis, THC specifically. Cannabidiol content decreases due to oxidation during storage as well, to form oxygen to form mono- and dimeric hydroquinones, especially for samples exposed to light at 22°C.[15]

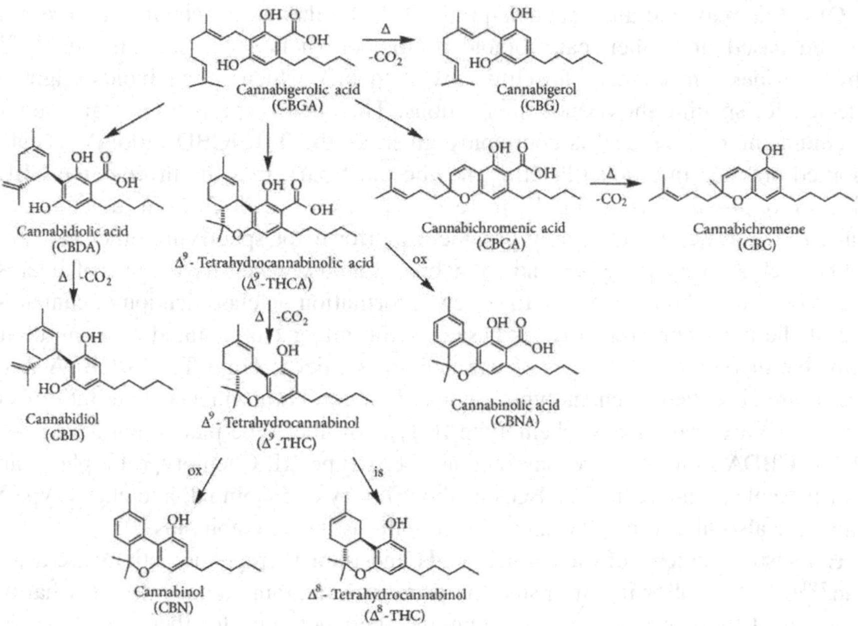

FIGURE 4.1 Chemical structure and synthetic pathways of phytocannabinoids.

Abbreviations: Δ = heating, ox = oxidation, is = isomerization

Source: Pellati F, Borgonetti V, Brighenti V, Biagi M, Benvenuti S, Corsi L. 2018. *Cannabis sativa* L. and Nonpsychoactive Cannabinoids: Their Chemistry and Role against Oxidative Stress, Inflammation, and Cancer. *Biomed Res Int*. 2018:1691428.

CANNABINOID MECHANISMS OF ACTION AND THERAPEUTIC ACTIVITY

Initially, cannabis, cannabinoids, endocannabinoids and research of their mechanisms of action centered around comparative functions relative to THC. In describing the action of cannabis, considering mainly THC, it is simplistic to explain that cannabinoid receptors bind to THC and to endocannabinoids, hence their interaction. Still today, the uninformed marketplace that promotes CBD sales touts cannabinoid receptors and their function to explain how CBD acts, which is inaccurate. Cannabinoid binding sites are diverse and complex, and while they are the most well researched for THC and endocannabinoids, other cannabinoids and other receptors exist and contribute greatly to physiological function.[8] Many cannabinoids act through CB1 and/or CB2 mechanisms (see Chapter 3). Because these are ubiquitous, their effects are summarized here and may be applied to all cannabinoids utilizing these mechanisms. "The most important pharmacological effects triggered by stimulation of CB receptors can be identified as the: (a) psychotropic effects, (b) analgesic effects, (c) immunomodulatory effects, and (d) cardiovascular effects."[8] There are many in-depth reviews about the mechanisms of action of cannabinoids.[11,16,17]

Often cannabinoid and cannabis products and cultivars (or chemovars) are designated based upon their cannabinoid profile, or chemotype (see Chapter 2).[18,19] This provides a mechanism for clinicians to specify which cannabinoids might be selected for specific therapeutic applications. The chemotype is often expressed as a "cannabinoid ratio" and is commonly given as the THC/CBD ratio. A recently adopted practice in product labeling, for the most part, lists the inverse, the CBD/THC ratio, possibly reflecting the increasing prominence of CBD in the consumer market. These descriptors rarely provide a platform for specifying other cannabinoids, such as propyl analogs and cannabinoid acids, which have come of interest in recent years. Should one seek to review information on classification of cannabis, one of the most comprehensive is based on the major cannabinoid concentrations with five different chemotypes of cannabis recognized: High THCA/CBDA ratio (≫1.0) are classified as chemotype I; plants that exhibit an intermediate ratio (usually 0.5–2) are classified as chemotype II; typical fiber-type plants that have a low THCA/CBDA ratio (≪1) are classified as chemotype III. Chemotype IV plants are fiber-type plants that contain CBGA as the primary cannabinoid; and chemotype V plants are also fiber-type plants, but contain almost no cannabinoids.[10,18]

Exhaustive reviews of the cannabinoids and their therapeutic actions are available.[7,10,12] In the following are listed the primary cannabinoids of interest, what we know about their mechanisms of action and their potential for therapeutic physiological effects. Physiological effects considered to be adverse are discussed in a later section (see Chapter 6). In addition, a detailed description of cannabis therapeutic action specific to individual conditions is given in Part III in each clinical chapter.

THC/Δ9-THC (D9-THC)

Δ9-Tetrahydrocannabinol, commonly referred to as THC, is the most well-known cannabinoid derived from the cannabis plant and is well-known for its "psychoactive" or psychomimetic effects such as feeling high, "stoned," euphoric or disoriented, depending upon one's familiarity with its effects – hence the designation of cannabis as a dangerous drug with potential for abuse. It has a host of other potentially therapeutic effects paralleling endocannabinoid function because THC is a CB1 and CB2 cannabinoid receptor agonist. Its effects include, but are not limited to, the following listed in Table 4.1.[8,6,16,17,24]

The mechanism of action of THC has been thought to be mediated primarily by binding cannabinoid receptors CB1 and CB2 (see Chapter 3 for CBr review). THC is a moderate partial agonist of CBrs. Among the phytocannabinoids, THC has been found to have the highest affinity for the CB1 receptor, rendering it the most psychoactive of all the phytocannabinoids.[8] The interaction with CB1 receptors is responsible for the psychoactive, and analgesic effects of THC, among a host of other effects. In particular, the psychoactive, memory and cognition effects are mediated by interaction with central CB1 receptors. Anti-seizure activity by THC is thought to be medicated in part by its partial agonist action on the CB1 receptor.[20] Furthermore, THC action at CB1 and CB2 underlies its activities in modulating pain, spasticity, sedation, appetite and mood.[6] The interaction with CB2 receptors is believed to have a role in immune cell function and considered to be involved in the processes of

TABLE 4.1
Therapeutic Effects of THC

Psychoactive
Euphoric
Analgesic/antinociceptive
Anti-inflammatory
Antispasmodic/muscle relaxant
Immunomodulatory
Bronchodilator
Antiemetic
Appetite stimulant
Neuroprotective
Anticonvulsant
Sleep-inducing
Antitumoral
Antibacterial

neuroinflammation, atherosclerosis and bone remodeling, thus explaining its immunomodulatory properties.[6,16] Additionally, it has strong anti-inflammatory effects, 20 times that of aspirin and twice that of hydrocortisone, due to its cascade of effects seen at multiple receptors.[21] While agonism at CB1 promotes pro-inflammatory responses through reactive oxygen species (ROS) production, CB2 activation leads to a decrease in ROS and tumor necrosis factor alpha (TNF-α) levels, which reduces oxidative stress and inflammation.[22] In response to the mechanism of inflammation or injury, the number of CB2 receptors is upregulated significantly. Activity of THC has been documented at additional receptors as it is a known multitarget ligand showing non-CB1, non-CB2 activity. Anti-inflammatory effects occur as well in a non-CB-dependent mechanism. At the molecular level, THC has also been shown to inhibit mRNA expression of interleukin (IL) sites: IL-1α, IL-1β, IL-6 and TNF-α, affecting transcription factors such as nuclear factor kappa B (NF-κB) and cytokine expression.[23] Additional receptors of the endocannabinoid system are known, including orphan GPCRs such as GPR55, GPR18, GPR119, all of which present binding sites for THC.[17] THC also activates nuclear peroxisome proliferators-activated receptors (PPARs) α and γ (as do endocannabinoids) with vascular relaxation and antitumor effects being linked to agonism at PPARγ.[17] Another important mechanism includes interaction with transient receptor potential cation channels (TRP)V 1,2,3,4 (also known as vanilloid channels) by receptor agonism and TRPM (melastin) 8 antagonism, in modulating pain and nociception. THC also inhibits multiple voltage-gated ion channels, including T-type calcium (Ca) v3, potassium (K) v1.2, sodium (Na) voltage-gated ion channels and conductance in gap junctions, thereby affecting neural conductance.[6] Other binding sites found with THC include 5-hydroxytryptamine (HT) receptors, α1-adrenoceptors, muscarinic receptors, glycine receptors (GlyRs) and α-amino-3-hydroxy-5-methyl-4- isoxazolepropionic acid (AMPA) glutamate receptors, GLUA1 and GLUA3.[1] The activity of THC at the glycine receptors may contribute to the cannabis-induced analgesia. Antiemetic effects are thought to occur due to 5HT3 antagonism. THC is also an allosteric modulator of opioid receptors leading to its synergistic action with opiates. The neuroprotection exhibited by THC is likely a multicomponent effect, mediated not only by interaction with CBrs but also with PPARα and 5-HT1a.[8] The antitumoral effects of cannabinoids have been ascribed to CB1-mediated inhibition of mitosis and to the induction of apoptosis following activation of TRPV1 and/or CB2 receptors.[24] The antimicrobial effects of THC against a variety of methicillin-resistant *Staphylococcus aureus* (MRSA) strains outperformed antibiotics.[8]

THCV/Δ9-THCV

Δ9-Tetrahydrocannabivarin (THCV) is a propyl analogue of THC and is of interest because its psychoactive effects are much less than those of THC, approximately 25%.[7] On a practical level, THCV cultivars are not readily available for consumer use. Its effects include, but are not limited to, the following listed in Table 4.2.[6,7,17,25]

As compared to THC, THCV has a more rapid onset of action with a briefer duration of activity. It is a partial CB2 agonist, with dose-related inverse agonism at the CB1 receptor.[11] At lower doses (<3 mg/kg), THCV acts as a CB1 antagonist, thereby increasing inhibitory neurotransmission in the central nervous system. CB1 antagonism has anti-seizure applications, decreases food intake acting as an appetite suppressant and opposes the effects of THC when coadministered. THCV may also be beneficial in the treatment of metabolic syndrome as it has been found to produce weight loss, decrease body fat and serum leptin concentrations and increase energy expenditure in obese mice.[6] At a higher dose (10 mg/kg), THCV acts as a CB1 agonist, although this dose range is not generally applied clinically. As a CB2 partial agonist, THCV is believed to stimulate mesenchymal stem cells with activity related to its anti-inflammatory and anti-hyperalgesic properties. THCV is also a partial agonist of GPR55 and can activate 5HT1A receptors as well as TRP channels.[7,17] Action at 5-HT$_1$A receptors is thought to contribute to antipsychotic or anxiolytic effects.[25] Research studies are examining its effects upon stress-induced

TABLE 4.2
Therapeutic Effects of THCV

Appetite suppressant
Bone stimulant
Anxiolytic
Modulate "fight or flight"
Neuroprotective
Anticonvulsant
Anti-inflammatory
Anti-hyperalgesic
Antagonist of THC

psychological conditions such as PTSD, potentially due to its antagonism of CB1-dependent functions, as well as its anxiolytic actions.

CBD

Cannabidiol (CBD) is the second most abundant cannabinoid derived from the cannabis plant and the primary one found in hemp strains. Since about 2010, cultivation of many varieties of hemp and cannabis with higher percentages of CBD have made CBD more widely available to consumers. Several comprehensive reviews highlight the pharmacological activities of CBD as well as its complex cannabinoid receptor-dependent and independent actions.[26,27] It is of interest as it lacks the typical "psycho-activity" produced by THC. Its effects include, but are not limited to, the following listed in Table 4.3.[6,8,16,24,26,30-35]

CBD does not act directly on cannabinoid receptors, rather it is a negative allosteric modulator of CB1 receptors, affecting the activity of THC and 2-AG, and it is an inverse agonist of CB2 receptors.[16,26] To say it is non-psychoactive is somewhat misleading as it is anxiolytic, antipsychotic and sedating, but it does not induce euphoria or disorientation. Its effects on the ECS seem to be indirect through different mechanisms that are mediated by eCBs and their enzymes FAAH, MAGL, and actions at PPARα and γ.[28] CBD increases AEA levels directly impacting endocannabinoid tone via its inhibition of cellular uptake of AEA and weak inhibition of FAAH. Cannabidiol also modulates multiple receptors outside the ECS producing a host of physiological effects. CBD modulates the pharmacokinetics of THC by three mechanisms, contributing to an entourage effect. These include inverse agonism at CB1, modulation of signal transduction by changing neuronal membranes increasing the penetration of THC into muscle cells, and/or promoting downstream intracellular signaling, and inhibition of CYP 450 metabolism of THC to 11-OH-THC.[2,29] This last property would reduce the unpleasant symptoms associated with the

TABLE 4.3
Therapeutic Effects of CBD

Anxiolytic
Antipsychotic
Anti-inflammatory
Antiemetic/antinausea
Bone stimulant
Neuroprotective
Anti-ischemic
Antioxidant
Immunomodulatory
Anticonvulsant
Muscle relaxant
Antitumoral
Antibacterial

11-OH-THC such as disorientation and loss of "euphoria." Overall CBD modulates multiple potential adverse effects of THC such as tachycardia, anxiety, sedation and hunger.[6]

The effects of CBD are widespread and complex acting as a multitarget ligand in non-CB1–CB2 receptor systems, including both agonism and antagonism at multiple GPCRs; agonism at PPARγ; agonism at the serotonin receptor 5-HT1A and antagonism at 5-HT3A; agonism of TRPA1, TRPV1,2,3,4 and antagonism of TRPM8; positive allosteric modulation of GABA and GlyRs; inhibition of nicotinic acetylcholine receptors (n-AChRs) and voltage-gated sodium channels; inhibition of lipoxygenases (LOXs); and antagonism of adenosine transport proteins.[28]

The effects of CBD on pain are anecdotally most prominent for inflammatory and neuropathic types, rather than acting as a direct analgesic. The efficacy of CBD in treating chronic pain as well as neuropathic pain has not been proven, although some benefit has been shown using CBD/THC combinations. "As a whole, these data indicate that CBD and its analogues may be beneficial for pain resulting from inflammation however, human studies on this topic are lacking."[30] CBD regulates the perception of pain by affecting multiple receptors, including 5-HT1A, agonism at TRPV1, TRPA1 and antagonism at TPRM8, as well as GlyR, adenosine receptors, opioid receptors and n-ACHRs.[31] Activation of TRPV1 followed by desensitization through receptor downregulation is thought to contribute to its analgesic and anti-inflammatory effects. CBD was shown to produce an anti-hyperalgesic effect in rats via the TRPV1 receptor.[32] Anti-inflammatory effects are mediated by multiple systems, including α-adrenoreceptors, TRPV-1, GPR55 and 5-HT1A. CBD inhibits release of pro-inflammatory cytokines TNF-α, IL-6, IL-1β acting as an antioxidant and free radical scavenger that is more potent than vitamin C or vitamin E. It is known to reduce ROS species.

CBD is currently being explored in human trials as an anticonvulsant. Effects on adenosine reuptake and antagonism of GPR55 have been suggested to play an role in anti-seizure activity.[33] The mechanism of neuroprotection is thought to be complex, mediated by interaction with the ECS in conjunction with PPAR-α, 5-HT1A and other receptors.[8] The antipsychotic and anxiolytic effects of CBD may function in part by its action as a CB1 antagonist but also through its capability to modulate TRPV1 and 5HT1A.[34] Antiemetic effects are mediated by agonism at 5-HT1A receptors.[35] Vasorelaxation has been associated with PPARγ activity. CBD had been found to have direct antitumor activity in multiple types of cancer. In several cancer cell lines, CBD acted as a more potent inhibitor of growth than THC. In vivo, CBD was found to inhibit tumor metastasis. Antitumoral effects occur through a combination of mechanisms that include activation of CB2 (indirectly) and TRPV1 receptors and induction of oxidative stress, all contributing to induction of apoptosis.[24] The antimicrobial effects of THC against a variety of MRSA strains have outperformed antibiotics.[8]

CBDV

Cannabidivarin (CBDV) is a propyl analogue of CBD that lacks psychoactive properties and is currently being researched for its potential in treating epilepsy. On a

---

TABLE 4.4
Therapeutic Effects of CBDV

Anticonvulsant
Bone stimulant
Anti-inflammatory
Antinausea

---

practical level, CBDV cultivars are not readily available for consumer use. Its effects include, but are not limited to, the following listed in Table 4.4.[17,33,36]

The mechanism of action of CBDV has not been well studied. We know that CBDV displays very weak affinity for CB1 and CB2 receptors. It may act as a CB1 agonist, thereby blocking the nausea response. One pharmacological function of CBDV is the inhibition of diacylglycerol lipase, which may decrease the activity of 2-AG. Molecular targets outside the ECS have also been found as CBDV interacts with GPR55. CBDV potently activates the TRPA1 channel, and is a weak agonist of the TRPV1, TRPV2 and TRPV3 cation channels.[17] CBDV has been found to act as an anticonvulsant in rat hippocampal brain slices, with potential therapeutic applications for epilepsy.[36] The mechanisms responsible for the anti-seizure effects of CBDV are not yet understood but do not seem to involve an action on cannabinoid receptors.[33] There are also some indications that CBDV can act as a bone stimulant as does CBD.

CBC

Cannabichromene (CBC) is the third primary cannabinoid derived from the cannabis plant. The cannabis cultivars that produce significant quantities of CBC are rarely encountered and have been unavailable to consumers until most recently. It is of interest due to its lack of psychoactivity. Its effects include, but are not limited to, the following listed in Table 4.5.[6,8,24,37–39]

CBC is a CB2 receptor agonist that acts as a weak AEA reuptake inhibitor, thereby inhibiting AEA degradation and affecting endocannabinoid tone.[37] CBC may exert anti-inflammatory effects through a CB2 mechanism.[38] Molecular targets outside the

---

TABLE 4.5
Therapeutic Effects of CBC

Analgesic/antinociceptive
Anti-inflammatory
Normalizes GI motility
Antitumoral
Antibacterial
Antifungal

ECS have also been found. CBC is a potent TRPA1 agonist suggesting a potential role in analgesia.[6] CBC selectively reduced inflammation-induced hypermotility in mice in a manner independent of CBrs or TRPA1.[37] CBC was found to have strong antitumoral effects when tested in a wide range of cell lines generally following the two primary cannabinoids, CBD and THC in the rank of potency.[24] As early as the 1980s, it was known that CBC has antibacterial and antifungal properties by in vitro testing.[39] The antimicrobial effects of CBC against a variety of MRSA strains outperformed antibiotics.[8] The pharmacological applications of CBC are just beginning to be explored.

CBG

Cannabigerol (CBG) is a non-psychoactive cannabinoid found in high concentration in its acid form in the plant, early in its life cycle, and is present only in minor amounts in mature cannabis varieties.[40] Cultivars are now being released with increased potential for production of CBG, especially from hemp strains. This has allowed some consumer availability in recent years. Its effects include, but are not limited to, the following listed in Table 4.6.[6,8,17,24,41,42]

CBG has multifold and potent effects. It is a weak partial agonist at CB1 and CB2 receptors; although it is thought to bind primarily with CB2 receptors, CBG acts as an AEA uptake inhibitor, thereby affecting endocannabinoid tone.[7,41] CBG also functions as a GABA uptake inhibitor exhibiting greater efficacy than THC and CBD in providing muscle relaxant and anxiolytic properties.[6] Molecular targets outside the ECS have also been found. CBG antagonizes TRPV8 receptors and stimulates TRPV1, TRPV2, TRPA1, TRPV3 and TRPV4 receptors, leading to its potent analgesic effects (shown to have greater activity than THC). Its ability to block LOX enzymes also surpasses that of THC leading to anti-inflammatory effects. CBG is also a low-level inhibitor of prostaglandin production. It has been

TABLE 4.6
Therapeutic Effects of CBG

Anti-inflammatory
Analgesic
Anxiolytic
Lowers intraocular pressure
Antiemetic
Muscle relaxant
Appetite stimulant
Neuroprotective
Bone stimulant
Immunomodulatory
Antitumoral
Antibacterial

demonstrated to reduce inflammation in inflammatory bowel disease.[42] CBG inhibits voltage-gated Na^+ ion channels contributing to analgesic effects. It is a PPARγ agonist, potentially providing neuroprotective effects. CBG may also antagonize the stimulation of serotonin 5-HT1A, bringing into question the validity of over-the-counter claims of its benefit as an antidepressant.[17] Additionally, CBG inhibits keratinocyte proliferation, which may benefit psoriasis.[6] CBG is found to have strong antitumoral effects (comparable to CBC) when tested in a wide range of cell lines and follows CBD and THC in the rank of potency.[24] The antimicrobial effects of CBG against a variety of MRSA strains outperformed antibiotics.[8]

CBN

Cannabinol (CBN) is an oxidized metabolite resulting from the degradation of THC and is known to have mild psychoactive effects. Its acid form (CBNA) is found in the plant from oxidation of THCA and the neutral CBN may also be formed upon heating of this acid. It was the first cannabinoid to be isolated from the cannabis plant with its structure elucidated as far back as 1940. It is of interest due to its lethargy-inducing effects as it is considered useful for insomnia. Its effects include, but are not limited to, the following listed in Table 4.7.[6,8,17]

CBN is a weak CB1 and CB2 partial agonist, with an estimated 10–25% of the activity of THC at CBrs.[6,7] The affinity of CBN for CB2 receptors is greater than its affinity for CB1 receptors, suggesting that it has a greater effect on immune function than on central nervous system function. It is a known potent agonist of TRPA1, an agonist of TRPV2 and antagonist of TPRM8 channels, providing a mechanism for analgesia.[17] It may also activate non-CB1, non-CB2 and non-TRPV1 peripheral neuronal receptors. CBN inhibits the activity of COX and LOX enzymes contributing to its anti-inflammatory effects as well as the inhibition of keratinocyte proliferation via CBr-independent mechanisms, suggesting benefit in treating psoriasis.[6] Contrary to the euphoric effects of THC, CBN may produce feelings of lethargy, potentially making it useful for sedation and sleep. This utility has not been confirmed in research studies, but rather comes from anecdotal reports, and its mechanism has not been elucidated. The antimicrobial effects of CBN against a variety of MRSA strains outperformed antibiotics.[8]

TABLE 4.7
Therapeutic Effects of CBN

Analgesic
Sedating
Anti-inflammatory
Anticonvulsant
Antibacterial

CANNABINOID ACIDS

These generally refer to the aforementioned plant cannabinoids in their acid form prior to decarboxylation – removal of the COOH terminal (which primarily is found at the 2- or sometimes 4- position on the phytocannabinoid aromatic ring). In reviewing the synthesis chart (Figure 4.1), we see that the "mother cannabinoid" in the cannabis plant is CBGA, which can then form THCA, CDBA or CBCA, with the addition of the propyl forms in some strains to form their acid counterparts, THCVA and CBDVA. There are also in vivo metabolites of cannabinoids that exist in acid form as well, not to be confused with the phytocannabinoid acids. These end products of metabolism such as $\Delta9$- THC-11-oic acid (11-nor-9-carboxy-$\Delta9$-THC, or THC-COOH) and CBD-7-oic acid (CBD-COOH), the acidic COOH group comes off of the 11- and 7-positions of the aromatic ring, respectively, and are excreted.[43,44] (The degradation of cannabinoids in vivo is discussed in "Drug Interactions" in Chapter 6). Nevertheless, while little research has been done on the physiological effects of these cannabinoid acid metabolites, some data has been collected on the actions of THC-COOH. It has shown anti-inflammatory and antinociceptive functions, and antagonized platelet-activating factor in animal studies.[43]

Following their discovery, the cannabinoid acids were thought to be biologically inactive and for some time little was reported to dispute this claim. Further investigation showed they participate in a number of physiological and pharmacological activities.[45] Subsequent reports have identified a family of endogenous counterparts of the acids that are structurally different but share many of the actions of the phytocannabinoids in acid form.[43] Such an endogenous substance is N-arachidonoyl glycine (NAgly), which is similar in structure to AEA and is hypothesized to be formed upon its carboxylation. Most of the therapeutic research on cannabinoid acids refers to the phytocannabinoid precursors upon which we will focus next.

A therapeutic advantage of all the cannabinoid acids is that they are non-psychoactive as they have little to no affinity for cannabinoid receptors. Evidence exists for significant therapeutic activity, yet cannabinoid acids have not been promoted as effective for therapeutic use until recently. Interestingly, anecdotal reports of the benefits of raw cannabis have fueled some of this interest – for example, a Mexican folkloric account of the anti-inflammatory benefits of cannabis extracted into unheated (therefore not decarboxylated) alcohol as a relief for joint pain. This preparation is applied directly to the affected areas and preceded the production of topical products. The benefits of cannabis tea, which has been shown to contain little THC and is primarily THCA, have been reported (see discussion of raw cannabis in the Chapter 7).[46] Consumers partaking of raw cannabis or hemp or products of cold extraction processes are actually getting acid forms of all the present cannabinoids.

In general, cannabinoid acids have shown anti-inflammatory activity, are analgesic and encompass a host of other functions that are just beginning to be delineated. Cannabinoid acids inhibit COX enzymes, but in a higher concentration range, as compared to anti-inflammatory drugs (i.e., indomethacin).[47] Research conducted with synthetic analogues has shown additional actions that include antineoplastic, suppression of osteoclastogenesis, reduction of spasticity in multiple sclerosis, antifibrotic and anticystic effects.[43]

CBGA

Cannabigerolic acid (CBGA) is known as the "mother of all cannabinoids." It is the first cannabinoid synthesized by the cannabis plant. All other cannabinoids are catalyzed from CBGA via enzymatic activity. As such, it is present ordinarily only in small amounts in the mature plant, although new cultivars have been genetically manipulated that lack the enzymes required to convert CBGA into other cannabinoids; thus, it is becoming more readily available for consumer use. Its effects include, but are not limited to, the following listed in Table 4.8.[47,49,50]

Very little research is available regarding the therapeutic applications or mechanism of action of CBGA. CBGA was found to inhibit COX-1 and COX-2 enzymes and weakly inhibited prostaglandin production contributing to its anti-inflammatory action.[47] It has been shown to act as a dual PPARα/γ agonist with the ability to stimulate lipid metabolism and reduce excess lipid accumulation, as well as contribute to neuroprotection.[48] CBGA greatly inhibits the enzyme aldose reductase, in a dose-dependent manner, with a potential to diminish oxidative stress that leads to heart disease and other problems especially in diabetes.[49] CBGA was shown to have cytotoxic activity with colon cancer cell lines in vitro.[50] The pharmacological applications of CBGA have not yet been fully explored.

TABLE 4.8
Therapeutic Effects of CBGA

Analgesic
Anti-inflammatory
May modulate lipid metabolism
Antiproliferative

THCA

Δ9-Tetrahydrocannabinolic acid (THCA) is the most abundant cannabinoid in the mature cannabis plant. As the plant is dried and exposed to heat, the THCA is converted into THC by decarboxylation. Consumers partaking of raw cannabis or products that result from cold extraction processes are actually utilizing THCA, not THC. Although not widely disseminated, products containing THCA are now becoming available for consumers. Its effects include, but are not limited to, the following listed in Table 4.9.[6,24,33,44,47,51]

THCA has been reported to be a weak agonist of CB1 and CB2 receptors, but this remains controversial as an in vivo mechanism. Some studies indicate that THCA can bind to CB receptors, but has restricted access to the central nervous system. In that case, THCA would be expected to bind to CBrs at peripheral sites.[44] THCA interacts with several molecular targets and is a weak inhibitor of endocannabinoid degradation enzymes such as FAAH and MAGL. This increases levels of endocannabinoids resulting in higher endocannabinoid tone.[6] THCA was found to inhibit COX-1 and COX-2 enzymes and weakly inhibit prostaglandin production in vitro, contributing to anti-inflammatory action.[47] Interaction

TABLE 4.9
Therapeutic Effects of THCA

Anti-inflammatory
Antispasmodic
Neuroprotective
Antinausea
Anticonvulsant
Immunomodulatory
Antiproliferative

with CB2 and the orphan receptor GPR18 as well as GPR55 has also been documented.[44] The anti-inflammatory activity of cannabis extracts on colon epithelial cells attributed to THCA activity is mediated, at least partially via the GPR55 receptor.[51] THCA is a potent TRPA1 agonist and TRPM8 antagonist, suggesting potential for analgesia.[44] THCA's antinausea effect was blocked by a PPARα antagonist in animal studies.[35] THCA has been found to possess anticonvulsant activity in preclinical investigations by a mechanism not yet identified.[33] THCA also reduces cell viability of various cancer cell lines, perhaps through TNF-α inhibition and was found to be more efficacious than THC for some cell lines.[6,24,44] THCA may modify the absorption and/or the metabolism of THC producing an entourage effect.

CBDA

Cannabidiolic acid (CBDA) is the most abundant cannabinoid in the mature hemp plant. As the plant is dried and exposed to heat, the CBDA is converted into CBD by decarboxylation. Consumers partaking of raw hemp or cold extraction processes are actually getting CBDA, not CBD. Products containing CBDA are not widely available for consumer use. Its effects include, but are not limited to, the following listed in Table 4.10.[4,7,10,35,52–54]

CBDA does not interact efficiently with CB1 receptors. It is thought to interact somewhat with CB2 and the orphan receptors GPR18 and GPR55. At higher concentrations, it can inhibit ECS degradation enzymes, especially FAAH, thereby

TABLE 4.10
Therapeutic Effects of CBDA

Anti-inflammatory
Decreases GI motility
Antinausea
Antiproliferative
Antimicrobial

increasing endocannabinoid tone.[43] CBDA interacts with several molecular targets. It has been found to possess an inhibitory effect on COX enzymes, through downregulation and enzyme inhibition. It has also been found to both inhibit and stimulate the prostaglandin production.[52] It is a TRPA1 and TRPV1 agonist and TRPM8 antagonist in the low micromolar range. These mechanisms contribute to its anti-inflammatory and analgesic functions. CBDA has been shown to act as dual PPARα/γ agonist with the ability to modulate lipid metabolism and inflammation. CBDA activates 5-HT1A receptors, suggesting a potential anxiolytic or antidepressant role, as well as promoting antiemetic effects in animal studies.[35,53] CBDA exerts antiproliferative actions in vitro in a non-CB-dependent manner, possibly related to its downregulation of oncogenes.[52] CBDA is said to portray antispasmodic actions, but this has only been substantiated by slowed gastrointestinal motility in animal studies.[54] It also has antimicrobial functions.[7]

CONCLUSION

This chapter has outlined the vast complexity of mechanism, function and therapeutic potential that cannabinoids offer. While the information available about cannabinoid therapeutics is considerable, much less is known about effective dosage, pharmacokinetics and formulations effective in clinical cannabis applications (see Chapter 7). In clinical cannabis practice, we start by identifying which therapeutic effects associated with which cannabinoids will best serve the patient's needs. It is becoming apparent that combinations of cannabinoids often bring more therapeutic advantage than single dominant cultivars or products. Cannabinoid interactions are capable of producing entourage effects and therapeutic regimens are augmented not only by utilizing cannabinoid combinations but also by considering the function of other plant constituents. One prime example is utilizing CBD or THCV to mitigate potentially impairing CB1-dependent functions of THC. Yet another example is the inclusion of both CBD and THC and/or cannabinoid acids and/or CBG in anticancer therapies. Clearly, cannabinoids act at multiple target receptors; thus, tolerance may be reduced by using lower amounts of individual cannabinoids in mixed or preferably full-plant regimens. The appreciation of non-THC and non-CBD dominant cannabinoid preparations is in their infancy. The more we learn about the clinical effects and appropriate dosing of cannabinoids, the more we enhance their utility as therapeutic agents. Research continues into the application of isolated, purified cannabinoids that may be more easily regulated by the FDA, especially those without psychoactive properties. The next chapter reviews the therapeutic functions of additional components of cannabis required for a more comprehensive understanding of entourage effects and product selection.

REFERENCES

1. Pertwee RG. Cannabinoid pharmacology: the first 66 years. *Br J Pharmacol.* 2006;147(Suppl 1):S163–S171.
2. Andre CM, Hausman JF, Guerriero G. Cannabis sativa: the plant of the thousand and one molecules. *Front Plant Sci.* 2016;7:19.

3. US Food and Drug Administration. FDA regulation of cannabis and cannabis-derived products, including cannabidiol (CBD). 2020. www.fda.gov/news-events/public-health-focus/fda-regulation-cannabis-and-cannabis-derived-products-including-cannabidiol-cbd Accessed December 15, 2020.

4. Mead A. Legal and regulatory issues governing cannabis and cannabis-derived products in the United States. *Front Plant Sci.* 2019;10:697.

5. Hanus LO. Pharmacological and therapeutic secrets of plant and brain (endo)cannabinoids. *Med Res Rev.* 2009;29(2):213–271.

6. Russo EB, Marcu J. Cannabis pharmacology: the usual suspects and a few promising leads. *Adv Pharmacol.* 2017;80:67–134.

7. Izzo AA, Borrelli F, Capasso R, Di Marzo V, Mechoulam R. Non-psychotropic plant cannabinoids: new therapeutic opportunities from an ancient herb. *Trends Pharmacol Sci.* 2009;30(10):515–527.

8. Appendino G, Taglialatela Scafati O. Cannabinoids: chemistry and medicine. In: Ramawat K, Mérillon JM, eds. *Natural Products.* Berlin, Heidelberg: Springer; 2013: 3417–3435. www.researchgate.net/publication/300516737_Cannabinoids_Chemistry_and_Medicine Accessed July 13, 2020.

9. Grotenhermen F. Cannabinoids and the endocannabinoid system. *Cannabinoids.* 2006;1(1):10–14.

10. Galal AM, Slade D, Gul W, et al. Naturally occurring and related synthetic cannabinoids and their potential therapeutic applications. *Recent Pat CNS Drug Discov.* 2009;4(2):112–136.

11. Turner SE, Williams CM, Iversen L, Whalley BJ. Molecular pharmacology of phytocannabinoids. *Prog Chem Org Nat Prod.* 2017;103:61–101.

12. Kogan NM, Mechoulam R. Cannabinoids in health and disease. *Dialogues Clin Neurosci.* 2007;29(4):413–430.

13. Formato M, Crescente G, Scognamiglio M, et al. (–)-Cannabidiolic acid, a still overlooked bioactive compound: an introductory review and preliminary research. *Molecules.* 2020;25(11):2638.

14. Gülck T, Møller BL. Phytocannabinoids: origins and biosynthesis. *Trends Plant Sci.* 2020;25(10):985–1004.

15. Trofn IG, Dabija G, Vaireanu DI, Filipescu L. The influence of long-term storage conditions on the stability of cannabinoids derived from cannabis resin. *Rev Chim Buchar.* 2012;63(4):422–427.

16. Pellati F, Borgonetti V, Brighenti V, et al. Cannabis sativa L. and nonpsychoactive cannabinoids: their chemistry and role against oxidative stress, inflammation, and cancer. *BioMed Res Int.* 2018;1–15.

17. Morales P, Hurst DP, Reggio PH. Molecular targets of the phytocannabinoids: a complex picture. *Prog Chem Org Nat Prod.* 2017;103:103–131.

18. Aizpurua-Olaizola O, Soydaner U, Öztürk E, et al. Evolution of the cannabinoid and terpene content during the growth of cannabis sativa plants from different chemotypes. *J Nat Prod.* 2016;79(2):324–331.

19. Berman P, Futoran K, Lewitus GM, et al. A new ESI-LC/MS approach for comprehensive metabolic profiling of phytocannabinoids in Cannabis. *Sci Rep.* 2018;8:14280.

20. Blair RE, Deshpande LS, DeLorenzo RJ. Cannabinoids: is there a potential treatment role in epilepsy? *Expert Opin Pharmacother.* 2015;16(13):1911–1914.

21. Formukong EA, Evans AT, Evans FJ. Analgesic and antiinflammatory activity of constituents of Cannabis sativa L. *Inflammation.* 1988;12(4):361–371.

22. Atalay S, Jarocka-Karpowicz I, Skrzydlewska E. Antioxidative and anti-inflammatory properties of cannabidiol. *Antioxidants.* 2020;9(1):21.

23. Nagarkatti P, Pandey R, Rieder SA, Hegde VL, Nagarkatti M. Cannabinoids as novel anti-inflammatory drugs. *Future Med Chem*. 2009;1(7):1333–1349.
24. Ligresti A, Moriello AS, Starowicz K, et al. Antitumor activity of plant cannabinoids with emphasis on the effect of cannabidiol on human breast carcinoma. *J Pharmacol Exp Ther*. 2006;318(3):1375–1387.
25. Cascio MG, Zamberletti E, Marini P, Parolaro D, Pertwee RG. The phytocannabinoid, Δ^9-tetrahydrocannabivarin, can act through 5-HT$_1$A receptors to produce antipsychotic effects. *Br J Pharmacol*. 2015;172(5):1305–1318.
26. Pisanti S, Malfitano AM, Ciaglia E, et al. Cannabidiol: state of the art and new challenges for therapeutic applications. *Pharmacol Ther*. 2017;175:133–150.
27. Zuardi AW. Cannabidiol: from an inactive cannabinoid to a drug with wide spectrum of action. *Rev Bras Psiquiatr*. 2008;30(3):271–280.
28. Nahler G, Jones TM. Pure cannabidiol versus cannabidiol-containing extracts: distinctly different multi-target modulators. *J Altern Complement Integr Med*. 2018;4:1–11.
29. Comelli F, Giagnoni G, Bettoni I, Colleoni M, Costa B. Antihyperalgesic effect of a Cannabis sativa extract in a rat model of neuropathic pain: mechanisms involved. *Phytother Res*. 2008;22(8):1017–1024.
30. Zhornitsky S, Potvin S. Cannabidiol in humans-the quest for therapeutic targets. *Pharmaceuticals (Basel)*. 2012;5(5):529–552.
31. McPartland JM, Duncan M, Di Marzo V, Pertwee RG. Are cannabidiol and Δ(9)-tetrahydrocannabivarin negative modulators of the endocannabinoid system? A systematic review. *Br J Pharmacol*. 2015;172(3):737–753.
32. Costa B, Giagnoni G, Franke C, Trovato AE, Colleoni M. Vanilloid TRPV1 receptor mediates the antihyperalgesic effect of the nonpsychoactive cannabinoid, cannabidiol, in a rat model of acute inflammation. *Br J Pharmacol*. 2004;143(2):247–250.
33. Perucca E. Cannabinoids in the treatment of epilepsy: hard evidence at last? *J Epilepsy Res*. 2017;7(2):61–76.
34. Fernández-Ruiz J, Hernández M, Ramos JA. Cannabinoid-dopamine interaction in the pathophysiology and treatment of CNS disorders. *CNS Neurosci Ther*. 2010;16(3):e72–91.
35. Rock EM, Sullivan MT, Pravato S, et al. Effect of combined doses of Δ9-tetrahydrocannabinol and cannabidiol or tetrahydrocannabinolic acid and cannabidiolic acid on acute nausea in male Sprague-Dawley rats. *Psychopharmacology*. 2020;237:901–914.
36. Hill AJ, Mercier MS, Hill TD, et al. Cannabidivarin is anticonvulsant in mouse and rat. *Br J Pharmacol*. 2012;167(8):1629–1642.
37. Izzo AA, Capasso R, Aviello G, et al. Inhibitory effect of cannabichromene, a major non-psychotropic cannabinoid extracted from Cannabis sativa, on inflammation-induced hypermotility in mice. *Br J Pharmacol*. 2012;166(4):1444–1460.
38. Udoh M, Santiago M, Devenish S, McGregor IS, Connor M. Cannabichromene is a cannabinoid CB2 receptor agonist. *Br J Pharmacol*. 2019;176(23):4537–4547.
39. Turner CE, Elsohly MA. Biological activity of cannabichromene, its homologs and isomers. *J Clin Pharmacol*. 1981;21(S1):283S–291S.
40. McPartland J, Russo E. Cannabis and cannabis extracts: greater than the sum of their parts? *J Cannabis Ther*. 2001;1:103–132.
41. Deiana S. Potential medical uses of cannabigerol: a brief overview. In: Preedy V, ed. *Handbook of Cannabis and Related Pathologies*, 1st ed. London, UK: Academic Press, Elsevier; 2017: Chapter 99. www.researchgate.net/publication/312153031_Chapter_99_Potential_Medical_Uses_of_Cannabigerol_A_Brief_Overview Accessed December 15, 2020.
42. Borrelli F, Fasolino I, Romano B, et al. Beneficial effect of the non-psychotropic plant cannabinoid cannabigerol on experimental inflammatory bowel disease. *Biochem Pharmacol*. 2013;85(9):1306–1316.

43. Burstein SH. The cannabinoid acids, analogs and endogenous counterparts. *Bioorg Med Chem.* 2014;22(10):2830–2843.
44. Moreno-Sanz G. can you pass the acid test? Critical review and novel therapeutic perspectives of δ9-tetrahydrocannabinolic acid A. *Cannabis Cannabinoid Res.* 2016;1(1):124–130.
45. Burstein SH. The cannabinoid acids: nonpsychoactive derivatives with therapeutic potential. *Pharmacol Ther.* 1999;82(1):87–96.
46. Hazekamp A, Bastola K, Rashidi H, Bender J, Verpoorte R. Cannabis tea revisited: a systematic evaluation of the cannabinoid composition of cannabis tea. *J Ethnopharmacol.* 2007;113(1):85–90.
47. Ruhaak L, Felth J, Karlsson P, et al. Evaluation of the cyclooxygenase inhibiting effects of six major cannabinoids isolated from Cannabis sativa. *Biol Pharm Bull.* 2011;34(5):774–778.
48. D'Aniello E, Fellous T, Fabio Iannotti FA, et al. Identification and characterization of phytocannabinoids as novel dual PPARα/γ agonists by a computational and in vitro experimental approach. *Biochim Biophys Acta.* 2019;1863(3):586–597.
49. Smeriglio A, Giofrè SV, Galati EM, et al. Inhibition of aldose reductase activity by Cannabis sativa chemotypes extracts with high content of cannabidiol or cannabigerol. *Fitoterapia.* 2018;127:101–108.
50. Nallathambi R, Mazuz M, Namdar D, et al. Identification of synergistic interaction between cannabis-derived compounds for cytotoxic activity in colorectal cancer cell lines and colon polyps that induces apoptosis-related cell death and distinct gene expression. *Cannabis Cannabinoid Res.* 2018;3(1):120–135.
51. Nallathambi R, Mazuz M, Ion A, et al. Anti-inflammatory activity in colon models is derived from Δ9-tetrahydrocannabinolic acid that interacts with additional compounds in cannabis extracts. *Cannabis Cannabinoid Res.* 2017;2(1):167–182.
52. Takeda S, Misawa K, Yamamoto I, Watanabe K. Cannabidiolic acid as a selective cyclooxygenase-2 inhibitory component in cannabis. *Drug Metab Dispos.* 2008;36(9):1917–1921.
53. Bolognini D, Rock EM, Cluny NL, et al. Cannabidiolic acid prevents vomiting in Suncus murinus and nausea-induced behaviour in rats by enhancing 5-HT1A receptor activation. *Br J Pharmacol.* 2013;168(6):1456–1470.
54. Cluny NL, Naylor RJ, Whittle BA, Javid FA. The effects of cannabidiolic acid and cannabidiol on contractility of the gastrointestinal tract of Suncus murinus. *Arch Pharm Res.* 2011;34:1509–1517.

5 Cannabis Secondary Metabolites

Cannabis is a complex plant able to produce more than 480 chemical entities. *Cannabis sativa* L. produces not only cannabinoids but also other kinds of secondary metabolites that may be grouped into six classes – terpenoids, flavonoids, stilbenoids, alkaloids, phytosterols and lignans. Little attention has been given to the pharmacology of these compounds in particular as they relate to cannabis.[1] Several reviews describing the chemistry, synthesis and medicinal effects of these compounds provide in-depth detail.[1-3] Therapeutic effects of these secondary metabolites in general are broad and include effects such as anti-inflammatory, antineoplastic, neuroprotective, cardiovascular protective, antioxidant, antimicrobial and longevity effects, with the ability to induce apoptosis. Of these, the terpenoids, or terpenes, have received the most attention for producing medicinal effects, although as investigation of this plant progresses, the flavonoids are also receiving attention. These two classes of compounds are discussed in depth in the following sections.

TERPENES

Terpenes are present in the form of volatile oils in many medicinal plants, including cannabis, and are responsible for its varied and pungent aroma, contributing to its chemotaxic classification and pharmacological effects. Some reports refer to these molecules as terpenoids. Though these names are often used interchangeably, terpenoids are actually terpenes that have been denatured by oxidation (i.e., from drying). Technically, a terpenoid contains oxygen, while a terpene is a hydrocarbon. Terpenes are small organic molecules that are derived from 5-carbon isoprene units. They are classified according to the number of repeating units of 5-carbon building blocks (isoprene units). Most of the common terpenes in cannabis are monoterpenes with 10 carbons, or sesquiterpenes with 15 carbons. Their relatively small size leads to volatility, allowing them to dissipate into the air, contributing to their aromatic characteristics. For the sake of uniformity when referring to the properties of the cannabis plant, the term terpene will be used, while the term terpenoid will be used when the plant matter has been processed, such as in product derivations.

Terpenes contribute to the full and unique array of medicinal properties associated with any particular cultivar and present a wide array of pharmacological properties, which have recently been described in several reviews.[2,4-7] They have been deemed generally as safe (GRAS) substances by the Flavor and Extract Manufacturers Association, reflecting a high-safety profile for consumption.[8] Terpenes are lipophilic compounds that easily cross membranes and the blood–brain barrier. Many terpenes act as natural defense mechanisms against insects as resins are often sticky providing

DOI: 10.1201/9781003098201-6

a natural barrier for invading predators. Terpenes are quite potent effecting animal and human behavior when inhaled, with results shown to in ng/ml serum levels.[2,4]

Mono- and sesquiterpenes have been detected in flowers, roots and leaves of cannabis, with the secretory glandular hairs or trichomes as the main production sites.[9] Monoterpenes tend to predominate in most plants; however, these terpenes will decrease in concentration during the drying and storage process, due to their high volatility resulting in a higher relative proportion of sesquiterpenoids, especially caryophyllenes. In addition, the extraction process involved in preparing many products such as concentrates and oils results in a selective loss of monoterpenes due to the use of heat in currently popular extraction processes.[10] This leads to heterogeneity in the final product, especially in samples that have not been stored properly, and thus have lost much of their volatile terpenoid content. Over 200 have been reported in the cannabis plant, but only a few are found in significant concentration. Terpenes in concentrations above 0.05% in the plant are considered of pharmacological interest. Terpenoids are usually present in dried cannabis flower buds in the 0.05–3.5% range by weight, although minor components are present at lower concentrations.[11,12] Research has shown the following:

> Monoterpenes [monoterpenoids], including D-limonene, β-myrcene, α- and β-pinene, terpinolene and D-linalool constitute the major terpene [terpenoid] profile from 3 to 28 mg/g of flower dry weight. Sesquiterpenes [Sesquiterpenoids], including β-caryophyllene and α-humulene constitute the remaining major terpenes [terpenoids] in cannabis, from 0.5 to 10 mg/g of flower dry weight.[12]

As is the case with cannabinoids, terpene biosynthesis is genetically determined. It has been said that the terpene content of a cultivar determines whether a cultivar is an "indica" or a "sativa." As previously discussed, these characterizations are not scientifically accurate, can be misleading, and represent an outdated way of categorizing cannabis (see Chapter 2). We do have some information regarding the association of terpenes with certain characteristics. One report found:

> "Mostly indica" strains were characterized by dominancy of β-myrcene, present in high relative contents, with limonene or α-pinene as second most abundant terpenoid, while "mostly sativa" strains were characterized by more complex terpene profiles, with some strains having α-terpinolene or α-pinene as dominant terpenoid, and some strains having β-myrcene as dominant terpenoid.[13]

Another report attempting to correlate leaf structure with terpene content found that narrow leaflet (higher in THC) and hemp strains (higher in CBD) both contained significantly more β-myrcene, while broad leaflet cultivars contained more linalool.[14] Clearly, with the crossbreeding that has occurred, leaflet structure no longer indicates sativa versus indica, and even the presence of β-myrcene is no longer the only determinant of "sedation," although it is definitely a primary component.

The mechanisms of action are varied, including interactions with neurotransmitter receptors, G protein receptors, muscle and neuronal ion channels, enzymes, cell membranes and other secondary messenger systems. The antimicrobial mode of action of terpenes includes a bacterial membranous disruption effect resulting in alterations of membrane permeability and leakage of intracellular materials.[5,11]

> Most terpenoids are able to inhibit two crucial processes which are essential to microbial survival, this includes oxygen uptake and oxidative phosphorylation. . . . Thus, terpene interaction leads to alteration in cellular respiration which later causes uncoupling of oxidative phosphorylation in the microbe.[15]

Some terpenes act as natural skin penetration enhancers, with mechanisms of action based on "(1) disintegration of the highly ordered intercellular lipid structure between corneocytes in stratum corneum, (2) interaction with intercellular domain of protein, which induces their conformational modification, (3) increase the partitioning of a drug."[16] This property contributes significantly to utility in transdermal application of cannabis.

The seven major terpenes found in cannabis and considered to be relevant in cannabis therapeutics with a presentation of the likely mechanisms of action are reviewed in the following sections. Clinical research regarding the effects of terpenes in human trials is scarce and there is yet much to be learned. Much of the mechanistic information comes from in vitro studies and animal experiments.

α-PINENE

α-Pinene is the most common terpene found in nature. Much as the name suggests, this terpene smells like pine trees (pine oil), appears in conifers and numerous other plants and is highly repellant to insects. It is a monoterpene (10 carbon atoms). Other sources include fresh sage, basil, parsley and dill as well. Its therapeutic effects include, but are not limited to, the following listed in Table 5.1.[2,5,17–19]

α-Pinene inhibits inflammatory cytokines such as IL1-β and the expression of inflammatory and catabolic genes contributing to anti-inflammatory and anti-catabolic effects. It also inhibits prostaglandin E1 (PGE-1), contributing to its

---

TABLE 5.1
Therapeutic Effects of α-Pinene

Bronchodilator
Promotes alertness
Memory enhancing
Anti-inflammatory
Antinociceptive
Antioxidant
Gastroprotective
Hypoglycemic
Chondroprotective
Antibacterial
Antifungal

---

anti-inflammatory, antioxidant and anticarcinogenic effects. It promotes mental alertness and memory retention by enhancing cholinergic activity via inhibition of acetylcholinesterase. It is one of several monoterpenes that have shown analgesic activity in animal studies.[17] α-Pinene is gastroprotective for ulcerated lesions in mice, reducing acidity and increasing gastric mucosa.[18] Antimicrobial actions are thought to occur by promoting antimicrobial efflux genes, decreasing bacterial membrane integrity and disrupting heat-shock responses. It is a bronchodilator at low concentrations with 60% uptake by inhalation in the lungs.[19]

Entourage effects: α-Pinene crosses the blood–brain barrier very easily, preserving acetylcholine levels and thereby limiting the memory loss effect of THC. It has synergy with the phytocannabinoids CBD, CBG and THC, and has also been suggested as a modulator of THC overdose supporting its use as an antidote to cannabis intoxication.[4] Cultivars with this terpenoid may be useful in attention deficit, asthma or dementia disorders.

β-MYRCENE

β-Myrcene is resinous and has a green balsamic, musky and slightly metallic odor. It is a component of the essential oil of several plants, including mangos, lemongrass, hops, black pepper bay, ylang-ylang, wild thyme, parsley, basil and bay leaves. It is a monoterpene (10 carbon atoms). Its therapeutic effects include, but are not limited to, the following listed in Table 5.2.[2,4,5,17,19]

β-Myrcene inhibits inflammatory cytokines such as IL-1β and the expression of inflammatory and catabolic genes contributing to anti-inflammatory and anticatabolic effects.[20] It inhibits nitric oxide (NO) production in human chondrocytes by an IL-1β mechanism, suggesting chondroprotective effects. Its anti-inflammatory effects occur in part via prostaglandin E2 (PGE-2) stimulation. It also blocks the cancer-causing effects of aflatoxins. It is one of several monoterpenes that have shown analgesic activity in animal studies.[17] β-Myrcene is hypnotic and sedating, making it useful as a sleep aid. A study in mice showed that it potentiates the

---

TABLE 5.2
Therapeutic Effects of β-Myrcene

Sedating
Anti-inflammatory
Analgesic
Antispasmodic/muscle relaxant
Anxiolytic
Antiseptic
Antioxidant
Chondroprotective
Antibacterial
Antifungal

---

sleep-inducing effects of barbiturates.[2,5] Its narcotic effect is likely mediated by α-2 adrenoreceptors. Its analgesic effect in mice was blocked by naloxone, an opioid antagonist, suggesting a mechanism of action through the opioid receptor. It also acted as a muscle relaxant in mice.[4] β-Myrcene inhibits biofilm formation of bacterial pathogens contributing to antimicrobial activity.[19]

Entourage effects: β-Myrcene helps cannabinoids and terpenes pass through cell membranes, thereby accelerating their effect and increasing saturation of THC at the CB1 receptor. It displays synergism with the neuroprotective antioxidant effects of THC and CBD. It may counteract excessive psychoactive adverse events produced by THC.[4] Cultivars with this terpenoid may be useful in sleep, muscle spasm, pain and inflammatory disorders.

D-LIMONENE

D-Limonene is the second most prevalent terpene found in nature. It has a citrus aroma and takes its name from the lemon and gives citrus its characteristic scent. It is prominent in the rinds of citrus fruits and in essential citrus oils. It is a monoterpene (10 carbon atoms). Its therapeutic effects include, but are not limited to, the following listed in Table 5.3.[2,4,5,16,19]

D-Limonene is highly bioavailable with 70% absorption after inhalation. It mildly inhibits inflammatory cytokines such as IL1-β and the expression of inflammatory and catabolic genes contributing to anti-inflammatory and anticatabolic effects.[20] It is one of several monoterpenes that have shown analgesic activity in animal studies.[17] It also inhibits IL-1β-induced nitrous oxide production in human chondrocytes, suggesting chondroprotective activity. It increases the metabolic turnover of dopamine and serotonin, especially at the 5-HT1A receptor, leading to anxiolytic and antidepressant effects. A study in which hospitalized depressed patients were exposed to

TABLE 5.3
Therapeutic Effects of D-Limonene

Anxiolytic
Antidepressant
Anticonvulsant
Immunomodulatory
Bronchodilator
Dissolves gallstones
Relieves reflux and heartburn
Chondroprotective
Muscle relaxant
Anticarcinogenic
Antibacterial
Antifungal

citrus fragrance resulted in an antidepressant outcome. It is also an agonist at α-2 adrenoreceptors, contributing to anesthetic and serotonin-boosting effects. It blocks the carcinogenesis induced by benz[α]anthracene (a component of tar), diminishing some of the adverse effects of smoking. D-Limonene also detoxifies carcinogens by inducing phase II carcinogen-metabolizing enzymes. It also induces apoptosis of cancer cells.[19] D-Limonene is a potent skin penetration enhancer promoting transdermal absorption.[16] Its inclusion in topical formulas helps skin inflammatory conditions.

Entourage effects: D-Limonene assists in the absorption of other terpenoids and cannabinoids through the skin, mucous membranes and the digestive tract. It has synergy with the phytocannabinoids CBD, CBG and THC, possibly by a low-affinity interaction with cannabinoid receptors.[2,4,5] Cultivars with this terpenoid may be useful in mood disorders, especially when anxiety and depression are codiagnosed.

D-LINALOOL

D-Linalool has a pleasant floral aroma, often associated with a lavender scent. It is found in many flowers and spices, including citrus, lavender, rosewood and birch trees. It is a monoterpene (10 carbon atoms). Its therapeutic effects include, but are not limited to, the following listed in Table 5.4.[2,4,5,17]

D-Linalool modulates glutamate and GABA neurotransmitters leading to sedative, anxiolytic and anticonvulsant properties.[2,5] D-Linalool is a PPARα agonist supporting energy homeostasis functions. It is antinociceptive at high doses via glutamate receptors. It is one of several monoterpenes that have shown analgesic activity in animal studies.[17] Interaction with opiodergic, adrenergic and cholinergic systems have also been implicated in analgesic function. It is an agonist at α-2 adrenoreceptors, contributing to potential anesthetic and serotonin-boosting effects. Its local anesthetic effects were equivalent to procaine and menthol.[4] It is one of several monoterpenes that have shown analgesic activity in animal studies.[17] D-Linalool improves immune function via the neuroendocrine system, by inhibition of the hypothalamic-pituitary-adrenal (HPA) axis, reducing the secretion of HPA

TABLE 5.4
Therapeutic Effects of D-Linalool

Anxiolytic

Antidepressant

Stress reduction

Sedating

Analgesic/antinociceptive

Anesthetic

Anticonvulsant

Antibacterial

stress hormones such as corticosterone. It also normalizes CD4–CD8 ratios providing immune modulation.[2,5]

Entourage effects: D-Linalool serves as an antidote to the potential anxiogenic effect of THC. It has synergy with the phytocannabinoids with CBD, THC, THCV, CBDV, and is proposed to interact synergistically with CBG as well.[4] It can also influence CYP enzymes, suggesting that it can alter the pharmacokinetics of cannabinoids. Cultivars with this terpenoid may be useful in pain or seizure disorders, as well as in mood disorders such as anxiety, depression and PTSD.

TERPINEOL

Terpineols found in cannabis include two isomeric forms, α-terpineol and 4-terpineol, referred to collectively as terpineol. It has a light aroma, often found in lilacs, pine trees, eucalyptus, tea tree, lime blossoms, apple, cumin, sage and rosemary. It is a monoterpene (10 carbon atoms). Its therapeutic effects include, but are not limited to, the following listed in Table 5.5.[5,16,17,21,22]

Terpineol inhibits inflammatory cytokines such as IL-1β and the expression of inflammatory and catabolic genes contributing to anti-inflammatory and anticatabolic effects. It is also a potent inhibitor (stronger than aspirin) of COX-2 enzymes, reducing the production of prostaglandins, providing anti-inflammatory and analgesic effects. It is one of several monoterpenes that have shown analgesic activity in animal studies.[17] An additional mechanism of the analgesic effect involves effects on 5-HT2A serotonin receptors. It was shown to reduce the development of tolerance to morphine analgesia and reduced hyperalgesia in a chronic muscle pain fibromyalgia model, presumably by affecting the opioid and serotonergic receptors.[19] α-Terpineol exerted a cytotoxic effect against six human cancer cell lines, such as prostate, breast, lung, leukemia and ovarian, potentially by IL-1β-regulated nuclear factor signaling.[21] In mice, inhalation of α-terpineol was found to reduce motility by 45% calming airway smooth muscle relaxation in asthma vasorelaxation and blood pressure reduction effects.[5] It has shown dose-dependent antibiotic efficacy. The mechanism of action of α-terpineol as an antifungal seems to be dependent

TABLE 5.5
Therapeutic Effects of Terpineol

Anti-inflammatory
Antioxidant
Antiproliferative
Vasorelaxant
Analgesic
Antibacterial
Antifungal
Antiviral
Antimalarial

upon disrupting the cytoplasm of the microbe.[16] It has also shown skin permeation enhancement effects.[22]

Entourage effects: Terpineol has possible synergy with phytocannabinoids in reducing opioid tolerance and withdrawal symptoms.[19] It may increase the transdermal absorption of cannabis constituents. Cultivars with this terpenoid may be useful in pain, asthma and inflammatory disorders.

β-CARYOPHYLLENE

β-Caryophyllene has a light spice aroma and is found in the essential oils of black pepper, copaiba, balsam, oregano, hops, rosemary, basil, cinnamon, clove and other spices. It is the most common sesquiterpene (15-carbon terpene) in cannabis, and is usually the most predominant terpenoid overall in cannabis after drying through heating. Its effects include, but are not limited to, the following listed in Table 5.6[2,4,5,19]

β-Caryophyllene is a selective CB2 agonist with the ability to bind directly to the peripheral CB2 receptor, making it the only primary terpene in cannabis that also acts as a direct regulator of endocannabinoid tone. It shows strong anti-inflammatory action (comparable to dexamethasone) resulting in anti-inflammatory analgesic activity at low doses in wild-type but not CB2 knockout mice, demonstrating a CB2-dependent mechanism. It also inhibits PGE-1, contributing to anti-inflammatory and analgesic effects. β-Caryophyllene is PPARα and γ agonist, reducing immunoinflammatory processes. It is a potent antagonist of nAChRs, thereby decreasing the action of acetylcholine, and potentially contributing to neuromodulatory effects.[19] Its activity at the CB2 receptor also contributes to immune-modulating effects. It has shown anxiolytic and antidepressant as well as neuropathic pain therapeutic involvement possibly in a CB2 receptor-mediated activity. Its synergy with μ-opioid receptor pathways also enhances analgesia.[2,5]

Entourage effects: β-Caryophyllene binds directly to the peripheral CB2 receptor as do cannabinoids, possibly amplifying some cannabinoid effects. β-Caryophyllene has synergy with the phytocannabinoids CBD, THC, CBG, THCA and CBGA.[4] Cultivars with this terpenoid may be useful in inflammatory, autoimmune and pain disorders.

TABLE 5.6
Therapeutic Effects of β-Caryophyllene

Anti-inflammatory
Immunomodulatory
Anxiolytic
Antidepressant
Analgesic
Gastroprotective
Antibacterial
Antifungal
Antimalarial

α-HUMULENE

α-Humulene, also known as α-caryophyllene, is most noted for giving beer its "hoppy" aroma. It is found in the essential oils of *Humulus lupulus* (hops), from which it derives its name, Vietnamese coriander, clove, basil, hops, sage, spearmint and ginseng, among others. It is a sesquiterpene (a 15-carbon terpene). Its effects include, but are not limited to, the following listed in Table 5.7.[5,11,22–25]

α-Humulene inhibits inflammatory cytokines such as IL-1β and the expression of genes contributing to anti-inflammatory and anticatabolic effects. It also inhibits TNF-α, potentially related to its effect in reduction of induced mouse paw edema, including that caused by histamine. It reduces the production of prostaglandin E synthase-2 (PGE-2) as well as inducible nitric oxide synthase and COX-2 expression. Similar to the anti-inflammatory effects of β-caryophyllene, α-humulene's anti-inflammatory effects were comparable to those observed in dexamethasone-treated animals.[23] In a murine model of allergic airway inflammation, it decreased the expression of P-selectin, and decreased allergic inflammation and mucus production in the lungs.[24] It is also an appetite suppressant and may be used as a weight loss aid.[5] Its antitumoral and cytotoxic affects are thought to be due to decreased glutathione and increased ROS production.[25]

Entourage effects: α-Humulene can antagonize the appetite-stimulating effect of THC. Cultivars with this terpenoid may be useful in allergic airways and anorectic disorders.

TABLE 5.7
Therapeutic Effects of α-Humulene

Anti-inflammatory
Antinociceptive
Appetite suppressant
Antitumoral
Antibacterial

FLAVONOIDS

Flavonoids are aromatic, polycyclic phenols prevalent in foods and provide health benefits in such foods as berries, red wine, soybeans, chocolate and broccoli, to name but a few. Flavonoids contribute to the color, aroma and pharmacologic properties of cannabis. Cannabis ranks among the plants with the highest flavonoid content, estimated to be 2.5% of the weight of leaves and flowers. It is reported that the greatest concentration is in the sprouts, with decreasing content as the plant ages.[3] Over 20 have been identified in cannabis. The primary ones include cannflavin A and cannflavin B (unique to cannabis), apigenin, quercetin, luteolin, kaempferol, β-sitosterol, vitexin, isovitexin and orientin.[11,26] Their chemistry and synthesis in the plant is not yet completely elucidated.

Flavonoids display a wide range of therapeutic pharmacological properties, such as activation or inhibition of LOX and COX enzymes, detoxification of carcinogens and chemoprevention.[3] In addition to potential anticancer activity, flavonoids are broadly reported to have antibacterial, antiviral, anti-inflammatory, antioxidant, cardioprotective, neuroprotective and hepatoprotective properties.[2,5] The contribution of the flavonoid components have yet to be appreciated within the context of cannabis medicine. Any entourage effects with cannabinoids or other constituents of the plant have barely been investigated. An example given for synergy in an article about phytopharmaceuticals was the use of polyphenols, in which the authors note that "The main targets were found to be COX 1+2, NF-κB, and membrane glycoproteins that belong to the ATP-binding cassette transporter family."[27] These are some of the same targets that are active with terpenes and cannabinoids, leading to the speculation that interactions may occur at these receptors. Characteristics of the primary cannabis flavonoids are as follows:

Cannflavin A and B – Both cannflavin A and B have been found to be potent inhibitors of PGE-2 in human rheumatoid synovial cells. In addition, cannflavin A inhibits COX and LOX enzymes to a greater extent than THC, contributing to the potent anti-inflammatory activity of cannabis.[1] As compared to aspirin, cannflavins are 30 times more potent as COX enzyme inhibitors.

Apigenin– Apigenin is the primary anxiolytic agent found in chamomile and acts through selective binding to central GABA receptors. In addition, apigenin inhibits the production of TNF-α thereby inhibiting inflammation. It also interacts with estrogen receptors and has been shown to inhibit estradiol-induced proliferation of breast cancer cells.[3]

Quercetin – Quercetin is a potent antioxidant that scavenges free radicals, super-oxide anions and chelates iron ions involved in free radical formation. It also inhibits NF-κB, influencing the expression of oncogenes, inflammation and apoptosis. It is postulated that it might synergize with CBN, which also downregulates NF-κB in a way that could counteract an increase in NF-κB caused by THC.[26]

A review of the properties of the remaining flavonoids in cannabis – luteolin, orientin, vitexin and isovitexin – focuses mainly on their anticarcinogenic properties in cell studies.[28] As for entourage, it has barely been studied with regard to cannabis flavonoids. Flavonoids may modulate the pharmacokinetics of THC, via inhibition of CYP 450 enzymes 3A11 and 3A4.[4,26]

CONCLUSION

The terpenoid content in cannabis is responsible for many of the characteristic physiological effects of specific cultivars. This content cannot be underestimated in providing consistency in reproduction of therapeutic effects. At this time, lab testing of cannabis products focuses on cannabinoid content and not as commonly on terpene profiles. Some products on occasion do list major terpenes, but often do not report a comprehensive profile of the cultivar from which products have been extracted. They may be listed in preparations to which terpenes have been specifically added, but the percentage of content is not ordinarily given. The flavonoid components are not currently measured or considered. Their potential therapeutic significance is as yet undetermined.

As the medicinal effects of the cultivar depend so greatly upon the terpene content, how are we to make informed decisions? I always advised my patients to choose full raw cannabis flower by selecting it based upon its aroma, to be used by vaporizing or smoking and making homemade topicals or edibles. This is especially useful for mood effects. As I told my patients, "If it makes you feel better when you smell it, choose that strain!" A recent cannabis use survey revealed that 60% of cannabis users rely on smelling the flower to select their cannabis.[29] Retention of the full terpene profile occurs not only in using raw flower, but cold extraction with alcohol as well as live rosin processing yields maximal retention. As more products are characterized by their full cannabinoid as well as terpenoid profile, better choices will be available for patient use as well as for research.

REFERENCES

1. Flores-Sanchez IJ, Verpoorte R. Secondary metabolism in cannabis. *Phytochem Rev.* 2008;7:615–639.
2. Andre CM, Hausman JF, Guerriero G. Cannabis sativa: the plant of the thousand and one molecules. *Front Plant Sci.* 2016;7:19.
3. Pollastro F, Minassi A, Fresu LG. Cannabis phenolics and their bioactivities. *Curr Med Chem.* 2018;25(10):1160–1185.
4. Russo EB. Taming THC: potential cannabis synergy and phytocannabinoid-terpenoid entourage effects. *Br J Pharmacol.* 2011;163:1344–1364.
5. Baron, EP. medicinal properties of cannabinoids, terpenes, and flavonoids in cannabis, and benefits in migraine, headache, and pain: an update on current evidence and cannabis science. *Headache.* 2018;58(7):1139–1186.
6. ElSohly MA, Radwan MM, Gul W, Chandra S, Galal A. Phytochemistry of Cannabis sativa L. *Prog Chem Org Nat Prod.* 2017;1031:36.
7. Gallily R, Yekhtin Z, Hanuš LO. The anti-inflammatory properties of terpenoids from cannabis. *Cannabis Cannabinoid Res.* 2018;3(1):282–290.
8. Adams TB, Gavin CL, McGowen MM, et al. The FEMA GRAS assessment of aliphatic and aromatic terpene hydrocarbons used as flavor ingredients. *Food Chem Toxicol.* 201;49(10):2471–2494.
9. Hruza S. Cannabis, the polypharmaceutical herb: a review of the endocannabinoid system and Cannabis plant constituents. www.academia.edu/28772390/Cannabis_the_polypharmaceutical_herb_A_review_of_the_endocannabinoid_system_and_Cannabis_plant_constituents Accessed July 23, 2020.
10. Sexton M, Shelton K, Haley P, West M. Evaluation of cannabinoid and terpenoid content: cannabis flower compared to supercritical CO2 concentrate. *Planta Med.* 2018;84(4):234–241.
11. Nahler G, Jones TM. Pure cannabidiol versus cannabidiol-containing extracts: distinctly different multi-target modulators. *J Altern Complement Integr Med.* 2018;4:1–11.
12. Fischedick JT, Hazekamp A, Erkelens T, et al. Metabolic fingerprinting of Cannabis sativa L., cannabinoids and terpenoids for chemotaxonomic and drug standardization purposes. *Phytochemistry.* 2010;71:2058–2073.
13. Casano S, Grassi G, Martini V, Michelozzi M. Variations in terpene profiles of different strains of Cannabis sativa L. *Acta Hortic.* 2011;925:115–122.
14. Lynch RC, Vergara D, Tittes S, et al. Genomic and chemical diversity in cannabis. *CRC Crit Rev Plant Sci.* 2016;35:5–6:349–363.
15. Mahizan NA, Yang SK, Moo CL, et al. Terpene derivatives as a potential agent against antimicrobial resistance (AMR) pathogens. *Molecules.* 2019;24(14):2631.
16. Herman A, Herman AP. Essential oils and their constituents as skin penetration enhancer for transdermal drug delivery: a review. *J Pharm Pharmacol.* 2015;67(4):473–485.

17. Guimarães AG, Quintans JS, Quintans LJ Jr. Monoterpenes with analgesic activity: a systematic review. *Phytother Res.* 2013;27(1):1–15.
18. Pinheiro Mde A, Magalhães RM, Torres DM, et al. Gastroprotective effect of alpha-pinene and its correlation with antiulcerogenic activity of essential oils obtained from Hyptis species. *Pharmacogn Mag.* 2015;11(41):123–130.
19. Russo EB, Marcu J. Cannabis pharmacology: the usual suspects and a few promising leads. *Adv Pharmacol.* 2017;80:67–134.
20. Rufino AT, Ribeiro M, Sousa C, et al. Evaluation of the anti-inflammatory, anti-catabolic and pro-anabolic effects of E-caryophyllene, myrcene and limonene in a cell model of osteoarthritis. *Eur J Pharmacol.* 2015;750:141–150.
21. Khaleel C, Tabanca N, Buchbauer G. α-Terpineol, a natural monoterpene: a review of its biological properties. *Open Chem.* 2018;16:349–361.
22. Kong Q, Zhang L, An P, et al. Antifungal mechanisms of α-terpineol and terpene-4-alcohol as the critical components of Melaleuca alternifolia oil in the inhibition of rot disease caused by Aspergillus ochraceus in postharvest grapes. *J Appl Microbiol.* 2019;126(4):1161–1174.
23. Fernandes ES, Passos GF, Medeiros R, et al. Anti-inflammatory effects of compounds alpha-humulene and (-)-trans-caryophyllene isolated from the essential oil of Cordia verbenacea. *Eur J Pharmacol.* 2007;569(3):228–236.
24. Rogerio AP, Andrade EL, Leite DF, Figueiredo CP, Calixto JB. Preventive and therapeutic anti-inflammatory properties of the sesquiterpene alpha-humulene in experimental airways allergic inflammation. *Br J Pharmacol.* 2009;158(4):1074–1087.
25. Legault J, Dahl W, Debiton E, Pichette A, Madelmont JC. Antitumor activity of balsam fir oil: production of reactive oxygen species induced by alpha-humulene as possible mechanism of action. *Planta Med.* 2003;69(5):402–407.
26. McPartland J, Russo E. Cannabis and cannabis extracts: greater than the sum of their parts? *J Cannabis Therapeutics.* 2001;1:103–132.
27. Wagner H. Synergy research: approaching a new generation of phytopharmaceuticals. *Fitoterapia.* 2011;82(1):34–37.
28. Tomko AM, Whynot EG, Ellis LD, Dupré DJ. Anti-cancer potential of cannabinoids, terpenes, and flavonoids present in cannabis. *Cancers (Basel).* 2020;12(7):1985.
29. Sexton M, Cuttler C, Finnell JS, Mischley LK. A cross-sectional survey of medical cannabis users: patterns of use and perceived efficacy. *Cannabis Cannabinoid Res.* 2016;1(1):131–138.

Part II

Patient Practice Management

6 Adverse Effects, Risks

ADVERSE EFFECTS, RISKS – AN OVERVIEW

Historically, in considering the benefit-to-risk ratio of cannabis use, especially prior to medical use, much information circulated about the risks of smoking "marijuana" due to the primary concerns of the effects of THC and smoke. It is instructive to recall that most of the studies on adverse effects (AEs) were designed to identify them, and not to present how to use cannabis in a safe and informed manner. As clinicians we are obligated to consider a risk/benefit ratio. Hence, this presentation of adverse effects is meant to be discerning, with a review of individual studies identifying confounders where possible, as well as critical examination of review articles.

Fortunately, the focus on smoking cannabis has shifted with the advent of alternative delivery systems as well as cultivars with greater percentages of CBD. The determination of AEs of cannabis intake is absolutely dependent on the content of the product, that is, the CBD/THC ratio, and the purity of the product – the presence of contaminants such as heavy metals, solvents, pesticides, mold and the route of delivery. Other factors that are critical to consider include the tolerance of the user – whether they are naive or chronic users, the age of the user and the duration of use. The literature provides few articles out of hundreds that present these points as primary. Most older reports evaluating the effects of only smoked cannabis have focused on effects of non-lab tested THC-rich materials used for recreational purposes. "It is important to note that the literature describing adverse events of cannabis including cardiovascular or cerebrovascular events is based on cannabis use from the black market without standardized quality control."[1] These analyses present a skewed picture to the non-discerning reader. One typical report such as this 1998 article listed AEs based purely upon smoked recreational cannabis. These effects included chronic bronchitis, impairments of attention and memory (that persist while the user remains chronically intoxicated) and the possibility of a cannabis dependence syndrome.[2]

The distinction between AEs and "risk" of cannabis use is not often defined and these terms are used interchangeably. Much of the literature on AEs focuses on the chronic effects of THC-rich cannabis such as changes in mood and cognition often viewed as behavioral effects. While behavioral effects vary among individuals, these are absolutely dependent upon the user's familiarity with cannabis (naive vs. experienced), their age, tolerance and cannabinoid content, so it is impossible to predict exactly what the overall behavioral effects of cannabis will be. Other AEs that have been reported include psychomotor impairment, poor judgment and memory effects. Most of these adverse effects occur in naive users, while chronic users who have developed a tolerance are not as strongly impacted. As stated in a review of cannabis risks, "Multiple regression analyses revealed that lower frequency of cannabis use predicted increased frequency of adverse reactions. Symptoms of cannabis use

DOI: 10.1201/9781003098201-8

disorder, conformity motives, and anxiety sensitivity were significant predictors of both the prevalence of, and distress caused by, adverse reactions."[3] On the other hand, AEs that are primarily acute may include disorientation, dizziness, rapid heart rate, chest pain, low blood pressure/ feeling faint, loss of physical coordination, dry mouth, agitation, anxiety, depression, hallucinations and/or psychosis.[4]

The results of a comprehensive review of the literature offer commentary on the quality of published studies: 731 articles were screened and only 68 studies were found that were considered to be adequate quality for inclusion in the analysis. Of the 68 identified reviews, 62 reported harm, 20 reported insufficient evidence of harm and 6 reported no evidence of harm for 6 outcomes. Harm was reported for multiple mental health outcomes that included psychosis, mania and suicide. Evidence for structural, functional and chemical brain changes was documented. There was also evidence for impaired driving ability and changes to memory and learning.[5] A meta-analysis published in 2008 spanning 30 years of research did not find a higher incidence of serious AEs associated with medical cannabinoid use. This review excluded studies of risk from recreational users and no trials of medical cannabis administered by smoking were included. Interestingly, researchers found that the rate of non-serious AEs was 1.86 times higher among medical cannabis users than among controls. These included nervous system, psychiatric, gastrointestinal and respiratory effects.[6] "The current review of evidence from clinical trials of cannabinoids and cannabis extracts for medical indications suggests that the adverse effects of their short-term use are modest."[4]

One recent review stresses that risks to vulnerable populations warrant particular attention, such as pregnant women, youth due to impacts on developing brains and those with a predisposition for psychosis or schizophrenia. It also reminded us of legal risks, "Social harms associated with cannabis include the impacts of impairment on driving, and financial impacts on health care and police, court and incarceration costs resulting from prohibition."[1]

A summary of the overall risks determined by literature review by the Committee on the Health Effects of Marijuana by the National Academy of Sciences, Engineering and Medicine (NASEM), published in 2017 is presented subsequently. *The literature review generally examined recreational, smoked, THC-rich cannabis, and is not translatable to medicinal use with other delivery methods.* Yet, as clinicians, we must be equipped to counsel patients who present with such use, as well as advise about potential risks. For brevity, I have included only those conclusions with substantial or moderate evidence for risk. Limited, no risk or non-adverse associations may also be found in the report.[7] NASEM found significant evidence of adverse effects associated with non-medicinal cannabis use across many health categories. Their findings for substantial or moderate evidence are summarized as follows:

1. Substantial evidence of a statistical association between cannabis smoking and worse respiratory symptoms and more frequent chronic bronchitis episodes (long-term cannabis smoking).
2. Substantial evidence of a statistical association between cannabis use and increased risk of motor vehicle crashes.

3. Substantial evidence of a statistical association between maternal cannabis smoking and lower birthweight of the offspring.
4. Substantial evidence of a statistical association between cannabis use and the development of schizophrenia or other psychoses, with the highest risk among the most frequent users.
5. Substantial evidence that risk factors for developing problem cannabis use include being male, smoking cigarettes, initiating cannabis use at an earlier age and increases in cannabis use frequency.
6. Moderate evidence of a statistical association between cannabis use and increased risk of overdose injuries, including respiratory distress, among pediatric populations in US states where cannabis is legal.
7. Moderate evidence of a statistical association between cannabis use and the development of substance dependence and/or a substance abuse disorder for substances, including alcohol, tobacco and other illicit drugs.
8. Moderate evidence of a statistical association between cannabis use and the impairment in the cognitive domains of learning, memory and attention (acute cannabis use).
9. Moderate evidence of a statistical association between cannabis use and increased symptoms of mania and hypomania in individuals diagnosed with bipolar disorders (regular cannabis use).

Furthermore, researchers found no evidence/no statistical association between cannabis use and the incidence of lung cancer, the incidence of head and neck cancers or worsening of negative symptoms of schizophrenia among individuals with psychotic disorders. What is notably absent from these associations are cardiovascular and immune adverse effects, which were listed as *none*. Other adverse health findings related to cannabis that were not described in the NASEM report include cannabis use disorder (CUD), cannabis withdrawal syndrome (CWS) and cannabinoid hyperemesis syndrome (CHS) (see Chapter 38 for CHS discussion).

Historically, the information gathered relates to research on recreational cannabis users for the most part, and not input from medical cannabis patients who have a different use profile, as there was little information available until recently. A review of adverse effects in medical cannabis patients stated:

> We also caution against assuming that the adverse effects of recreational cannabis use can be expected to occur with medical cannabinoid use. The amounts used, the existence of comorbidities and the methods of drug delivery are different in the two populations, which should therefore be evaluated separately.[6]

In a study oriented toward acute effects (positive and adverse), responses from medical as well as recreational study participants were reported. "Relative to recreational users, medical users were less likely to report undesirable acute effects but were more likely to report undesirable withdrawal symptoms. Older (50+) individuals reported fewer undesirable acute effects and withdrawal symptoms compared with younger users."[8]

As opposed to the vast amount of risk research attributed to "marijuana," not as much is known about the risk, if any, of use of CBD-rich cannabis or hemp-derived CBD. Few studies have been done that employ low doses of CBD, as would be used by most medical cannabis patients. Studies with higher dose extracts generally find that CBD or the addition of CBD content actually mitigates the risk posed by THC.[9,10] This is as would be expected from our knowledge of CBD as a pharmacokinetic modulator of THC function. As far as the primary AEs of CBD are concerned, these include dry mouth, somnolence, decreased appetite and diarrhea.[4,11] In some cases, the opposite of somnolence but rather insomnia was noted. Adverse effects associated with CBD appear to be dose dependent. Much of the aforementioned risk predictions, however, have been based upon studies involving extremely high levels of CBD, in the range of 10–20 mg/kg. The average dose for medicinal use is more often in the 10 mg per dose range, well under 0.5 mg/kg. Adverse effects from CBD are rarely encountered with medicinal CBD from cannabis or hemp extracts, but rather are more likely with purified CBD, which is used at much higher doses. Currently, the proliferation of CBD use by mainstream populations suggests the importance of educating the public about the risk/benefit ratio of use of different forms of CBD.

Studies of AEs from Sativex use, a mixed CBD/THC extract, have shown the rate of significant events was low. The most common AEs reported from a large multicenter study of patients using Sativex for multiple sclerosis were cognitive/psychiatric effects, fatigue and drowsiness, all at a rate of 4% or less.[12] There was no evidence of addiction, abuse, misuse or impairment of memory, and no loss of driving ability was observed.[13] Sativex use in a study of patients with chronic pain resulted in minimal AEs and the authors report that the THC:CBD treatment was well tolerated. AEs were related to the "bad" taste of the THC:CBD spray (noted by 6.6%) and 6.3% had increased appetite. Other AEs were in the 1% range.[14]

In light of the complex and conflicting study data and with the advent of cannabis medicinal use, we will address the relevant aforementioned issues in several main sections, including pulmonary and cardiovascular risks, risks in pregnancy, in driving, risks to cognition, psychosis, cannabis use disorders and drug interactions. Specific consideration of risks to children, youth and the elderly are covered in the relevant cannabis practice chapters.

REFERENCES

1. Lucas P, Baron EP, Jikomes N. Medical cannabis patterns of use and substitution for opioids & other pharmaceutical drugs, alcohol, tobacco, and illicit substances: results from a cross-sectional survey of authorized patients. *Harm Reduct J.* 2019;6(1):9.
2. Hall W, Solowij N. Adverse effects of cannabis. *Lancet.* 1998;352(9140):1611–1616.
3. LaFrance E, Stueber A, Glodosky N, Mauzay D, Cuttler C. Overbaked: assessing and predicting acute adverse reactions to cannabis. *J Cannabis Res.* 2020;2:3.
4. Degenhardt L, Hall WD. The adverse effects of cannabinoids: implications for use of medical marijuana. *CMAJ.* 2008;178(13):1685–1686.
5. Memedovich KA, Dowsett LE, Spackman E, Noseworthy T, Clement F. The adverse health effects and harms related to marijuana use: an overview review. *CMAJ Open.* 2018;6:E339–E346.

6. Wang T, Collet J, Shapiro S, Ware MA. Adverse effects of medical cannabinoids: a systematic review. *CMAJ*. 2008;178(13):1669–1678.
7. National Academies of Sciences, Engineering, and Medicine. *The Health Effects of Cannabis and Cannabinoids: The Current State of Evidence and Recommendations for Research*. Washington, DC: The National Academies Press (US); 2017: Summary. www.ncbi.nlm.nih.gov/books/NBK425741/ Accessed November 8, 2020.
8. Sexton M, Cuttler C, Mischley LK. A survey of cannabis acute effects and withdrawal symptoms: differential responses across user types and age. *J Altern Complement Med*. 2019;25(3):326–335.
9. Solowij N, Broyd S, Greenwood LM, et al. A randomised controlled trial of vaporised Δ9-tetrahydrocannabinol and cannabidiol alone and in combination in frequent and infrequent cannabis users: acute intoxication effects. *Eur Arch Psychiatry Clin Neurosci*. 2019;269(1):17–35.
10. Niesink RJ, van Laar MW. Does cannabidiol protect against adverse psychological effects of THC? *Front Psychiatry*. 2013;4:130.
11. Brown JD, Winterstein AG. Potential adverse drug events and drug-drug interactions with medical and consumer cannabidiol (CBD) use. *J Clin Med*. 2019;8(7):989.
12. Patti F, Messina S, Solaro C, et al. Efficacy and safety of cannabinoid oromucosal spray for multiple sclerosis spasticity. *J Neurol Neurosurg Psychiatry*. 2016 September;87(9):944–951.
13. Rekand T. THC:CBD spray and MS spasticity symptoms: data from latest studies. *Eur Neurol*. 2014;71(Suppl 1):4–9.
14. Ueberall MA, Essner U, Mueller-Schwefe GHH. Effectiveness and tolerability of THC:CBD oromucosal spray as add-on measure in patients with severe chronic pain: analysis of 12-week open-label real-world data provided by the German Pain e-Registry. *J Pain Res*. 2019;12:1577–1604.

6.1 Pulmonary Risks

SMOKING

Cannabis consumed by smoking poses several health risks. Cannabis smoke produces carbon monoxide, acetaldehyde, ammonia, nitrosamines and polycyclic aromatic hydrocarbons (tars), which may be carcinogenic. A poorly designed study compared the tar and carboxyhemoglobin levels after smoking a filtered tobacco cigarette as compared to an unfiltered cannabis cigarette. They reported five times the carboxyhemoglobin level in the blood, a threefold increase in inhaled tar and retention of one-third more inhaled tar in the respiratory tract in the subjects who smoked cannabis.[1] This study is quoted in pulmonary risk literature, but it is misleading as no correction was made for the reduction of tar by the filter in the tobacco group, but not in the cannabis group. In a recent review of the harms of cannabis smoke, it was concluded that, "the addition of tobacco to cannabis, in most cases, resulted in increased tar content when samples were smoked as cigarettes," and the addition of tobacco may actually increase carbon monoxide (CO) levels.[2] The retention of CO is complicated as well by depth of inhalation, as with a greater inhalation such as may be seen with cannabis smoking, increased CO retention is likely to result.

Damage to central airways and changes in local immune response pose greater respiratory risk. Chronic cannabis smoking increases the risk for developing chronic bronchitis with associated wheezing, cough, chest tightness and sputum production.[3] Fortunately, these symptoms usually resolve after cessation of use.[4] In a review of studies on the effect of smoking cannabis, "All 14 studies noted an association with increased respiratory symptoms, including cough, phlegm, and wheeze. Yet no consistent association was found between long-term marijuana smoking and airflow obstruction measures."[5] Cannabis use may result in some changes to pulmonary function tests, but it does not result in increased risk for chronic obstructive pulmonary disease (see Chapter 17).[6]

What about the projected risk for increasing the incidence of lung cancer? A 2006 case-controlled study of 1,200 participants demonstrated that even heavy smoking of cannabis is not associated with lung cancer and other types of upper aerodigestive tract cancers.[4] Some studies have attempted to show smoked cannabis as a cancer risk, but confounders such as concomitant tobacco use were not excluded.[6] A 2015 pooled meta-analysis of six case-control studies in the United States, Canada, the United Kingdom and New Zealand that included data on 2,159 lung cancer cases and 2,985 controls found little evidence for an increased risk of lung cancer among habitual or long-term cannabis smokers.[7] These authors do suggest a possible association for adenocarcinoma. In fact, there is no strong evidence of a direct link between chronic cannabis use and lung cancer or any other type of cancer. It is hypothesized that cannabis provides antitumoral as well as anticarcinogenic protection to which is a property of several phytocannabinoids as well as some of the other secondary metabolites.

DOI: 10.1201/9781003098201-9

Regarding the risks of smoking cannabis, the NASEM report concludes that there is substantial evidence of only one measure, worse respiratory symptoms, and more frequent chronic bronchitis episodes with long-term cannabis smoking. The category of moderate evidence includes improved airway dynamics with acute use, but not with chronic use, and higher forced vital capacity. Upon cessation of smoking, moderate evidence points to improvements in respiratory symptoms.[8] Overall, the risks of respiratory complications of cannabis smoking appear to be relatively small and to be far lower than those of tobacco smoking. While heavy cannabis users may be at a higher risk for developing chronic bronchitis or a potential increased risk of exacerbating COPD and asthma, current studies do not provide sufficient evidence for a link. As far as the overall risk is concerned, the pertinent question is how much smoking poses a measurable risk? Are occasional users at risk, and what is the level at which harm is a likely outcome? The Coronary Artery Risk Development in Young Adults study, a cohort study of 5,115 adults, found no effect of occasional low marijuana use on pulmonary function.[9] A survey of 878 adults older than 40 in Vancouver found that cannabis smokers had no more COPD or respiratory symptoms than non-smokers.[10] Some answers may come from a cross-sectional study using National Health and Nutrition Examination Survey (NHANES) data. They found that up to 20 joint-years (the equivalent of one smoked joint per day for 20 years) of smoked cannabis caused no adverse changes in lung function.[11] It is tenable to predict that occasional smokers, perhaps even up to a few puffs/day, will not cause respiratory distress.

VAPORIZING

What are the pulmonary risks, if any, of inhalation by vaporization. Many cannabis smokers have switched from smoking to vaporizing. Studies show that this reduces respiratory symptoms. Analysis of vapor from a vaporizer recovered 9.5% smoke toxins; in contrast, cannabis smoke from a pipe recovered 87% smoke toxins. Vaporization, compared to smoking, generates less carbon monoxide.[12] A survey of 6,883 cannabis users found that vaporizing, compared with smoking, caused fewer respiratory symptoms such as coughing, wheezing, shortness of breath and mucus production.[13] A pilot study documenting change from smoking to vaporizing found improvements in forced expiratory volumes 1 month after the introduction of the vaporizer.[14] Table top vaporizers carry less risk than the ever-popular vaporizer pens. Aside from the risk of contamination by petrochemicals such as butane used in the extraction of some oils (used in vape pens), the presence of other diluents has called their safety into question. A new lung disease associated with heavy vaping (mostly e-cigarettes) emerged in late 2019. Vitamin E acetate, an additive in some e-cigarettes, or vaping products are linked to lung injury. As per the Centers for Disease Control and Prevention, as of December 27, 2019, nearly 2,561 cases of lung injury (EVALI) have been identified caused by inhalation of vitamin E acetate.[15] Other diluents may include polypropylene glycol, propylene glycol, polyethylene glycol, vegetable glycerin and ethylene glycol. One article on risk states:

> To date, it remains unclear whether the risk is limited to specific types of vaping products or oils, or with specific use patterns. For patients who choose to vape, providers

should recommend avoiding products purchased outside of registered facilities (i.e., from a street dealer) and should monitor for changes in breathing.[6]

It is clear that this type of lung disease comes from poorly regulated vaping diluents. Vaping full flower cannabis avoids these risks.

CONTAMINANTS

There are other risks to inhaling cannabis, whether by smoke or by vapor. This has to do with various kinds of contaminants that may result from the growing conditions of the plant or the extraction process in preparing oils. Fungal contamination (*Aspergillus* and *Penicillium* species) in cannabis samples has been demonstrated. Contamination with fungal or bacterial pathogens could increase risk of pneumonia and other respiratory problems.[16] There are concerns that pesticides may pose risks in cannabis products. Pesticides and other impurities are more likely to be found at potentially unsafe levels in concentrated cannabis products (vaping cartridges, carbon dioxide, extractions, etc.).[17] A large concern for a time when hemp-generated products (as hemp is a bioaccumulator) and metal coils from vape cartridges were being routinely imported from other countries was the risk for heavy metal contamination. Now that hemp is legal to grow in the United States, heavy metal levels are not as likely a contaminant. An important solution that addresses most of these potential hazards is to use only lab-tested products, supplied with a Certificate of Analysis listing cannabinoid and terpene content as well as contaminants such as additives, pesticides, mold and heavy metals.

CONCLUSION

Smoking cannabis can be an entrenched habit with some consumers. Many patients are unwilling to stop smoking cannabis, even though the smoke is bad for their health. Usually this is manageable with smart advice, that is, vaporize more, smoke less, or smoke less of cannabis with a higher potency, and use a water-pipe. Suggesting the patient try other delivery methods appears a reasonable approach. In my experience, patients are willing to moderate their smoking, especially as they become older in age. However, there are some cases where this simply does not happen. As clinicians, we know that patients are often their own worst enemy. A case in point, one 71-year-old patient, a 50-pack year tobacco smoker who developed lung cancer, stopped tobacco, and replaced it with smoking cannabis for 15 years. The lung cancer recurred, and he was advised again to stop smoking cannabis. He did not comply, but switched to a water pipe. He still complained of daily phlegm. Oftentimes keeping the level of smoking minimal is the best we can achieve.

REFERENCES

1. Wu TC, Tashkin DP, Djahed B, Rose JE. Pulmonary hazards of smoking marijuana as compared with tobacco. *N Engl J Med.* 1988;318:347–351.

2. Gowing L, Ali RL, White JM. DASC Monograph No 8 Research Series, Drug and Alcohol Services Council, South Australia. Respiratory harms of smoked cannabis. 2021. www.researchgate.net/publication/237781380_Respiratory_harms_of_smoked_cannabis Accessed February 8, 2021.

3. McInnis OA, Plecas D. Canadian Center on Substance Abuse 4th in Series. Clearing the Smoke on Cannabis. Respiratory effects of cannabis smoking – an update. 2016. www.ccsa.ca/sites/default/files/2019-10/CCSA-Clearing-Smoke-on-Cannabis-Highlights-2019-en.pdf Accessed November 8, 2020.

4. Tashkin DP. Effects of marijuana smoking on the lung. *Ann Am Thorac Soc*. 2013; 10(3):239–247.

5. Tetrault JM, Crothers K, Moore BA, et al. Effects of marijuana smoking on pulmonary function and respiratory complications: a systematic review. *Arch Intern Med*. 2007;167:221–228.

6. Slawek D, Meenrajan SR, Alois MR, et al. Medical cannabis for the primary care physician. *J Prim Care Community Health*. 2019;10:1–7.

7. Zhang LR, Morgenstern H, Greenland S, et al. Cannabis smoking and lung cancer risk: pooled analysis in the International Lung Cancer Consortium. *Int J Cancer*. 2015;136(4):894–903.

8. National Academies of Sciences, Engineering, and Medicine. *The Health Effects of Cannabis and Cannabinoids: The Current State of Evidence and Recommendations for Research*. Washington, DC: The National Academies Press, US; 2017: Respiratory Disease. www.ncbi.nlm.nih.gov/books/NBK425753/www.ncbi.nlm.nih.gov/books/NBK425753/ Accessed November 8, 2020.

9. Pletcher MJ, Vittinghoff E, Kalhan R, et al. Association between marijuana exposure and pulmonary function over 20 years. *JAMA*. 2012;(2):173–181.

10. Tan WC, Lo C, Jong A, et al. Marijuana and chronic obstructive lung disease: a population-based study. *CMAJ*. 2009;180(8):814–820.

11. Kempker JA, Honig EG, Martin GS. The effects of marijuana exposure on expiratory airflow. A study of adults who participated in the U.S. National Health and Nutrition Examination Study. *Ann Am Thorac Soc*. 2015;12(2):135–141.

12. Abrams D, Vizoso H, Shade S, et al. Vaporization as a smokeless cannabis delivery system: a pilot study. *Clinical Pharm*. 2007;82:572–578.

13. Earleywine M, Barnwell SS. Decreased respiratory symptoms in cannabis users who vaporize. *Harm Reduct J*. 2007;4(1):11.

14. Van Dam NT, Earleywine M. Pulmonary function in cannabis users: support for a clinical trial of the vaporizer. *Int J Drug Policy*. 2010;21(6):511–513.

15. Centers for Disease Control. Outbreak of lung injury associated with the use of e-cigarette, or vaping, products. February 25, 2020. www.cdc.gov/tobacco/basic_information/e-cigarettes/severe-lung-disease.html Accessed November 8, 2020.

16. Punja ZK, Collyer D, Scott C, Lung S, Holmes J, Sutton D. Pathogens and molds affecting production and quality of Cannabis sativa L. *Front Plant Sci*. 2019;10:1120.

17. McPartland JM, McKernan KJ. Contaminants of concern in cannabis: microbes, heavy metals and pesticides In: Chandra S, Lata H, ElSohly MA, eds. *Cannabis Sativa L. – Botany and Biotechnology*. Cham, Switzerland: Springer; 2017:457–474.

6.2 Cardiovascular Risks

Cannabinoids have complex effects on the cardiovascular system. A detailed discussion of these effects, some of which may be therapeutic, is presented in Chapter 24. A review of the cardiovascular effects of cannabinoids summarizes, "Cannabinoids, through central and local mechanisms, affect key cardiovascular parameters in health and disease, such as heart rate, blood pressure, vascular and cardiac contractility and inflammation."[1] Because the endocannabinoid system is intimately involved in cardiovascular function, these effects will vary from person to person, sometimes be beneficial and rarely pose risk. In considering the risks of cannabis, only THC-rich forms pose any recorded risk, and of these, only inhalation in non-tolerant subjects causes variable responses. Once tolerance is achieved with chronic use, cardiovascular variability becomes compensated with less pronounced physiological effects. "The acute effects of THC including intoxication and tachycardia are quite subject to tachyphylaxis, and will often diminish with chronic administration."[2] Indeed, in acute use by naive subjects, inhaled THC-rich cannabis results in an initial increase in heart rate and blood pressure with long-term use leading to a decrease in heart rate and blood pressure. The risk literature provides mixed results as often the reviewers do not analyze the studies they cite, resulting in no correction for bias, leading to conclusions such as stated here: "From a cardiovascular perspective, evidence shows that marijuana is associated with increased sympathetic drive, risk for myocardial infarction and acute coronary syndrome, decreased time to angina, and increased mortality."[3] But is this true? Many of the studies from which cardiovascular risk conclusions are drawn did not exclude tobacco smokers as study subjects, contributing to low-validity results. One discerning author noted that concurrent tobacco smoking increases the risk for cardiac events.

> Cannabis consumption has been shown to cause arrhythmia including ventricular tachycardia, and potentially sudden death, and to increase the risk of myocardial infarction (MI). These effects appear to be compounded by cigarette smoking and precipitated by excessive physical activity, especially during the first few hours of consumption.[4]

As far as risk for arrhythmias is concerned, only 3% of cannabis users had arrhythmias in a study even without correction for tobacco confounders.[5] A study conducted in a middle-aged US population cannabis use was not associated with increases in electrocardiogram abnormalities. "This contributes to the growing body of evidence that has supported that occasional cannabis use and cardiovascular markers of subclinical atherosclerosis and disease are not associated."[6] Another review that included six studies found mixed outcomes, some potentially beneficial and some potentially adverse, but all with insufficient evidence. "Evidence examining the effect of cannabis on dyslipidemia, acute MI, stroke, or cardiovascular all-cause mortality and diabetes was insufficient."[7] It has been suggested that cannabis

DOI: 10.1201/9781003098201-10

use may increase the risk for stroke. In the Personality and Total Health Through Life retrospective study, a 3.3-fold risk of stroke/transient ischemic attack was found in past year cannabis users.[8] In an American College of Cardiology review, myocardial infarction (MI), stroke, peripheral artery disease, arrhythmia and cardiomyopathy were listed as potential cardiovascular risks with cannabis use. The authors comment, "Unfortunately, most of the available data are short term, observational, and retrospective in nature; lack exposure determination; exhibit recall bias; include minimal cannabis exposure with no dose or product standardization; and typically evaluate low-risk cohorts."[9] The authors go on to point out that major confounding factors include access to health care and tobacco use variables.

As far as increased risk for MI or mortality from heart disease is concerned, the risk attributed to cannabis use was again generated from poorly designed studies having low validity. In the Determinants of Myocardial Infarction Onset Study, the authors found an elevated risk up to 4.8 times for MI within 1 hour of use of cannabis. The risk declined rapidly after 1 hour. The authors concluded that a calculated annual risk of 1.5–3% of acute cardiovascular event was seen in daily cannabis users.[10] However, tobacco smokers (68%) were not excluded in the study group, while in the "matched" cannabis abstainer group, only 32% smoked. One critical review of this report concludes, "This study did not examine subsequent cannabis use patterns, and no significant differences in cardiac mortality were observed on 18-year follow-up of the same cohort. More recent epidemiological investigation places cannabis MI risk at 0.8%."[2] This author's conclusion was as follows:

> Cardiovascular adverse events were seen occasionally in early studies [of Sativex] in which rapid titration and high doses (up to 130 mg of THC/day) were allowed. These have become quite rare with conventional dosing (to 32.4 mg/day) and slower escalation: tachycardia, hypertension, both well under 2% incidence; and orthostatic hypotension 0.1–0.2%.[2]

It is possible then that there may be a less than 1% increase in risk for an acute myocardial event as a result of cannabis use, particularly within the first hour of use by naive users with low tolerance to THC. Studies have shown no statistically significant association between cannabis use and mortality. A multicenter cohort study of 3,886 MI survivors that followed patients for up to 18 years found an increased, although not statistically significant, mortality rate among marijuana users.[11] While the possibility exists that individuals with cardiovascular risks could be adversely affected by cannabis intake, a study of 65,171 subjects over the course of 49 years showed no significant difference in mortality rate between cannabis users and non-users.[12] It is concluded now that the risk for increased mortality from MI due to cannabis use is unsubstantiated.[7]

Yet another category of at-risk patients has been proposed, a younger group, not otherwise at risk for cardiovascular events. In the Partners YOUNG-MI retrospective study of patients who presented with first MI under the age of 50 years, they determined that cannabis use was associated with twice the risk of death among these patients after correction for tobacco use. But researchers noted that the retrospective study had a larger percentage of subjects using tobacco, so once again tobacco presents as a confounder with unclear correctability.[13,14] In a 15-year longitudinal follow-up of 3,617 adults in the CARDIA (Coronary Artery Risk Development in Young Adults) study, 84% reported history of cannabis use. Cumulative lifetime and recent cannabis use did not show an association with incidence of cardiovascular disease, coronary heart disease or cardiac mortality.[15,16]

What about CBD-rich forms of cannabis? Here the picture is completely reversed. No cardiovascular risk has been documented. In fact, oral CBD at doses of up to 800 mg produced no significant cardiovascular effects as measured by heart rate and blood pressure.[17] In fact, CBD has been shown to be protective in cases of myocardial ischemia and cardiomyopathies.

CONCLUSION

The effects of cannabis on cardiovascular function should, by rights, not be reviewed in the risks section. With judicious use, cannabis appears to be more protective than result in AEs. In fact, the National Academy of Sciences, Engineering and Medicine 2017 report found no evidence for cardiovascular risk.[18] Nevertheless, patients should be counseled about acute versus chronic cardiovascular effects. The clinician should inform the patient of the potential for tachycardia and increased blood pressure specifically with inhaled THC-rich cannabis. Current medical opinion continues to promote risk assessment. "Cardiovascular specialists should have open discussions with patients acknowledging the limited scientific data, but potential cardiovascular hazards of marijuana use, especially when used via smoking/inhalation routes."[13] We must keep in perspective that medical cannabis protocols rarely involve acute dosage regimens, with most patients achieving tolerance within a few weeks, and mixed combinations of CBD and THC are becoming more prevalent. Low doses of THC, as well as CBD, may be cardioprotective. The inclusion of cardiovascular effects in this section is not really about risk, so much as a potential for non-serious adverse events from inhaled THC-rich cannabis in naive users.

REFERENCES

1. Bondarenko AI. Cannabinoids and cardiovascular system. *Adv Exp Med Biol.* 2019;1162:63–87.
2. Russo E. Synthetic and natural cannabinoids: the cardiovascular risk. *Br J Cardiol.* 2015;22:7–9.
3. Kaufman TM, Fazio S, Shapiro MD. Brief commentary: marijuana and cardiovascular disease: what should we tell patients? *Ann Intern Med.* 2019;170:119.
4. Goyal H, Awad HH, Ghali JK. Role of cannabis in cardiovascular disorders. *J Thorac Dis.* 2017;9(7):2079–2092.
5. Desai R, Patel U, Deshmukh A, Sachdeva R, Kumar G. Burden of arrhythmia in recreational marijuana users. *Int J Cardiol.* 2018;264:91–92.
6. Jakob J, Stalder O, Syrogiannouli L, et al. Association between marijuana use and electrocardiographic abnormalities by middle age The Coronary Artery Risk Development in Young Adults (CARDIA) study. *Addiction.* 2021;116(3):583–595.

7. Ravi D, Ghasemiesfe M, Korenstein D, Cascino T, Keyhani S. Associations between marijuana use and cardiovascular risk factors and outcomes: a systematic review. *Ann Intern Med.* 2018;168:187–194.
8. Hemachandra D, McKetin R, Cherbuin N, Anstey KJ. Heavy cannabis users at elevated risk of stroke: evidence from a general population survey. *Aust N Z J Public Health.* 2016;40:226–230.
9. Page II RL, Allen LA, Kloner RA, et al. Medical marijuana, recreational cannabis, and cardiovascular health: a scientific statement from the American Heart Association. *Circulation.* 2020;142:e131–e152.
10. Mittleman MA, Lewis RA, Maclure M, Sherwood JB, Muller JE. Triggering myocardial infarction by marijuana. *Circulation.* 2001;103(23):2805–2809.
11. Frost L, Mostofsky E, Rosenbloom JI, Mukamal KJ, Mittleman MA. Marijuana use and long-term mortality among survivors of acute myocardial infarction. *Am Heart J.* 2013;165:170–175.
12. Sidney S, Beck J, Tekawa I, Quesenberry C, Friedman G. 1997. Marijuana use and mortality. *Amer J Pub Health.* 87(4):585–590.
13. DeFilippis EM, Singh A, Divakaran S, et al. Cocaine and marijuana use among young adults with myocardial infarction. *J Am Coll Cardiol.* 2018;71(22):2540–2551.
14. DeFilippis EM, Bajaj NS, Singh A, et al. Marijuana use in patients with cardiovascular disease. *J Am Coll Cardiol.* 2020;75(3):320–332.
15. Rodondi N, Pletcher MJ, Liu K, Hulley SB, Sidney S. Coronary Artery Risk Development in Young Adults (CARDIA) Study. Marijuana use, diet, body mass index, and cardiovascular risk factors (from the CARDIA study). *Am J Cardiol.* 2006;98:478–484.
16. Auer R, Sidney S, Goff D, Vittinghoff E, et al. Lifetime marijuana use and subclinical atherosclerosis: the Coronary Artery Risk Development in Young Adults (CARDIA) study. *Addiction.* 2018;113:845–856.
17. Haney M, Malcolm RJ, Babalonis S, et al. Oral cannabidiol does not alter the subjective, reinforcing or cardiovascular effects of smoked cannabis. *Neuropsychopharmacology.* 2016;41(8):1974–1982.
18. National Academies of Sciences, Engineering, and Medicine. *The Health Effects of Cannabis and Cannabinoids: The Current State of Evidence and Recommendations for Research.* Washington, DC: The National Academies Press (US); 2017: Summary. www.ncbi.nlm.nih.gov/books/NBK425741/ Accessed December 15, 2020.

6.3 Pregnancy and Breastfeeding Risks

Cannabis use during pregnancy and breastfeeding ranges in prevalence from rare to high, depending largely upon the population surveyed. The rate of use in pregnancy was 7.1% in 2016 in a Kaiser population, by self-report with over half of the women using cannabis identified only by toxicology testing.[1] A 2013 National Survey on Drug Use and Health (NSDUH) found that over 4% of women surveyed admitted to drug use during pregnancy, inclusive of any drug, of which cannabis was the most prevalent. A 2015 report of Women's Infants and Children (WIC) Program clients in Colorado (a state with adult use decriminalization) revealed that 7.4% of mothers aged 30 years or less and 4% of those over age 30 were current cannabis users. "Of all marijuana users (past, ever, current), 35.8% said that they used at some point during pregnancy, 41% since the baby was born, and 18% while breastfeeding."[2] Another survey has recorded up to 65% of medical cannabis patients in Canada use during pregnancy.[3] Another review concluded that use values during pregnancy varied from 4% to 28% overall, occurring highest during the first trimester and lowest during the third trimester.[4] Most pregnant users reported using cannabis to treat nausea early in their pregnancy. Usage was higher in the first trimester than in the last, presumably due to a higher incidence of nausea at the beginning, and/or due to the fact that pregnancy had not yet been confirmed.[5] Thus, we can estimate that perhaps cannabis use may affect an average of 4–10% of all pregnant women, with a higher incidence in younger individuals, that is, those 25 and under, a cohort in which cannabis use is elevated. More studies need to be done on prevalence in recreational versus medical cannabis populations with a recording of types and amounts of cannabis consumed.

The question of whether cannabis use during pregnancy and breastfeeding carries risk has long been debated, with reported clinical studies back to the 1990s. To this day, most official government agencies and many reviews minimally advise caution, while others conclude total contraindication. There are several good reviews that have evaluated the quality of evidence and summarize the findings.[1,6–9] It is useful to recall that until the past decade, cannabis was primarily used by smoking, and to the best of my knowledge, all of the published studies on the risks of cannabis use in pregnancy have been done with smoking as the delivery method. Some were published with no correction for confounders, such as the mother's use of tobacco, alcohol or socioeconomic status – known to affect nutrition and prenatal health care. One can get lost in the morass of variable evidence, opposing conclusions and confounders that have not been adjusted.

DOI: 10.1201/9781003098201-11

RISK FOR THE MOTHER AND THE BIRTH

The conclusion from most studies is that risks to the health of the mother, the outcome of the birth and for prenatal influence of cannabis on gestation cannot be proven, although some studies have proposed that risk must be considered. Several reviews that affirm the risks have not adjusted for confounders, such as maternal use of other substances, cited here for reference.[10,11] Others dissent, saying, "No associations were found between in utero exposure to cannabis and other maternal complications."[12] Or, "Maternal cannabis use during pregnancy is not an independent risk factor for adverse neonatal outcomes after adjusting for confounding factors. The association between maternal cannabis use and adverse outcomes appears attributable to concomitant tobacco use and other confounding factors."[13] A recent large, population-based cohort study found that self-reported cannabis use, without concomitant use of nicotine and/or tobacco, was not associated with pregnancy complications, preterm birth or changes in neonatal outcomes such as Apgar scores and growth parameters.[14] The NASEM 2017 report, a review of more than 10,000 studies found only limited evidence of a statistical association between maternal cannabis smoking and pregnancy complications for the mother, including anemia, hypertension, diabetes, preeclampsia, duration of labor and premature labor.[15]

RISK FOR OFFSPRING EARLY DEVELOPMENT

There remains the possibility that cannabis smoking during pregnancy may cause alteration in the physical or emotional attributes of neonates. For example, decreased birth length, birthweight and increased irritability or arousal have been reported. The alterations were slight and correct with time, and come from low-validity studies. No correction for maternal nutrition or concurrent substance use were done, and many subjects were of lower socioeconomic class. Most of the information on the long-term consequences of prenatal exposure to cannabis comes from longitudinal studies of the Ottawa Prenatal Prospective Study (OPPS) and Maternal Health Practices and Child Development Study (MHPCD).[16–19] However, neither study excluded polysubstance use, or considered environmental and demographic factors. The OPPS interviewed low-risk, middle-class mothers for substance use during pregnancy, and the MHPCD measured the effects of multiple substances on pregnancy and child development in a cohort of low socioeconomic status mothers. It should be noted that the majority of the MHPCD subjects reported no cannabis use, (60–80%), some light use (10–20%) and very few moderate to heavy use (5–15%), more in the first trimester, when they may not have known about the pregnancy and/or had more nausea. Notably, those reporting no tobacco use were in the minority, comprising 45%, so tobacco was a major confounder.[20] Another study, the Generation R (Gen R) study, was a population-based study from the Netherlands and the United Kingdom of over 12,000 pregnant women. This study did take into account potentially confounding factors, including maternal social background and other substance use during pregnancy. After adjustment for confounding factors, the association between cannabis use and birthweight failed to be statistically significant. The adjusted mean birthweights for babies of women using cannabis at least once per week before and throughout pregnancy were 90 g lighter than the offspring of other women. No significant effects were seen for birth length and head circumference.[21] Other studies found that cannabis-exposed babies, on average, were less than two-tenths of one inch shorter than babies not exposed to cannabis.[18] Two studies showed an increase in odds of having a low birthweight baby, while five studies reported no association. Babies exposed to cannabis in utero were also more likely to be placed in the neonatal ICU compared to non-exposed infants.[12] Another concluded that prenatal cannabis use was not independently associated with lower average birthweight. When adjusted for smoking tobacco, an association between cannabis exposure and small for gestational age was eliminated.[22] A retrospective cohort study found a modestly increased risk of birthweight less than the 10th percentile among cannabis users after adjusting for confounders among tobacco non-users.[13] A recent review concluded that cannabis exposure was not correlated with changes in body weight and foot length at birth, and head circumference was reportedly larger in the exposed cohort at 8 months. "These anthropometric measurements were used as an indication of normal fetal development, which correlates with brain development."[23] An oft-quoted study of cannabis use in Jamaica where this medicine was culturally accepted found, "The newborns of heavy cannabis using mothers had better scores on autonomic stability, quality of alertness, irritability, and self-regulation and were judged to be more rewarding for caregivers."[24]

RISKS FOR OFFSPRING COGNITIVE DEVELOPMENT

The area of greatest concern has been the cognitive development of the offspring, where prevailing thought had been that cannabis use led to reduced cognitive development as exposed children matured. There are multiple reports of cognitive deficits from studies such as the OPPS and the MHPCD that have confounding errors that result in flawed conclusions, as aforementioned. A review of three large longitudinal studies (the preceding two and the Gen R) states that, "There is also no preponderance of evidence that PCE [prenatal cannabis exposure] causes lifelong cognitive, behavioral, or functional abnormalities, and/or susceptibility to subsequent addiction." Yet they conclude that "Young women who become pregnant should immediately take a 'pregnant pause' from using marijuana."[25] Several existing reviews on the subject report variable conclusions. These discrepancies alone represent limited evidence.

> By comparing data from the cohorts, a pattern emerges where maternal cannabis use is associated with impaired high-order cognitive function in the offspring, including attention deficits and impaired visuoperceptual integration. In summary, cannabis consumption during pregnancy has profound but variable effects on offspring in several areas of cognitive development.[23]

The NASEM report states, "There is insufficient evidence to support or refute a statistical association between maternal cannabis smoking and: • Later outcomes in the offspring (e.g., sudden infant death syndrome, cognition/academic achievement, and later substance use)."[15]

RISK IN BREASTFEEDING

Cannabinoids have been shown to cross the placenta and be present in breast milk. "Cannabis concentration in the breastmilk is likely related to maternal dose, frequency of dosing, simple diffusion, and trapping within the breastmilk due to lipophilicity. The bioavailability of marijuana metabolites ingested by neonates in the breastmilk is largely unknown."[1] One study estimated that within 4 hours after inhalation of cannabis, 2.5% of the maternal dose of THC is transferred to the infant during breastfeeding.[5] Inhaled THC is nearly completely metabolized into inactive metabolites in about 3 hours. Oral forms can transfer to breast milk for many hours, perhaps up to 10 hours. The estimated half-life of THC in milk has been estimated to be 20 days, with a projected time to elimination of greater than 6 weeks, with transferred amounts in the nanogram range.[26] One study found the median concentration of THC in the breast milk was 9.47 ng/ml.[27] "There is no information about how the amount transferred is related to the concentration of THC in the marijuana, the frequency of use, or the concentration in maternal plasma."[6] Due to these dynamics, strategies used by nursing medical cannabis patients include inhalation, preferably by vaporization immediately after breastfeeding, then waiting approximately 3 hours or more before the next feeding.

Several reviews of the sparse literature about the effect of cannabis use during breastfeeding did not conclude poor health outcomes for the child.[28] Two early studies faced the same confounders that most of the aforementioned studies did, including data from subjects who also used other substances. Again, we are faced with poor evidence with inconclusive or non-significant results. Daily or near daily use of smoked cannabis during the first month of lactation showed a dose-dependent slight reduction in the infant's motor development, but not growth or intellectual development. Infants whose mothers used cannabis while breastfeeding during the third month of life had no difference in mental or motor development at 1 year.[28] It was concluded that occasional maternal cannabis use during breastfeeding did not have any discernable effects on breastfed infants, but the studies were inadequately designed to rule out all long-term harm.

In general, professional guidelines recommend that cannabis use should be avoided by nursing mothers, and nursing mothers should be informed of possible adverse effects on infant development from exposure to cannabis compounds in breastmilk.

CONCLUSION

There is no one conclusion about the risks of cannabis use during pregnancy and breastfeeding. Most reviewers accept the published findings of poorly validated studies that show risk, albeit that they have almost exclusively been done with THC-rich smoked cannabis. The reviewers who recognized and acknowledged bias in the design of these studies proceeded to draw conclusions from them and promote the concept that cannabis risk may be determined by limited studies! For example, the conclusion from the Public Health Advisory Report in Colorado found moderate evidence that use of cannabis during pregnancy is associated with risks to the offspring, including cognitive function, IQ, attention and decreased growth. They further qualify however:

> [T]he available research evaluated the association between marijuana use and potential adverse health outcomes. This association does not prove that the marijuana use alone caused the effect. Despite the best efforts of researchers to account for confounding factors, there may be other important factors related to causality that were not identified.[9]

They aptly point out that most studies were done when cannabis was illegal. "Research funding, when appropriated, was commonly sought to identify adverse effects from marijuana use. This legal fact introduces both funding bias and publication bias into the body of literature related to marijuana use."[9]

Some prevalent opinions that currently inform physicians who seek guidance are presented here. The American College of Obstetricians and Gynecologists opines:

> Pregnant women or women contemplating pregnancy should be encouraged to discontinue use of marijuana for medicinal purposes in favor of an alternative therapy for which there are better pregnancy-specific safety data. There are insufficient data to evaluate the effects of marijuana use on infants during lactation and breastfeeding.[29]

The American Academy of Pediatrics concludes:

> In summary, the evidence for independent, adverse effects of marijuana on human neonatal outcomes and prenatal development is limited, and inconsistency in findings may be the result of the potential confounding caused by the high correlation between marijuana use and use of other substances such as cigarettes and alcohol, as well as sociodemographic risk factors.[6]

And the Canadian Centre on Substance Use and Addiction position is, "Until the effects of prenatal cannabis exposure are well understood, the safest option available to pregnant women is to avoid using cannabis. Medical cannabis use for therapeutic purposes during pregnancy or lactation is also contraindicated."[8] And,

> There is currently, however, a concern expressed in the literature that the medical community does not have sufficient guidance for addressing maternal cannabis use during pregnancy, and there is a strong need for training in the management of cannabis use during pregnancy.[8]

Consumer perceptions about cannabis use in pregnancy does not necessarily follow provider recommendations. Despite recommendations to abstain from cannabis use, its use is increasing during the perinatal period. Seventy percent of both pregnant and non-pregnant cannabis users surveyed responded that they perceived slight or no risk.

A lack of communication with health care providers regarding the health aspects of cannabis was evident. Women perceived this lack of counseling as an indication that adverse outcomes associated with cannabis use are not significant. A discussion about health concerns surrounding cannabis use may influence women's perceptions of risk and help them to make informed choices.[4]

We are faced with limited and inconsistent evidence on the effects of cannabis exposure during pregnancy and breastfeeding. Although evidence is limited, clinical guidelines for cannabis use during pregnancy provide consistent recommendations for pregnant women to abstain. How is a clinician to give advice to a pregnant patient? My point of view as a cannabis clinical specialist is to weigh the risks and benefits, especially in consideration of cannabis as a medicine, not as a drug of abuse. The benefits include treatment of nausea and appetite, especially in the first trimester; management of mood disorders such as stress, anxiety or depression; and help with sleep and discomfort as the pregnancy advances. It is way past time to investigate the risk/benefit ratio of cannabis use in pregnancy and breastfeeding by other delivery methods and with a lower THC content. There are, of course, several studies that have been done to explore and validate the efficacy of various forms of cannabis containing CBD, THC or cannabinoid acids, all of which can be combined for non-psychoactive effects for symptom relief during pregnancy, such as for nausea, lack of appetite, sleep, muscle spasm, pain and depression or anxiety. The risk profile for CBD or CBD/THC mixed cannabis on pregnancy and breastfeeding is unknown, although neurobehavioral effects on adults suggest no anticipation of impairment. THC-rich cannabis is not necessary for any of these outcomes, and smoking as a delivery method is of course to be avoided.

REFERENCES

1. Metz TD, Borgelt LM. Marijuana use in pregnancy and while breastfeeding. *Obstet Gynecol.* 2018;132(5):1198–1210.
2. Wang GS. Pediatric concerns due to expanded cannabis use: unintended consequences of legalization. *J Med Toxicol.* 2017;13(1):99–105.
3. Westfall RE, Janssen PA, Lucas P, Capler R. 2006. Survey of medicinal cannabis use among childbearing women: patterns of its use in pregnancy and retroactive self-assessment of its efficacy against 'morning sickness.' *Complement Ther Clin Pract.* 12(1):27–33.
4. Bayrampour H, Zahradnik M, Lisonkova S, Janssen P. Women's perspectives about cannabis use during pregnancy and the postpartum period: an integrative review. *Prev Med.* 2019;119:17–23.
5. Baker T, Palika D, Rewers-Felkins K, et al. Transfer of inhaled cannabis into human breast milk. *Obstet Gynecol.* 2018;131(5):783–788.
6. Ryan SA, Ammerman SD. O'Connor ME. Marijuana use during pregnancy and breastfeeding: implications for neonatal and childhood outcomes. *Pediatrics.* 2018;142(3): e20181889.
7. Carsley S, Leece P. Ontario Agency for Health Protection and Promotion (Public Health Ontario). *Evidence Brief: Health Effects of Cannabis Exposure in Pregnancy and Breastfeeding.* Toronto, ON: Queen's Printer for Ontario; 2018. www.publichealthontario.

ca/-/media/documents/E/2018/eb-cannabis-pregnancy-breastfeeding.pdf?la=en Accessed July 1, 2020.

8. Porath-Waller AJ, Konefal S, Kent P. Canadian Ctr on Substance Abuse 2nd in Series Clearing the Smoke on Cannabis. Maternal cannabis use during pregnancy: an update. 2018. www.ccsa.ca/sites/default/files/2019-04/CCSA-Cannabis-Maternal-Use-Pregnancy-Report-2018-en.pdf Accessed July 1, 2020.

9. Colorado Department of Public Health and Environment, Retail Marijuana Public Health Advisory Committee, Monitoring Health Concerns Related to Marijuana in Colorado. Changes in marijuana use patterns, systematic literature review, and possible marijuana-related health effects. 2016. https://drive.google.com/file/d/0B0tmPQ67k3NVQlFnY3VzZGVmdFk/view Accessed July 10, 2020.

10. Hayabatsh M, Flenady V, Gibbons K, et al. Birth outcomes associated with cannabis use before and during pregnancy. *Pediatr Res*. 2012;71:215–219.

11. Warshak CR, Regan J, Moore B, et al. Association between marijuana use and adverse obstetrical and neonatal outcomes. *J Perinatol*. 2015;35:991–995.

12. Gunn JK, Rosales CB, Center KE, et al. Prenatal exposure to cannabis and maternal and child health outcomes: a systematic review and meta-analysis. *BMJ Open*. 2016;6(4):e009986.

13. Conner SN, Bedell V, Lipsey K, et al. Maternal marijuana use and adverse neonatal outcomes: a systematic review and meta-analysis. *Obstet Gynecol*. 2016;128(4):713–723.

14. Chabarria KC, Racusin DA, Antony KM, et al. Marijuana use and its effects in pregnancy. *Am J Obstet Gynecol*. 2016;215(4):506.e1–506.e7.

15. National Academies of Sciences, Engineering, and Medicine. *The Health Effects of Cannabis and Cannabinoids: Current State of Evidence and Recommendations for Research*. Washington, DC: The National Academies Press (US); 2017. www.ncbi.nlm.nih.gov/books/NBK425741/ Accessed July 1, 2020.

16. Fried PA. The Ottawa Prenatal Prospective Study (OPPS): methodological issues and findings: it's easy to throw the baby out with the bath water. *Life Sci*. 1995;56(23–24):2159–2168.

17. Fried PA. 1998. Postnatal consequences of maternal marijuana use. Ottawa Prenatal Prospective Study. https://archives.drugabuse.gov/sites/default/files/061-072_Fried.pdf Accessed July 1, 2020.

18. Day N, Cornelius M, Goldschmidt L, et al. The effects of prenatal tobacco and marijuana use on offspring growth from birth through 3 years of age. *Neurotoxicol Teratol*. 1992;14(6):407–414.

19. Day NL, Leech SL, Goldschmidt L. The effects of prenatal marijuana exposure on delinquent behaviors are mediated by measures of neurocognitive functioning. *Neurotoxicol Teratol*. 2011;33(1):129–136.

20. Maternal Health Practices and Child Development Project. www.michigan.gov/documents/PEA_long-term_Day_104254_7.pdf Accessed July 1, 2020.

21. El Marroun H, Tiemeier H, Steegers EA, et al. Intrauterine cannabis exposure affects fetal growth trajectories: the Generation R Study. *J Am Acad Child Adolesc Psychiatry*. 2009;48(12):1173–1181.

22. Leemaqz SY, Dekker GA, McCowan LM, et al. Maternal marijuana use has independent effects on risk for spontaneous preterm birth but not other common late pregnancy complications. *Reprod Toxicol*. 2016;62:77–86.

23. Wu CS, Jew CP, Lu HC. Lasting impacts of prenatal cannabis exposure and the role of endogenous cannabinoids in the developing brain. Medscape website. July 18, 2014. www.medscape.org/viewarticle/745279 Accessed July 1, 2020.

24. Dreher MC, Nugent K, Hudgins R. Prenatal marijuana exposure and neonatal outcomes in Jamaica: an ethnographic study. *Pediatrics*. 1994;93:254–260.
25. Richardson KA, Hester AK, McLemore GL. Prenatal cannabis exposure: The "first hit" to the endocannabinoid system. *Neurotoxicol Teratol*. 2016;58:5–14.
26. Wymore E, Bunik M, Claire Levek, et al. 2018. Duration of marijuana excretion in human breast milk. *Breastfeed Med*. 2018;13(S-2):S-40.
27. Bertrand KA, Hanan NJ, Honerkamp-Smith G, Best BM, Chambers CD. Marijuana use by breastfeeding mothers and cannabinoid concentrations in breast milk. *Pediatrics*. 2018;142(3):e20181076.
28. Garry A, Rigourd V, Amirouche A, et al. Cannabis and breastfeeding. *J Toxicol*. 2009: 596149.
29. American College of Obstetricians and Gynecologists. Committee Opinion No. 722: marijuana use during pregnancy and lactation. *Obstet Gynecol*. 2017;130(4):e205–e209.

6.4 Driving Risks

It is an undisputed conclusion that the effects of THC in naive or occasional subjects (those who are inexperienced and have not developed a tolerance) can alter perception, impede psychomotor functioning and influence judgment. The outcome of these observations warrants and has resulted in a stringent caution to not drive or operate machinery while impaired due to the influence of cannabis. This is written into the laws of all the states that have approved some legal form of cannabis intake. Among young drivers, driving after using cannabis now exceeds the rate of driving after drinking. The reported prevalence of driving after using cannabis was higher among young people and males outnumbering females by three to one.[1] THC may impair driving psychomotor skills, divide attention, lane tracking and cognitive functions and therefore is thought to impair driving in a dose-dependent manner.[2] However, its contribution to the occurrence of motor vehicle crashes remains less clear. We've come a long way from placing culpability for motor vehicle accidents upon drivers who happen to test positive for the presence of THC metabolites. The mere presence of THC metabolites in a urine test provides no information about how impaired the person was while driving. Tolerance, duration of use, mode of delivery and the presence of other confounding substances, especially alcohol, but other pharmaceutical drugs as well, all contribute to the level of impairment that may or may not be present in the driver. And in recent years, many more cannabis users are incorporating CBD into their dose, which is known to mitigate the psychoactive effects of THC. Drivers with a CBD/THC mix in their system, while testing positive for THC, will not suffer from the same level of altered psychomotor performance or perception.

The maximum influence of THC-rich cannabis on performance typically manifests in subjects some 20–40 minutes following inhalation. These maximum concentrations decline rapidly after inhalation, often falling below 5 ng/ml in non-chronic users within 1–4 hours.[3,4] With oral ingestion, THC blood concentrations rise slowly over time, resulting in maximal concentrations 60–120 minutes after dosing.[3,4] THC blood concentrations then decline slowly over a period of several hours. While consumers of low levels of cannabis will likely test negative for the presence of THC in blood within 12 hours following inhalation, THC's lipid solubility and storage in fatty tissues may cause some chronic users to potentially test positive for residual concentrations of THC even after several days of abstinence long after any behavioral influence has worn off.[4,5] "It is difficult to establish a relationship between a person's THC blood or plasma concentration and performance impairing effects."[6]

One study reported on the effects of Sativex, a mixed CBD/THC oromucosal spray on driving. A randomized, placebo-controlled long-term follow-up clinical trial with a CBD/THC spray showed no association with cognitive decline, depression or significant mood changes after 12 months of treatment. Additionally, another study further evaluated the usage of Sativex in patients with multiple sclerosis spasticity did not adversely influence standard driving ability in this patient population.

                    DOI: 10.1201/9781003098201-12

At the final visit, the overall mean score for five driving tests improved by approximately 2%. There were no statistically significant changes versus baseline in mean scores for four of the five driving tests. A statistically significant improvement versus baseline in favor of Sativex (nabiximols) spray was recorded for the stress tolerance determination test +6.1%.[7]

Previous research studies on cannabis and driving have focused on the effects on driving performance. These studies have been almost exclusively experimental, involving laboratory tasks, driving simulator and on road real driving experiments. Many of the early studies were designed to accurately take into account many of the variable factors already given.[4] There are, as might be expected, some contradictory findings. Some of the relevant studies implicating risk in driving follow. A study of the acute effects of smoked cannabis over a 6-hour period was done with two doses of THC, 17.5 and 35 mg. Cognition, impulse control and psychomotor function impairment was induced in a dose-dependent manner. Impairments were most pronounced in the 2 two hours after smoking but were still measurable at 6 hours post dosing.[8] THC was administered at 10–20 mg doses to 18 male participants. A reduction of average speed (from 1 to 6 mph) on simulated motorway driving was seen for both doses. "This strongly suggests that the participants as drivers are aware of their impairment, but attempt to compensate for their impairment by driving more cautiously." In simulator tracking tasks, participants drove less accurately on the higher dose, suggesting that steering control was affected. "Overall, it is possible to conclude that cannabis has a measurable effect on psycho-motor performance, particularly tracking ability. Its effect on higher cognitive functions, for example divided attention tasks associated with driving, appear not to be as critical."[9] Subjects in most of the simulator and instrumented vehicle studies following smoked cannabis typically drive slower, follow other cars at greater distances and take fewer risks than when sober. "These effects appear to suggest that the drivers are attempting to compensate for the subjective effects of using marijuana. In contrast, subjects dosed with alcohol typically drive faster, follow at closer distances, and take greater risks."[6] One recent meta-analysis assessing the risk of road accident associated with drivers' use of cannabis concluded that although consumption was nominally associated with greater accident risk, this risk was comparable to that associated with motorists' consumption of penicillin or anti-histamines.[10] Conversely, a systematic review and meta-analysis of nine observational studies found that acute cannabis consumption *is* associated with an increased risk of motor vehicle crashes, especially for fatal collisions.[11]

Using cannabis and driving under its influence are behaviors more common among young adults and males, groups with higher crash risks irrespective of use. Risk assessment typically declines after adjustments for such factors.[12] When the odds ratio was adjusted for age, gender and race/ethnicity, the increased risk of crash involvement associated with THC (previously calculated to be at least 2.5) was reduced by about half to 1.2–1.4.[13] As compared to an odds ratio risk of crash (1 = normal attentive driver), 1.4 was found for interacting with a passenger, 1.9 for listening to the radio and 6.1 for texting, the risk ratio of crash for cannabis is very low.[6,14] Population level studies have not shown a relationship between medical cannabis laws and an increase in motor vehicle accidents or traffic fatalities. One such report concludes, "Our study suggests that, on average, medical marijuana laws are associated with reductions in traffic fatalities, particularly pronounced among those aged 25 to 44 years, a group representing a great percentage of all registered patients for medical marijuana use."[15] This decline may be due to other research that shows that cannabis is used by some as a substitute for alcohol (see Chapter 30).

CONCLUSION

Although cannabis use in naive users may mildly impair psychomotor skills, this impairment is typically manifested by subjects decreasing their driving speed and requiring greater time to respond to emergency situations.[16] "Cannabis alone, particularly in low doses, has little effect on the skills involved in automobile driving. Cannabis leads to a more cautious style of driving. However, it has a negative impact on decision time and trajectory. This in itself does not mean that drivers under the influence of cannabis represent a traffic safety risk."[17] The most important consideration in the risk of cannabis on driving skills has to do with the user's tolerance. If a naive user, psychomotor impairments may be expected, while in chronic users, no or little impairment will be noted. Caution should be advised to naive users to defer from driving until they become adjusted to the effects of cannabis. The caveat is that driving "impaired" is a risk, and is illegal. Without impairment, the risk of driving under the influence of THC remains low, while there is no recorded risk for CBD or balanced CBD/THC combinations (such as Sativex), and presumably for any CBD/THC product with a higher percentage of CBD.

REFERENCES

1. Douglas J. Beirness DJ, Porath A. Canadian Center on Substance Abuse 3rd in Series. Clearing the smoke on cannabis: cannabis use and driving – an update. 2019. www.ccsa.ca/sites/default/files/2019-04/CCSA-Cannabis-Use-Driving-Report-2017-en.pdf Accessed July 1, 2020.
2. Hartman RL, Huestis MA. Cannabis effects on driving skills. *Clin Chem.* 2013;59: 478–492.
3. Huestis MA, Henningfield JE, Cone EJ. Blood cannabinoids. 1. Absorption of THC and formation of 11-OH-THC and THCCOOH during and after smoking marijuana. *J Analytical Toxicol.* 1992;16:276–282.
4. Armentano P. Should per se limits be imposed for cannabis? Equating cannabinoid blood concentrations with actual driver impairment: practical limitations and concerns. *Humboldt J Soc Relat.* 2013;35:45–55.
5. Karschner EL, Schwilke EW, Lowe RH, et al. Do Delta-9-tetrahydrocannabinol concentrations indicate recent use in chronic cannabis users? *Addiction.* 2009;104:2041–2048.
6. Compton, R. A report to Congress. (DOT HS 812 440). Washington, DC: National Highway Traffic Safety Administration. Marijuana-Impaired Driving. July 2017. www.nhtsa.gov/sites/nhtsa.dot.gov/files/documents/812440-marijuana-impaired-driving-report-to-congress.pdf Accessed July 1, 2020.
7. Rekand T. THC:CBD spray and MS spasticity symptoms: data from latest studies. *Eur Neurol.* 2014;71(Suppl 1):4–9.

8. Ramaekers JG, Kauert G, van Ruitenbeek P, et al. High-potency marijuana impairs executive function and inhibitory motor control. *Neuropsycopharmacology*. 2006;31(10): 2296–2303.

9. Sexton BF, Tunbridge RJ, Brook-Carter N (TRL Limited), Jackson PG (DETR), Wright K. 2000. Prepared for Road Safety Division, Department of the Environment, Transport and the Regions. TRL Report 477. The influence of cannabis on driving. https://docplayer. net/9053645-The-influence-of-cannabis-on-driving.html Accessed June 15, 2020.

10. Elvik R. Risk of road accident associated with the use of drugs: a systematic review and meta-analysis of evidence from epidemiological studies. *Accid Anal Prev*. 2013;60:254–267.

11. Asbridge M, Hayden J, Cartwright J. Acute cannabis consumption and motor vehicle collision risk: systematic review of observational studies and meta-analysis. *BMJ*. 2012;344. e536.

12. Rogeberg O, Elvik R. The effects of cannabis intoxication on motor vehicle collision revisited and revised. *Addiction*. 2016;111(8):1348–1359.

13. Rogeberg O. A meta-analysis of the crash risk of cannabis positive drivers in culpability studies: avoiding interpretational bias. *Accid Anal Prev*. 2019;123:69–78.

14. Dingus TA, Guo F, Lee S, et al. Driver crash risk factors and prevalence evaluation using naturalistic driving data. *Proc Natl Acad Sci*. 2016;113(10):2636–2641.

15. Santaella-Tenorio J, Mauro CM, Wall MM, et al. US traffic fatalities, 1985–2014, and their relationship to medical marijuana laws. *Am J Public Health*. 2017;107:336–342.

16. National Organization for the Reform of Marijuana Laws. Marijuana and driving. A review of the scientific evidence. http://norml.org/library/item/marijuana-and-driving-a-review-of-the-scientific-evidence Accessed June 15, 2020.

17. Canadian Senate Special Committee on Illegal Drugs. Cannabis: Summary Report: Our Position for a Canadian Public Policy. Ottawa. Chapter 8: driving under the influence of cannabis. 2002. www.druglibrary.org/schaffer/library/studies/canadasenate/table_of_contents.htm Accessed June 15, 2020.

6.5 Cognitive Function Risks

Most of the research on cognition and potential risk has been reported for actions of THC or THC-rich cannabis as smoked by recreational users. Distinction between acute and chronic users is essential as effects differ widely between the two. We now know that chronic administration of THC leads to tolerance, with accommodation to many of its psychoactive effects. It has been determined that effects are dose related within populations as well as within the same user. One author tries to account for differences as follows:

> Compelling data have shown that memory is also affected in a biphasic fashion. THC modulates memory and cognition in a biphasic and age-dependent manner: in old animals, low concentrations improve memory and cognition while high concentrations impair these functions; in young animals, even a low concentration is detrimental.[1]

Yet, even these conclusions are too simplistic.

Reports of cognition risk have been contradictory, in no small part due to poor research design, uncontrolled for bias, inconsistent dosing and lack of consideration for the tolerance of subjects. Generally, an important issue affecting most studies was the lack of documentation of subject's baseline or premorbid neurocognitive abilities (pre-onset of regular cannabis usage). Many studies also had insufficient information about other potential confounding factors. These factors include time of last cannabis exposure, extent of exposure to drugs of abuse, presence of confounding neuropsychiatric factors or other neurological risks that can independently affect brain function.[2]

Generally accepted conclusions about the effects of THC, especially in naive users in the short term, include dose-related cognitive impairments in attention, executive function, verbal learning and memory functions.[1,3] Heavy users have also been predicted to have escalating effects. Paradoxically, although not surprisingly, once cannabinoid receptor regulation is considered after tolerance has developed, many of these functions improve. Studies vary in the definition of "heavy" use, but the term has been used to refer to those who use cannabis at least three times weekly, up to daily use and typically will have consumed cannabis for years. This frequency of regular use has been associated with lower scores on tests of memory, attention, planning and decision-making.[4] Conversely, acute cannabis use induces robust and dose-dependent episodic memory effects with more mixed reports of impaired working memory, attention, psychomotor control, inhibition and abstract reasoning.[5] Clearly, what is missing from all of these assessments is a consideration of the subject's intrinsic endocannabinoid tone, in order to make an accurate projection of what the effects of THC on cognition will be in an individual. A recent review concludes:

> There was evidence of changes to functional and structural integrity, memory and learning, and increased anhedonia. There was inconsistent evidence regarding learning, attention, forgetting/retrieval, executive function, motor and perceptual motor

DOI: 10.1201/9781003098201-13

function, [and] sleep. There was no evidence of changes in reaction time, verbal/language skills or visual spatial function.[6]

The author also relates that cannabis use in those with psychosis did not lead to reduced cognitive function. The consensus remains: "There is little evidence, however, that long-term cannabis use causes permanent cognitive impairment, nor is there is any clear cause and effect relationship to explain the psychosocial associations."[7]

EFFECTS ON INTELLIGENCE AND AGE OF USE ONSET

Cognitive function has been measured by intelligence quotient (IQ), with much debate about the effects of cannabis. Associations between poorer performance and a range of cannabis use parameters, including detriments due to a younger age of use onset, are frequently reported. In a much-quoted study of the effect of cannabis use on IQ, it was reported that a decline of up to 6 points was recorded for adolescent study subjects diagnosed with cannabis dependence.[8] This study was heartily debunked by several reviewers. It is interesting that the study cohort was made up of diagnosed cannabis-dependent subjects, yet widely reported as translatable to adolescents in general. A review by the Director of the National Institute of Drug Abuse (NIDA) alleged that cannabis use, particularly by adolescents, is associated with brain alterations and lower IQ. The basis of her claim was later questioned in a separate analysis. That paper suggested that socioeconomics, not subjects' cannabis use, was responsible for differences in IQ and that the plant's true effect (on intelligence quotient) could be zero.[9] Also,

> Correlations between cannabis use and IQ change in the Dunedin cohort [the above referenced study] are consistent with confounding from socioeconomic status. . . . Although it would be too strong to say that the results have been discredited, the methodology is flawed and the causal inference drawn from the results premature. [10]

On the other hand, a 2016 study of 2,235 teenagers from the Avon Longitudinal Study of Parents and Children showed that those who had used cannabis ⩾50 times did not differ from never-users on IQ or educational performance. Adolescent cannabis use was not associated with poorer outcome once adjusted for potential confounds, in particular adolescent cigarette use.[5] Another study found that cannabis use in adolescent subjects was correlated in a dose-dependent manner with a decline in IQ scores. Upon stopping use, the IQ change was reversed. The authors concluded that cannabis does not have a long-term effect on global intelligence.[11]

Nevertheless, there is support for age of onset effects regarding "executive function." In a 2012 study of recreational cannabis users, the early-onset group (prior to age 16) performed more poorly than controls. But this group also smoked cannabis twice as often and nearly three times as much compared to the late-onset smokers. The authors concluded that age of onset, frequency and magnitude of marijuana use were all shown to impact cognitive performance.[12] They point out, and rightly so:

> It is possible that MMJ [medical marijuana] use may not lead to the same neurocognitive consequences that have been observed in recreational users. . . . MMJ users

primarily initiate MMJ use as a means of symptom alleviation, and as such are likely to seek products for their therapeutic potential rather than to experience the psychoactive effects.[12]

They further suggest that MMJ patients may demonstrate some improvement on measures of executive functioning. There are some reports of changes to the white matter in brains of adolescent cannabis users.[13] This appears to be reversible and dependent upon type of use and age of onset.

> Just as a quick refresher, we see lower white matter integrity in those with earlier onset of cannabis use. The earlier you start, the lower the white matter integrity. Then we saw this relationship between lower white matter integrity, higher impulsivity. In our medical cannabis users, we're actually seeing increases in white matter integrity between baseline and three months and baseline six months.[14]

EFFECTS AFTER WITHDRAWAL

Multiple studies have shown that negative effects on cognition do not persist after abstinence from cannabis. This applies to acute effects, such as short-term memory loss, and long-term effects, such as postulated decline in IQ scores. In a study of 7.5 and 15 mg THC given orally to naive users, only the 15 mg dose impaired performance on two memory tasks while performance on an implicit memory task was preserved. No effects of THC were found at 24 or 48 hours following ingestion.[15] It's imperative to really evaluate the literature, such as the following review that reports the opposite result:

> We systematically review[ed] the empirical research published (from January 2004 to February 2015) on acute and chronic effects of cannabis and cannabinoids and on persistence or recovery after abstinence. After 12 to 24 hours of abstinence, heavy users performed worse than non-users and less-frequent users on tasks that assessed verbal learning and memory.[3]

Here the results of chronic long-term use may be considered to pose a risk in reduced memory function, but chronic users will be in a phase of withdrawal that is likely to last more than 72 hours, so what is really being evaluated here is how memory functions during withdrawal. In looking at exactly this distinction, a meta-analysis review including only studies that tested users after at least 25 days of abstinence indicated:

> No significant effect of cannabis use on global neurocognitive performance or any effect on the eight assessed domains. Overall, these meta-analyses demonstrate that any negative residual effects on neurocognitive performance attributable to either cannabis residue or withdrawal symptoms are limited to the first 25 days of abstinence.[16]

EFFECTS OF CBD

A significant question remains as to whether CBD or CBD-rich cannabis has effects on cognitive function, and whether to classify these effects as risk or benefit. A review of studies that have investigated the effect of cannabis on cognition indicate that CBD alone shows no effect, but when administered in a mixed cannabis extract, it prevents some of the detrimental effects of THC as measured by a Short Orientation Memory Concentration test.[17] Studies of high-dose CBD utilized in pediatric seizure therapy have indicated sedation as an adverse effect, but cognition has not been adequately measured.

CONCLUSION

There is no convincing evidence that heavy long-term cannabis use permanently impairs memory or other cognitive functions. Regarding THC-rich cannabis use, the risks to cognition have been summarized: (1) mild cognitive difficulties may result from regular cannabis use; (2) use beginning prior to the age of 16 is a predictor of cognitive impairment; (3) altered brain structure and function is associated with regular cannabis use, but causality has not been proven; (4) cognitive deficits associated with heavy cannabis use are recovered after abstinence; (5) cannabis use does not produce long-term cognitive impairment.[18] I would add the caveat that the risk to short-term cognitive function is the more relevant consideration. To reiterate, especially in naive users, these may be dose-related impairments in attention, executive function, verbal learning and memory functions on a temporary basis. These are expected to reverse once the acute effects of cannabis have ended. The risks to cognition from CBD-rich cannabis use have not been adequately studied, yet are expected to be insignificant.

REFERENCES

1. Calabrese EJ, Rubio-Casillas A. Biphasic effects of THC in memory and cognition. *Eur J Clin Invest*. 2018;48(5):e12920.
2. Grant I, Gonzalez R, Carey CL, Natarajan L, Wolfson T. Non-acute (residual) neurocognitive effects of cannabis use: a meta-analytic study. *J Int Neuropsychol Soc*. 2003;9(5):679–689.
3. Broyd SJ, van Hell HH, Beale C, Yücel M, Solowij N. Acute and chronic effects of cannabinoids on human cognition-a systematic review. *Biol Psychiatry*. 2016;79(7):557–567.
4. Sohn E. Weighing the dangers of cannabis. *Nature*. 2019;572(7771):S16–S18.
5. Mokrysz C, Landy R, Gage SH, et al. Are IQ and educational outcomes in teenagers related to their cannabis use? A prospective cohort study. *J Psychopharmacol*. 2016;30(2):159–168.
6. Memedovich KA, Dowsett LE, Spackman E, Noseworthy T, Clement F. The adverse health effects and harms related to marijuana use: an overview review. *CMAJ Open*. 2018;E339–E346.
7. Iversen L. Long-term effects of exposure to cannabis. *Curr Opin Pharmacol*. 2005;5(1): 69–72.
8. Meier M, Caspi A, Ambler A, et al. Persistent cannabis users show neuropsychological decline from childhood to midlife. *Proc Natl Acad Sci USA*. 2012;109:E2657–2664.
9. Armentano, P. Study: cannabis use not associated with deficits in intelligence quotient. NORML website. https://norml.org/blog/2014/10/22/study-cannabis-use-not-associated-with-deficits-in-intelligence-quotient Accessed September 10, 2020.

10. Rogeberg O. Correlations between cannabis use and IQ change in the Dunedin cohort are consistent with confounding from socioeconomic status. *Proc Natl Acad Sci USA*. 2013;110(11):4251–4254.

11. Fried P, Watkinson B, James D, Gray R. Current and former marijuana use: preliminary findings of a longitudinal study of effects on IQ in young adults. *CMAJ*. 2002;166:887–891.

12. Gruber SA, Sagar KA, Dahlgren MK, Racine M, Lukas SE. Age of onset of marijuana use and executive function. *Psychol Addict Behav*. 2012;26:496–506.

13. Price JS, McQueeny T, Shollenbarger S, et al. Effects of marijuana use on prefrontal and parietal volumes and cognition in emerging adults. *Psychopharmacology (Berl)*. 2015;232(16):2939–2950.

14. Gruber S. How does marijuana affect the brain? Harvard Magazine website. September 13, 2019 podcast. www.harvardmagazine.com/2019/podcast/staci-gruber Accessed July 7, 2020.

15. Curran HV, Brignell C, Fletcher S, Middleton P, Henry J. Cognitive and subjective dose-response effects of acute oral delta 9-tetrahydrocannabinol (THC) in infrequent cannabis users. *Psychopharmacology*. 2002;164(1):61–70.

16. Schreiner AM, Dunn ME. Residual effects of cannabis use on neurocognitive performance after prolonged abstinence: a meta-analysis. *Exp Clin Psychopharmacol*. 2012;20(5):420–429.

17. Colizzi M, Bhattacharyya S. Does cannabis composition matter? differential effects of delta-9-tetrahydrocannabinol and cannabidiol on human cognition. *Curr Addict Rep*. 2017;4(2):62–74.

18. Gabrys R, Porath A. Canadian Center on Substance Abuse 6th in Series. Clearing the Smoke on Cannabis. Regular use and cognitive functioning. 2019. www.ccsa.ca/sites/default/files/2019-09/CCSA-Cannabis-Use-Cognitive-Effects-Report-2019-en.pdf Accessed July 7, 2020.

6.6 Psychosis Risks

One of the risks routinely listed for cannabis is a risk for psychosis, or induction of a psychotic episode. THC is well-known for its "psychoactive" properties, but what does this mean? We know that THC-rich cannabis can stimulate cannabinoid receptors in the brain, affecting many perceptual and mood-altering processes, including memory, cognition, orientation, stress responses and neurotransmitter levels. The state of one's own endocannabinoid tone is an important feature in understanding psychosis and an individual's response to THC. In most subjects, the stimulatory effect of THC is experienced as a mild, transient, somewhat disorienting, possibly euphoric state. It is only in vulnerable populations that the risk for psychosis is usually of importance. In general, this population has been identified as adolescents who are at risk for developing schizophrenia at an earlier age than otherwise would be evidenced. THC also has the potential to induce transient psychotic experiences in healthy individuals, especially those with no tolerance, and worsen existing symptoms in patients with pre-existing psychosis. Overdose from high doses of THC with the use of concentrates in particular elevates the potential for adverse effects.[1] The effects of CBD are quite the opposite, with CBD having documented antipsychotic properties. The effect of cannabis on the risks and benefits associated with schizophrenia in particular is discussed in detail elsewhere (see Chapter 44). A deeper exploration of risk is presented here.

The evidence for cannabis acting as a causal factor for schizophrenia or psychosis has not been clearly established. There are populations thought to be at-risk for earlier onset of psychosis with use of THC-rich cannabis, based on polymorphisms at the CNR1 gene that encodes cannabinoid receptors implicated in schizophrenia pathophysiology.[2,3] History of cannabis use has been shown to be associated with an earlier age of onset of psychosis by almost 3 years. In a study of inpatients with a psychosis diagnosis, those who started using cannabis before age 15 had an increased probability of experiencing an earlier psychotic onset. A correlation between type of cannabis used, frequency of use and onset of psychosis was also found. As is often the case, the cannabis using population in this study was more likely to use tobacco and other illicit drugs, for which no correction was made.[4] Continued cannabis users were shown to have a greater increase in relapse of psychosis than did both non-users and discontinued users.[5] A review of the effects of cannabinoids on schizophrenia concludes:

> Cannabis sativa [use] is associated with increased risk of developing psychotic disorders, including schizophrenia, and earlier age at which psychotic symptoms first manifest. Cannabis exposure during adolescence is most strongly associated with the onset of psychosis amongst those who are particularly vulnerable. . . . [G]enetic polymorphisms may modulate the relationship between cannabis use and psychosis.[6]

DOI: 10.1201/9781003098201-14

Regarding the negative effects of cannabis on psychosis outcomes, a literature review concluded:

> [A]ssociations between cannabis and psychotic symptoms or other psychopathology scores were more inconsistent, with only three studies presenting evidence of association with increased positive symptoms and one study reporting an association with decreased negative symptoms. . . . [F]ew studies adjusted for baseline illness severity, and most made no adjustment for alcohol, or other potentially important confounders.[7]

Another review concluded that the studies are conflicting, and while

> cannabis use may trigger the onset of psychosis in vulnerable individuals in whom a psychotic disorder otherwise may not have developed. As a result, these patients have a better prognosis, exhibit fewer negative symptoms, have better social skills, and have an enhanced treatment response compared with nonusers. In addition, a recent meta-analysis demonstrated that patients with lifetime cannabis use disorders have superior cognitive function compared with nonuser counterparts.[8]

In fact, the positive correlation between cannabis and improved cognitive function in schizophrenics has been reported elsewhere.[9]

As far as the risk for an acute psychotic episode is concerned, this would most likely result from a THC overdose, which might be diagnosed as cannabis intoxication delirium or cannabis-induced psychotic disorder. Cannabis intoxication is discussed in the next section under "Cannabis Use Disorders." A brief preview includes the criteria that "Clinically significant maladaptive behavioral or psychological changes that developed during, or shortly after, cannabis use."[10] If delirium is added to that criteria, we have Cannabis Intoxication Delirium, a DSM-V diagnosis with the code F12.121 or 12.921.[10] When cannabis is smoked, acute effects may occur within minutes; if cannabis is ingested orally, intoxication may take a few hours to develop. These effects usually dissipate once abstinence occurs. Cannabis-induced psychotic disorder (CIP) is a DSM-V diagnosis with the code F12.959. As opposed to intoxication, the symptoms can onset as early as a few hours up to a week after use.

> CIP is commonly precipitated by a sudden increase in potency (e.g., percent of THC content or quantity of cannabis consumption; typically, heavy users of cannabis consume more than 2 g/d). Criteria for CIP must exclude primary psychosis, and symptoms should be in excess of expected intoxication and withdrawal effects.[11]

CIP often includes multiple mood symptoms, including social phobia, hypomania, agitation with a potential for visual hallucinations.[11] One author reports on two cases of emergent psychosis after "dabs" (a method of inhaling highly concentrated oil, discussed in the next section with "Cannabis Intoxication"). "Although 'dabbing' with cannabis wax is becoming increasingly popular in the US for both recreational and 'medicinal' intentions, our cases raise serious concerns about its psychotic liability."[1] The clinical manifestation of an acute psychotic episode induced by cannabis is rare, although intoxication (without delirium) poses a more common risk. In either event, psychotic symptoms generally resolve with abstinence unless an underlying psychotic disorder is present.

Of course, none of the aforementioned reviews and conclusions have addressed the effects of CBD-rich cannabis on psychosis, because that does not pose a risk. The effect of CBD on schizophrenia is reviewed in detail elsewhere (see Chapter 44). In brief review, several studies have shown the antipsychotic effect of purified CBD.[12] In comparing the efficacy of CBD to an antipsychotic drug, while both reduced psychosis, CBD showed a superior side effect profile and was associated with increased anandamide levels.[13] The therapeutic use of CBD as an antipsychotic extends to its diminishing action on the psychoactivity induced by THC.[14] "Although the observed effects are subtle, using high cannabidiol content cannabis was associated with significantly lower degrees of psychotic symptoms providing further support for the antipsychotic potential of cannabidiol."[15]

CONCLUSION

To recap, the potential risks of frequent use of THC-rich cannabis can include triggering a psychotic episode, bringing on an earlier age of onset of a psychotic condition, and/or increasing the risk for relapse. How prevalent or valid these risks are has not been established by valid comprehensive studies that have corrected for confounding variables, type of cannabis used or consideration of tolerance. In clinical practice, it is important to advise any patients vulnerable to developing schizophrenia or any other psychosis to avoid THC-rich cannabis. CBD-rich cannabis may, in fact, reduce the expression of psychosis and may be used to mitigate the acute psychoactive effects of THC.

REFERENCES

1. Pierre JM, Gandal M, Son M. Cannabis-induced psychosis associated with high potency "wax dabs". *Schizophr Res.* 2016;172(1–3):211–212.
2. Gouvêa ES, Santos Filho AF, Ota VK, et al. The role of the CNR1 gene in schizophrenia: a systematic review including unpublished data. *Braz J Psychiatry.* 2017;39(2):160–171.
3. Ujike, H, Takaki M, Nakata K, et al. CNR1, central cannabinoid receptor gene, associated with susceptibility to hebephrenic schizophrenia. *Mol Psychiatry.* 2002;7:515–518.
4. Di Forti M, Sallis H, Allegri F, et al. Daily use, especially of high-potency cannabis, drives the earlier onset of psychosis in cannabis users. *Schizophr Bull.* 2014;40:1509–1517.
5. Schoeler T, Monk A, Sami MB, et al. Continued versus discontinued cannabis use in patients with psychosis: a systematic review and meta-analysis. *Lancet Psychiatry.* 2016;3(3):215–225.
6. Manseau M, Goff D. Cannabinoids and schizophrenia: risks and therapeutic potential. *Neurotherapeutics.* 2015;12(4):816–824.
7. Zammit S, Moore THM, Lingford-Hughes A, et al. Effects of cannabis use on outcomes of psychotic disorders: a systematic review. *Br J Psychiatry.* 2008;193:357–363.
8. Lynch MJ, Rabin RA, George TP. The cannabis psychosis link. *Psychiatric Times.* January 12, 2012. www.psychiatrictimes.com/schizophrenia/cannabis-psychosis-link#sthash.en52agT0.dpuf Accessed June 20, 2020.

9. Løberg EM, Hugdahl K. Cannabis use and cognition in schizophrenia. *Front Hum Neurosci.* 2009;3:53.
10. American Psychiatric Association. *Diagnostic and Statistical Manual of Mental Disorders, DSM-V.* 5th ed. Arlington, VA: American Psychiatric Association; 2013.
11. Grewal RS, George TP. Cannabis-induced psychosis: a review. *Psychiatric Times.* 34:7. July 14, 2017. www.psychiatrictimes.com/view/cannabis-induced-psychosis-review Accessed June 20, 2020.
12. Rohleder C, Müller JK, Lange B, Leweke FM. Cannabidiol as a potential new type of an antipsychotic. A critical review of the evidence. *Front Pharmacol.* 2016;7:422.
13. Leweke, FM, Piomelli, D, Pahlisch, F, et al. 2012. Cannabidiol enhances anandamide signaling and alleviates psychotic symptoms of schizophrenia. *Transl Psychiatry.* 2012;20;2(3):e94.
14. Morgan CJ, Curran HV. Effects of cannabidiol on schizophrenia-like symptoms in people who use cannabis. *Br J Psychiatry.* 2008;192(4):306–307.
15. Schubart C, Sommer I, van Gastel W, et al. Cannabis with high cannabidiol content is associated with fewer psychotic experiences. *Schizophr Res.* 2011;130:216–221.

6.7 Cannabis Use Disorders

Cannabis use disorders comprise a broad category of risk about which much has been written, often with confusing language and unclear criteria. This chapter will review three DSM-V (Diagnostic Manual – Fifth Edition) diagnosed disorders: cannabis use disorder (CUD), cannabis withdrawal syndrome (CWS) and cannabis intoxication.

CANNABIS DEPENDENCE AND CANNABIS ABUSE

Cannabis is often cited as having a risk for addiction and overuse. Of course, this pertains to the effects of THC-rich cannabis used recreationally, a topic of many studies since the 1970s through the present. "Addiction" has been allied with a potential for cannabis abuse or dependence, loosely together comprising a cannabis use disorder, terms frequently employed in much of the literature. Upon the release of the new DSM-V in 2013, diagnoses of cannabis abuse or cannabis dependence were discontinued and a single new diagnosis was defined: cannabis use disorder, modeled in accordance with other substance use disorder categories, and evaluated by much the same criteria. The topic of diagnosed disorders originating from cannabis use holds a lot of evolving history, terms and bias. Being informed about the actual risks for these adverse outcomes as well as knowing how to screen for them is essential for clinicians whether in primary care or in a cannabis specialty practice.

Reference to cannabis dependence or cannabis abuse appears in the literature through 2013 and beyond. These have been characterized by symptoms of craving, tolerance, withdrawal and continued use despite adverse social, vocational or legal consequences associated with use.[1] As a clinician interested in helping my patients use cannabis as a medicine, I am not oriented toward describing the use of cannabis as a component of addiction. Quite often the prevailing bias has been to diagnose a cannabis abuse disorder where none exists.

An illustrative case: A 22-year-old female presented to my practice for nausea, depression and anxiety. She had been seen by a psychiatrist in the past year, referred for a panic attack when seen at the emergency room for shortness of breath (SOB). She smoked cannabis using a bong 2×/day and smoked about five tobacco cigarettes per day. She presented to my practice diagnosed with panic disorder and cannabis dependence. She had been advised to discontinue cannabis. It turned out that her SOB was due to an upper respiratory infection, not panic disorder. I advised her to decrease or stop smoking cigarettes and to switch to CBD-rich cannabis by a vape pen, which she did. She did not follow-up with the psychiatrist. She did not have cannabis dependence, but this diagnosis remained in her medical record.

That is not to say that in certain circumstances an overuse of THC-rich cannabis problem does not exist, but it is difficult to diagnose someone with a substance use problem, who seeks daily use of their substance if they are using it as a medicine.

DOI: 10.1201/9781003098201-15

Perspective, intention and bias bring much confounding into this topic. A 2019 review article on the dangers of cannabis use opines:

> As many as 30% of people who use cannabis develop symptoms consistent with addiction. They develop cravings, damage relationships and give up other activities they once enjoyed. . . . But as cannabis becomes more readily available, one concern is that more people at risk of developing an addiction will try it.[2]

The vast majority of subjects recruited for study and/or diagnosed with cannabis dependence or cannabis abuse have been those smoking THC-rich cannabis. At the outset, we must restrict the risk profile to those using THC-rich cannabis only, as these projections would not be expected to apply to non-psychoactive forms of cannabis, nor necessarily to medical cannabis patients. As rightly pointed out by long-standing researchers of cannabis dependence, "We know nothing of the risks of incidence of cannabis dependence in the context of long-term, supervised medical use."[3] The statistics evaluating these concepts have varied depending upon the parameters of the study and the bias of the author. A wide range of dependence levels have been reported, between 9% and 50%, among recreational cannabis users with prevalence peaking in the 20–24-year age group decreasing with age.[4,5] Other estimates suggest the peak to be among 18- to 29-year-olds (4.4% of this age group overall) and lowest at age 65 years and older (0.01%).[6,7] Approximately 10% of self-reported users experience dependency, increasing with chronic use.[8] In a survey of the perception of "addiction" among medical cannabis patients, the majority of respondents reported believing that cannabis is not addictive. Only 17% reported believing it is addictive and had difficulty stopping cannabis. Interestingly, in this survey, a lower percentage of the older cannabis users reported believing that cannabis is addictive than younger and middle-age users, likely associated with lower use of a THC-rich product.[9]

CANNABIS USE DISORDER

Current studies refer specifically to the designation of cannabis use disorder (CUD), a diagnosis characterized by craving, tolerance, withdrawal and continued use despite adverse social, vocational, or legal consequences of use. Substance use disorders are measured on a continuum from mild to severe: mild – 2–3 symptoms, moderate – 4–6 symptoms or severe – 7 or more symptoms. The DSM-V symptom criteria for Cannabis Use Disorder (ICD-9 305.20 mild ICD-10, F12.10, or ICD-9 304.30 moderate to severe ICD-10, F12.20) may be summarized as follows: cravings to use cannabis with excessive time spent in acquisition, use in hazardous situations, problems in fulfilling obligations, continued use despite problems or negative effects with important activities given up, tolerance and withdrawal.[10]

Diagnosis of CUD shows a wide prevalence range, as was the case for cannabis abuse and cannabis dependence from the prior classification system, discussed earlier. According to the National Survey on Drug Use and Health (NSDUH) statistics from 2005 to 2013, cannabis use prevalence among adults has increased slightly from 16–17% in the early 2000s to 19.8% in 2015 among those aged 18–25 years;

and from 4% to 6.5% among adults 26 years old or older, yet the overall CUD prevalence appeared to remain stable or showed a decrease. In fact, estimates from NSDUH 2002–2017 data showed adult cannabis users past year prevalence of CUD: overall decreased from 14.8% to 9.3%, moderate (4–5 criteria) decreased from 4.3% to 3.1% and severe (6+ criteria) from 2.4% to 1.3%.[11] The prevalence of cannabis-specific treatment use was consistent with the result from the 2012–2013 National Epidemiologic Survey on Alcohol and Related Conditions – III (NESARC-III), which found 7.16% of adults with CUD utilizing cannabis-specific treatment services in the past year.[12] While another 2019 report chose to display similar data with differing conclusions. They reported, according to NESARC,

> Among survey participants with past-year cannabis use, 36% met criteria for CUD; the incidence of CUD 7 to 8 years later was 25%. . . . Indeed, the risk of CUD was up to 50% greater among individuals who used daily and initiated use in adolescence.[1]

Note that these authors used the terms "met the criteria" and "risk of CUD" rather than actual diagnosis. With so much bias in reporting, it is difficult to know the actual risk. All of these estimates are gleaned, yet again, from surveys of populations using recreational cannabis. What do we know about the prevalence of CUD in medical cannabis patients? Nothing has been published yet.

A tool has been developed that is used to identify those at risk for CUD. An updated, revised Cannabis Use Disorder Identification Test (CUDIT-R) is an eight-item screening tool that is 73% sensitive and 95% specific.[13] The CUDIT-R is given in Figure 6.1.

Upon attaining a high score, the patient would then be referred for further evaluation using DSM-V criteria. Paradoxically, the action of using cannabis regularly, as one would a medicine, is more likely to lead to the diagnosis of CUD. Examples include a medical cannabis patient in pain, or experiencing insomnia, who will most likely use THC-rich cannabis daily, may not stop for 6 months and may be "stoned" (an extremely biased, non-medical term) daily even if it is only overnight. Such patients would achieve a high score using this tool; that is, YES to daily use for greater than 6 hours, YES to not being able to stop (or symptoms would recur), YES to a potential problem with concentration, especially prior to bed for insomnia, and, potentially, YES to thoughts of cutting down. Furthermore, such a patient might then score YES to 4–5 DSM-V criteria and may be diagnosed as having moderate to severe CUD. In fact, one study found that the risk of CUD was significantly higher in those with pain (4.2% vs. 2.7%).[14] These results are not surprising as cannabis use is known to be greatest among those experiencing chronic pain leading to a higher prevalence of CUD diagnosis in this population. Distinctions between recreational and medical cannabis users was addressed in a study of two community samples of cannabis users. Sample 1 was recruited from a medical cannabis dispensary in the United States and sample 2 was recruited from a community sample of past year recreational cannabis consumers in Australia, questionably comparable groups. Subjects were interviewed using the CUDIT-R. In comparing medical versus recreational subjects, the average number of DSM-V symptoms for medical subjects was 1.84, for recreational patrons this score showed a small increase to 2.27, actually

The Cannabis Use Disorder Identification Test - Revised (CUDIT-R)

Have you used any cannabis over the past six months?   YES / NO

If YES, please answer the following questions about your cannabis use. Circle the response that is most correct for you in relation to your cannabis use *over the past six months*

1. How often do you use cannabis?

Never	Monthly or less	2-4 times a month	2-3 times a week	4 or more times a week
0	1	2	3	4

2. How many hours were you "stoned" on a typical day when you had been using cannabis?

Less than 1	1 or 2	3 or 4	5 or 6	7 or more
0	1	2	3	4

3. How often during the past 6 months did you find that you were not able to stop using cannabis once you had started?

Never	Less than monthly	Monthly	Weekly	Daily or almost daily
0	1	2	3	4

4. How often during the past 6 months did you fail to do what was normally expected from you because of using cannabis?

Never	Less than monthly	Monthly	Weekly	Daily or almost daily
0	1	2	3	4

5. How often in the past 6 months have you devoted a great deal of your time to getting, using, or recovering from cannabis?

Never	Less than monthly	Monthly	Weekly	Daily or almost daily
0	1	2	3	4

6. How often in the past 6 months have you had a problem with your memory or concentration after using cannabis?

Never	Less than monthly	Monthly	Weekly	Daily or almost daily
0	1	2	3	4

7. How often do you use cannabis in situations that could be physically hazardous, such as driving, operating machinery, or caring for children:

Never	Less than monthly	Monthly	Weekly	Daily or almost daily
0	1	2	3	4

8. Have you ever thought about cutting down, or stopping, your use of cannabis?

Never	Yes, but not in the past 6 months	Yes, during the past 6 months
0	2	4

This scale is in the public domain and is free to use with appropriate citation:

Adamson SJ, Kay-Lambkin FJ, Baker AL, Lewin TJ, Thornton L, Kelly BJ, and Sellman JD. (2010). An Improved Brief Measure of Cannabis Misuse: The Cannabis Use Disorders Identification Test – Revised (CUDIT-R). *Drug and Alcohol Dependence* 110:137-143.

FIGURE 6.1   The Cannabis Use Disorder Identification Test (CUDIT-R).

Source: Adamson SJ, Kay-Lambkin FJ, Baker AL, et al. 2010. An Improved Brief Measure of Cannabis Misuse: The Cannabis Use Disorders Identification Test-Revised (CUDIT-R). *Drug Alc Depend*. 110: 137–143.

both low numbers.[15] Even so, many medical cannabis patients using THC-rich cannabis could achieve a high score.

In a rare discussion of how physicians should deal with the abuse potential of patients using cannabis, the question that often comes up is, as the prevalence of medical cannabis use has been increasing, are we increasing the risk for CUD? With the broader availability of cannabis in current times, concern that cannabis use disorders will increase has been promoted.[16] In a 2007 review, it was found that while usage went up in states (including Colorado, Washington, Alaska and Oregon) that pass medical cannabis laws, the cannabis dependence rate did not differ between states that have approvals versus those that do not.[17] Another report confirmed that no increase in CUD was found in adults aged 18 and above in states with RML (recreational marijuana law) enactment.[18] The projected increased risk for CUD with increased cannabis exposure does not seem to be well founded.

CANNABIS WITHDRAWAL SYNDROME

Cannabis withdrawal syndrome (CWS) is another diagnosis that is listed in the DSM-V, and is not uncommon in chronic users. The constellation of symptoms that may occur after cannabis users undergo abstinence, or stop, even for a tolerance break (discussed in Chapter 7) all fall under the purview of cannabis withdrawal. All of the studies about this have been done with THC-rich cannabis. "Abstinence from THC causes prominent behavior and affective changes. The decrease in mesolimbic dopamine function [affected by CB1 activation] is considered to play the central role in development of cannabis withdrawal."[19] Thus far, no withdrawal syndrome from CBD or CBD-rich cannabis has been identified. Cannabis withdrawal symptoms are an inherent aspect of chronic use of THC-rich cannabis, for which patients need informative guidance. Even though it is listed as a medical condition, with its own code in the DSM-V, it may best be considered as a risk to be managed for such patients.[10]

The criteria for Cannabis Withdrawal Syndrome (ICD-9 292.0, ICD 10 F12.288), a DSM-V designated diagnosis, may be summarized as follows: cessation of cannabis use that has been heavy and prolonged, cessation causes distress in functioning, symptoms of withdrawal may include irritability, anger, aggression, anxiety, insomnia, decreased appetite, restlessness, depressed mood, physical symptoms including abdominal pain, physical symptoms may include shakiness/tremors, sweating, fever, chills, or a headache, and symptoms are not due to another disorder or substance.[10,20] Symptoms appear 1–2 days after cessation and usually resolve within 1–2 weeks, although chronic high-dose usage may require a longer withdrawal period. Increased use and more recent use may predict the severity of withdrawal.[21,22] Determining whether or not a cannabis withdrawal syndrome exists and whether it is part of the reason cannabis users have difficulty quitting has become increasingly important. According to the NESARC-III in 2012–2013, the prevalence of CWS was 12.1% in frequent cannabis users.[23] It has been noted that withdrawal symptoms occur more frequently with heavy use such as that found for those who have been diagnosed with cannabis dependence or CUD.[6]

A survey published in 2006 of adults seeking treatment for cannabis abuse/dependence, found that 51–95% experienced cannabis withdrawal during the past year.[21] It has been estimated that 42% of adult non-treatment seeking cannabis smokers experience withdrawal.[24] Keep in mind that prevalence estimates would be expected to be greatest with patients using oral higher dosage forms of cannabis for which greater tolerance may have developed. In one survey of cannabis consumers (not limited to medical cannabis patients) in Washington State from 2013–2018, 65% noted a problem with withdrawal. The most commonly reported withdrawal symptoms were irritability (33.7%), insomnia (30.3%) and anxiety (22.7%). Older participants were significantly less likely than middle-age and younger individuals to report these symptoms, most likely due to the lower level of usage of THC-rich cannabis that is seen in this cohort.[9]

What does the introduction of CBD do to withdrawal symptoms, if anything? A six-day treatment with Sativex (a mixed CBD/THC extract) has been shown to reduce the magnitude of withdrawal effects, such as withdrawal-related irritability, depression and cannabis cravings. It also showed therapeutic benefit for sleep disturbance, anxiety, appetite loss, physical symptoms and restlessness.[25] As the composition of Sativex is approximately 50% THC, and 50% CBD, what is happening here is not only the inclusion of CBD, but also the THC dose is much reduced. This study supports the conclusion that weaning, rather than abrupt withdrawal as well as the presence of CBD, can attenuate withdrawal symptoms.

CANNABIS INTOXICATION AND TOXICITY

Cannabis intoxication is not synonymous with cannabis toxicity, and these concepts are often confused. Cannabis can produce what has been defined as intoxication symptoms, yet rarely can be termed toxic. The lethality of any drug in the present US Pharmacopoeia is measured by a value known as the lethal dose 50 (LD50), defined as the dosage amount that causes death in 50% of the animals or humans taking the drug. No LD50 for cannabis exists as it cannot be determined (ingestion of too great an amount would be required). The toxicity of a drug may also be estimated by a value called the "therapeutic ratio" (TR) defined as the lethal dose divided by the effective dose. For cannabis, this has been extrapolated to be approximately 40,000 – even though the LD50 cannot be determined (as compared to a TR of about 10 for alcohol). The only case in which toxicity is discussed in terms of cannabis is associated with the presence of contaminants such as pesticides or petrochemicals. Cannabis itself is not toxic. Clearly, intoxication implies overuse due to a "desire to be intoxicated." With medical cannabis, this is typically not seen. Yet, intoxication has been associated with overuse of THC-rich cannabis, either acutely or in chronic users. If an acute episode of overuse occurs in a naive user, for example, there may be a transient exhibition of overuse symptoms, similar to what have been commonly listed for "toxicity." The most commonly encountered signs and symptoms of cannabis toxicity in adults have been described as paranoia, psychosis and decreased judgment, perception and coordination.[5]

The criteria for Cannabis Intoxication (ICD-9 292.89, ICD-10 various F12.1xx, 12.2xx, 12.9xx), a DSM-V designated diagnosis, may be summarized as follows: recent use of cannabis after which behavioral or psychological changes occur, including impaired motor coordination, euphoria, anxiety, sensation of slowed time, impaired judgment, social withdrawal, signs of conjunctival injection, increased appetite, dry mouth or tachycardia, and that these symptoms are not due to another disorder.[10]

Intoxication occurs in a matter of minutes after smoking cannabis, but can take longer, up to a few hours, with oral consumption. The effects last 3–4 hours when smoked, but can last for many hours when cannabis is consumed orally. Treatment of cannabis toxicity/overdose is supportive and based on serial reassessment of the airway and neurological signs.[26] The phenomenon of toxicity or overuse in chronic users is somewhat different, as these individuals have likely already developed a tolerance to THC-rich cannabis, so effects may be due to higher doses not likely to dissipate rapidly.

An illustrative case #1: A 47-year-old female using cannabis for 35 years presented to my medical cannabis practice. She was experiencing anxiety with increased usage of THC-rich cannabis up to doses of a 65 mg of an edible 5×/day for the past 2 years. She had a stated goal of "needing to get off THC," which is why she came in. She also had skin itching with high liver function tests (LFTs), yet a normal liver ultrasound. I agreed that she needed to "get off THC" and lower her cannabinoid usage entirely, that it may be contributing to her itching symptoms. It is of note that increased LFTs have been noted as a potential adverse effect of high doses of CBD (see Chapter 6.8). I advised a weaning protocol of CBD/THC 1:1 at a dose of 30 mg of each daily. She did not follow-up. This case demonstrates use of one the highest dosages of THC I've encountered, 325 mg/day. She was likely experiencing cannabis intoxication as expressed by a chronic-use, high-tolerance patient.

These overuse effects are also seen in patients or recreational users who do "dabbing." Dabbing may be described as inhalation of a vapor created by rapidly heating a cannabis concentrate to 300–400°C on a titanium or glass rod. Dabs contain THC concentrations up to 23–80%, compared to the 10–25% seen in traditionally smoked cannabis. Up to 40% of the THC can be inhaled.[27] This can provide an extremely concentrated dose in one inhalation, up to 25–50 mg THC per dab. The effects generally last for 3 hours or less dependent upon the individual and the amount consumed. In a survey of cannabis users who have experienced dabbing, "[P]articipants did report that 'dabs' led to higher tolerance and withdrawal (as defined by the participants), suggesting that the practice might be more likely to lead to symptoms of addiction or dependence."[28] Clinical practice experience shows that regular use of highly concentrated cannabis absolutely does lead to a higher tolerance development, for which a tolerance break is mandated (see Chapter 7 for tolerance reduction strategies).

An illustrative case #2: This is a 17-year-old male who came in with his mother for complaints of anxiety, depression and insomnia. It was a very instructive case for me, and I'm afraid, not atypical for some young adults. He had been under the care of a psychiatrist for 6 months. He was taking 1 mg of Klonapin in the evenings. He said he felt paranoid at night and was afraid to fall asleep. He was an honor student, doing well in school. Apparently, he had been using cannabis for 3 years, now excessively. He was dabbing wax 6–7 times/day and smoking in-between. He even admitted to dabbing in the middle of the night because he thought it would help him sleep better. He was restless, thin and seemed "wired." I advised them both that he was likely suffering from cannabis intoxication. That the THC in concentrate form was way too high a dose, done practically every 2 hours, and he could also be having a toxic reaction to butane in the wax preparation. He needed to stop dabbing and use of concentrates immediately. On 6-month follow-up, he was sleeping better, had less anxiety and was smoking cannabis (not dabbing) twice a day, after school and in the evening. One year later he was in college, had gained 30 pounds and still smoked

2×/day. I advised him to switch to a CBD-rich strain for ongoing anxiety, which he did, finding that it worked better for him than the THC-rich strains.

Young people especially may overuse cannabis, and in this case, the patient's use was excessive. He was actually causing his insomnia from using too much THC-rich product that caused paranoia, restlessness and difficulty with sleep. This is clearly a case in which the side effects of cannabis outweighed the benefits. That's why professional guidance is so important. With the proper use of cannabis, he was able to appropriately treat anxiety, eliminate insomnia and decrease toxicity. I use the term toxicity loosely, because it was likely a combination of butane and THC excess by dabbing that caused these negative effects. Should I have denied him a medical cannabis approval because he abused the substance in the past? No, not if teaching him how to use it properly brought positive results.

In their zeal for finding a quick shift in consciousness, and being products of a society that leads them to think more might be better, consumers who may overuse cannabis completely overshoot the mark of creating endocannabinoid balance. This overuse unwittingly causes their system to depend upon cannabis for normal functions, such as sleep, appetite and mood regulation. These are the exact symptoms that become prominent during cannabis withdrawal. Hence, do anxiety, depression, insomnia and lack of appetite come before cannabis overuse, or as a result of it? The answer in practice is both.

CONCLUSION

As has already been evidenced, the entire arena of cannabis medicinal use is in transition from consideration as a "disorder" to becoming a therapeutic intervention. One author applies the term "medicalization" to this process.

> The term "medicalisation" refers to a development whereby a medical vocabulary is expanded to define a new problem – a problem that previously had been regarded as a form of deviance (for example, alcohol problems, opiate addiction) or normal life events (menopause, infertility).[29]

It has been argued that we are now witnessing a medicalization of cannabis. New guidelines need to be adopted that set forth the risks of overuse as one would with any medication, along with measures for appropriate dose escalation, dose weaning and the acquisition of quality ensured, safe, lab-tested products.

The treatment, professional advice and diagnosis of medical cannabis abuse must be fundamentally different for patients using it medically than that of recreational cannabis users. This dilemma has yet to be resolved in professional guidance thus far. As with all substance use evaluations, including daily use of pharmaceutical medicines, the risk/benefit ratio is of primary importance. It is suggested that providers should monitor for symptoms and recommend tapering off of cannabis should they develop CUD. A summary of prevailing literature regarding treatment of CUD is represented by the following quotation:

> Clinical trials of various treatments for cannabis use disorder have likewise increased, focusing primarily on psychotherapy treatments, specifically, motivational

enhancement therapy, cognitive behavioral therapy, and contingency management. Their findings suggest that a combination of these three modalities produces the best abstinence outcomes, although abstinence rates remain modest and decline after treatment.[30]

It is imperative to first determine whether there actually is a disorder, of dependence, or overuse, or whether a medical cannabis patient is taking properly dosed cannabis, albeit regularly. Tolerance reduction strategies may be more useful than abstinence.

The problem exists that there remain real and valid risks of overuse, with attendant adverse effects in a significant number of users, most, but not all of them, associated with a more youthful age (see Chapter 10). Keeping in mind that *all* of the overuse effects have occurred from use of THC-rich cannabis, with little documentation of how many patients are currently using CBD-rich and/or CBD/THC mixed varieties, we really don't know the prevalence of overuse or abuse disorders within the medical cannabis population.

REFERENCES

1. Kansagara D, Becker WC, Ayers C, et al. Priming primary care providers to engage in evidence-based discussions about cannabis with patients. *Addict Sci Clin Pract.* 2019;14:42.
2. Sohn E. Weighing the dangers of cannabis. *Nature.* 2019;572(7771):S16–S18.
3. Degenhardt L, Hall WD. The adverse effects of cannabinoids: implications for use of medical marijuana. *CMAJ.* 2008;178(13):1685–1686.
4. Degenhardt L, Ferrari AJ, Calabria B, et al. the global epidemiology and contribution of cannabis use and dependence to the global burden of disease: results from the GBD 2010 study. *PLoS One.* 2013;8(10):e76635.
5. Volkow ND, Baler RD, Compton WM, Weiss SR. Adverse health effects of marijuana use. *N Engl J Med.* 2014;370(23):2219–2227.
6. Ramesh D, Schlosburg JE, Wiebelhaus JM, Lichtman AH. Marijuana dependence: not just smoke and mirrors. *ILAR J.* 2011;52(3):295–308.
7. Patel J, Marwaha R. Cannabis use disorder. [Updated June 24, 2020]. In: *StatPearls* [Internet]. Treasure Island, FL: StatPearls Publishing; 2020. www.ncbi.nlm.nih.gov/books/NBK538131/ Accessed July 10, 2020.
8. Memedovich KA, Dowsett LE, Spackman E, Noseworthy T, Clement F. The adverse health effects and harms related to marijuana use: an overview review. *CMAJ Open.* 2018;6:E339–E346.
9. Sexton M, Cuttler C, Mischley LK. A survey of cannabis acute effects and withdrawal symptoms: differential responses across user types and age. *J Altern Complement Med.* 2019;25(3):326–335.
10. American Psychiatric Association. *Diagnostic and Statistical Manual of Mental Disorders, DSM-V.* 5th ed. Arlington, VA: American Psychiatric Association; 2013.
11. Compton WM, Han B, Jones CM, Blanco C. Cannabis use disorders among adults in the United States during a time of increasing use of cannabis. *Drug Alcohol Depend.* 2019;204:107468.
12. Wu LT, Zhu H, Mannelli P, Swartz MS. Prevalence and correlates of treatment utilization among adults with cannabis use disorder in the United States. *Drug Alcohol Depend.* 2017;177:153–162.

13. Adamson SJ, Kay-Lambkin FJ, Baker AL, et al. An improved brief measure of cannabis misuse: the cannabis use disorders identification test: revised (CUDIT-R). *Drug Alc Depend.* 2010;110:137–143.

14. Hasin DS, Shmulewitz D, Cerdá M, et al. U.S. adults with pain, a group increasingly vulnerable to nonmedical cannabis use and cannabis use disorder: 2001–2002 and 2012–2013. *Am J Psychiatry.* 2020;177(7):611–618.

15. Bonn-Miller MO, Heinz AJ, Smith EV, Bruno R, Adamson S. Preliminary development of a brief cannabis use disorder screening tool: the cannabis use disorder identification test short-form. *Cannabis Cannabinoid Res.* 2016;1(1):252–261.

16. Budney AJ, Roffman R, Stephens RS, Walker D. Marijuana dependence and its treatment. *Addict Sci Clin Pract.* 2007;4(1):4–16.

17. Looby A, Earlywine M. Negative consequences associated with dependence in daily cannabis users. *Subst Abuse Treat Prev Policy.* 2007;10(2):3.

18. Cerdá M, Mauro C, Hamilton A, et al. Association between recreational marijuana legalization in the united states and changes in marijuana use and Cannabis Use Disorder from 2008 to 2016. *JAMA Psychiatry.* 2020;77(2):165–171.

19. Katz G, Lobel T, Tetelbaum A, Raskin S. Cannabis withdrawal: a new diagnostic category in DSM-5. *Isr J Psychiatry Relat Sci.* 2014;51(4):270–275.

20. Gorelick DA, Levin KH, Copersino ML, et al. Diagnostic criteria for cannabis withdrawal syndrome. *Drug Alcohol Dep.* 2012;123(1–3):141–147.

21. Budney AJ, Hughes JR. The cannabis withdrawal syndrome. *Curr Opin Psychiatry.* 2006;19:233–238.

22. Lichtman AH, Martin BR. Cannabinoid tolerance and dependence. *Handb Exp Pharmacol.* 2005;698:691–717.

23. Livne O, Shmulewitz D, Lev-Ran S, Hasin DS. DSM-5 Cannabis withdrawal syndrome: demographic and clinical correlates in U.S. adults. *Drug Alcohol Depend.* 2019;195:170–177.

24. Levin KH, Copersino ML, Heishman SJ, et al. Cannabis withdrawal symptoms in non-treatment-seeking adult cannabis smokers. *Drug Alcohol Depend.* 2010;111(1–2):120–127.

25. Allsop DJ, Copeland J, Lintzeris N, et al. Nabiximols as an agonist replacement therapy during cannabis withdrawal: a randomized clinical trial. *JAMA Psychiatry.* 2014;71(3):281–291.

26. Wang T, Collet J, Shapiro S, Ware MA. Adverse effects of medical cannabinoids: a systematic review. *CMAJ.* 2008;178(13):1669–1678.

27. Raber JC, Elzinga S, Kaplan C. Understanding dabs: contamination concerns of cannabis concentrates and cannabinoid transfer during the act of dabbing. *J Toxicol Sci.* 2015;40(6):797–803.

28. Loflin M, Earleywine M. A new method of cannabis ingestion: the dangers of dabs? *Addict Behav.* 2014;39(10):1430–1433.

29. Pedersen W, Sandberg S. The medicalisation of revolt: a sociological analysis of medical cannabis users. *Sociol Health Illn.* 2013;35(1):17–32.

30. Sherman BJ, McRae-Clark AL. Treatment of cannabis use disorder: current science and future outlook. *Pharmacotherapy.* 2016;36(5):511–535.

6.8 Drug Interactions

The assessment of drug–drug interactions (DDIs) with cannabis and cannabinoids and exogenous (pharmaceutical) drugs has been fraught with several misassumptions, clouding the issue of what actual effects are likely to take place with commonly used cannabis therapeutic regimens. There is a bidirectional action of cannabinoids with other drugs – the effect on cannabinoid levels by exogenous drugs, as well as the reverse, the effect of cannabinoids on the action of the drugs. This is primarily related to the metabolism of both by the cytochrome P (CYP) 450 system, a phase I metabolic pathway. As such, it should be noted that orally ingested cannabis and cannabinoids have the greatest potential for interaction, as they are metabolized by the liver before entering the bloodstream (first-pass metabolism). Many other delivery methods, including inhalation, oromucosal, transdermal and rectal, enter hepatic metabolism to lesser degrees, thus first-pass metabolism is reduced or eliminated, resulting in lower likelihood of interactions with non-cannabinoid substances, and are less likely to have DDIs. Second, the levels at which cannabis and cannabinoids are dosed (in most cases) are not high enough to produce a measurable effect on other drugs, exceptions of high dose strategies including treatment for seizure disorders and cancers.

Most DDI studies have been done at doses greater than normally seen in medicinal use. For example, in a recent study designed to predict the potential for CBD and THC to participate in CYP-mediated drug interactions, the determined doses appropriate for testing were based upon untutored (my opinion) calculations of average patient use. CBD oral doses ranged from 70 mg (average low dose) to 700 mg (average high dose) to 2,000 mg (maximum dose). For THC, the range predicted was 20 mg (average low dose) to 130 mg (average high dose) to 160 mg (maximum dose). Inhaled doses of THC were estimated at 25 mg (average low dose) to 70 mg (average high dose) to 100 mg (maximum dose).[1] In fact, in my practice and others, the average full extract CBD or THC cannabis dose was in the range of 25 mg of cannabinoids or less orally, while the average amount in a whole joint (multiple doses) after correction for pyrolysis and loss in sidestream smoke may be approximately 20 mg total (see Chapter 7).[2] In cases where greater amounts of cannabis are consumed, such as in individuals who have developed tolerance and in conditions that require high doses, there is also the confounding supposition that induction of the CYP system occurs not as a result of DDIs but also as a measure of homeostatic regulation.

DDIs of a pharmacodynamic nature involve synergistic or antagonistic interactions on the same drug targets, while pharmacokinetic interactions involve alterations of the drug's absorption, distribution, metabolism and excretion.[3] Most reported drug interactions are pharmacokinetic ones, via affecting drug metabolism enzymes such as the those of CYP 450 system.[4] Sixty percent of drugs are metabolized by the CYP 450 pathways, providing a plethora of substrates for potential interaction with concomitant cannabinoid consumption. There has been little research oriented toward the effect of other drugs on the action of cannabinoids, although this could be a

DOI: 10.1201/9781003098201-16

prevalent effect. At the low doses of cannabinoids in most medical cannabis protocols, effects of cannabinoids upon exogenous drugs are less likely to be a problem than the effects of higher doses of pharmaceuticals on cannabinoids. The notion that cannabis is a medicine that may be adversely affected by the concomitant use of other medications has had scant attention in the literature. Lastly, there is very little information on the interaction of other components, such as terpenes in cannabis on other drugs, although these would be expected to have relevance even at the low nanomolar doses at which they are circulated.

REVIEW OF PREDICTED DDIS WITH CANNABINOIDS AND THEIR METABOLITES

Important metabolites occur with the ingestion of THC and CBD. Commonly, these metabolites have been detected in the systemic circulation at higher concentrations than THC after oral administration has occurred.[1] THC is metabolized to an active metabolite – 11-hydroxy-THC (11-OH-THC), and CBD is metabolized primarily to 7-hydroxy-CBD (7-OH-CBD) as well as to 6-OH and 4-OH-CBD.[5,6] 11-OH-THC is then primarily catalyzed to 11-nor-9-carboxy-tetrahydrocannabinol, aka THC-11-oic acid (11-COOH-THC) by CYP2C19 and 2C9 pathways.[7] The metabolism of CBD involves the 3A4 and 2C19 pathways where 7-OH-CBD is further metabolized by CYP3A4 to CBD-7-oic acid (7-COOH-CBD).[8] CBN metabolism involves the CYP 450 3A4 and 2C9 pathways.

CBD and THC have both been shown to inhibit CYP activity in a concentration-dependent manner.[9] As one author points out, "[I]nterindividual differences in the expression and function of CYP450 enzymes may considerably affect the pharmacokinetics of CBD and its metabolites, and this could be relevant in the therapeutic action and any possible adverse effects of CBD-containing preparations."[8] This is true for THC as well. Genetic variation in the expression of these pathways affect the metabolism of cannabinoids. "Patients who are poor metabolizers of CYP2C9 have THC concentrations that are about 3-fold higher than those of extensive metabolizers of CYP2C9."[10] Compared to CBD, THC was an approximately 7.5 and 14 times more potent inhibitor of CYP1A2 and 2C9, respectively, but was approximately 3.5 times less potent an inhibitor of CYP3A activity. CBD and THC showed comparable inhibitory potency toward CYP2C19 and 2D6. 11-OH THC was a strong inhibitor of CYP2C9 and a relatively weak inhibitor of CYP2C19, 2D6 and 3A4.1. CYP interactions are listed in detail in Table 6.1. *Note:* Inducers decrease substrate levels and inhibitors increase substrate levels.[5,7,10]

CYP 450 inhibition is usually instantaneous leading to increased drug effects, while a longer period of time, several days, is usually required for the induction of CYP 450, which may lead to decreased drug effects.[4] All of these factors affect the decision as to whether DDIs will be clinically relevant, either with cannabinoids or exogenous drugs as victim. In the pharmacokinetic study mentioned earlier, designed to predict the potential for cannabinoids to participate in CYP-mediated drug interactions, all tested CBD oral doses (70, 700 and 2,000 mg) were predicted to participate in pharmacokinetic interactions with theophylline, diclofenac, omeprazole and midazolam, all CYP 450 substrates.[1] THC was predicted to participate in interactions

TABLE 6.1
CYP Drug Interactions

CYP Pathway	Substrates	Inducers	Inhibitors
CYP3A4	THC, CBN, CBD	Enzalutamide	CBD, THC
	Immunosuppressants	Phenytoin	Protease inhibitors
	Chemotherapeutics		Ketoconazole Loperamide
	Antihistamines		Nefazodone
	Statins		
	Antipsychotics		
	Benzodiazepines		
	Opioids		
	Macrolides		
	Antiretrovirals		
	Sildenafil		
	Antidepressants		
	z-Hypnotics		
	Ca channel blockers		
CYP2C19	CBD	Rifampin	CBD
	Antidepressants antiepileptics	Carbamazepine	Fluvoxamine
	Proton pump inhibitors	Phenobarbital	Fluoxetine
	Clopidogrel	Phenytoin	
	Propranolol		
	Carisoprodol		
	Warfarin		
	Cyclophosphamide		
CYP2C9	THC, CBN	Barbiturates	CBD, THC
	NSAIDs	Carbamazepine	Amiodarone
	Warfarin	Rifampin	Fluorouracil
	Oral antidiabetic agents		Metronidazole
	Angiotensin II receptor		Miconazole
	blockers		Sulfamethoxazole
CP1A2	Duloxetine	THC	
	Naproxen		
	Olanzapine		
	Cyclobenzaprine haloperidol		
	Clozapine		
	Theophylline		
	Chlorpromazine		
CYP2D6	SSRIs		CBD, THC
	Tricyclic Antidepressants		
	Antipsychotics		
	Opioids		
	Beta blockers		

with CYP substrates at high oral doses (130 and 160 mg). They found that unlike CBD, neither THC nor 11-OH-THC showed inactivation of any of CYP function. As they pointed out, predictions are not always what is found. Possible induction of CYP pathways may have been a compensating mechanism.[1] Fortunately, as mentioned earlier, and reiterated strongly here, no DDIs are expected with THC at commonly used medical cannabis doses, and for CBD, some of the following studies show that DDIs may begin to have relevance only at 40 mg or greater doses.

The phase II metabolic pathways of cannabinoids implicate potential for DDIs, but this has not been well studied. Oxidation of THC to THC-COOH results in final glucuronidation before excretion. Both CBN and CBD may also be directly glucuronidated by several uridine 5'-diphospho-glucuronosyltransferase (UGT) enzymes.[8,11] UGT enzymes catalyze glucuronidation of pharmaceuticals as well as cannabinoids. Inhibition of UGTs decreases excretion of substrates and increases their bioavailability, while activation increases excretion of substrates. While some UGTs are inhibited by CBD and CBN, others have been activated by CBN.[12] DDIs between CBD and secondary metabolism or transport proteins may also occur.[13]

DDIS RELEVANT TO CANNABINOID LEVELS

There are a few studies aimed at measuring the effect of exogenous drugs on cannabinoid metabolism. Most have had the reverse objective. But now, as medicinal use of cannabis is gaining prominence, these studies are sorely needed. These scant results are as follows:

1. CBD bioavailability increased by 89% while no effect was observed for THC, when THC/CBD spray (10.8 mg/10 mg) was coadministered with ketoconazole (400 mg), an inhibitor of CYP3A4.[9]
2. THC levels were reduced by 20–40%, and CBD levels reduced by 50–60% when THC/CBD spray (10.8/10 mg) was coadministered with rifampin (600 mg), a CYP3A4 inducer.[9]
3. No significant changes in cannabinoid levels were recorded when THC/CBD spray (10.8 mg/10 mg) was coadministered with omeprazole (40 mg), a CYP2C19 inhibitor.[9]
4. The DDI potential between CBD and coadministered clobazam, which is metabolized extensively by CYP3A4, CYP2C19 and CYP2B6, showed CBD to be a victim of this DDI with increases in C_{max} of 73%.[14]
5. The COX inhibitors indomethacin, acetylsalicylic acid and other NSAIDS may antagonize THC effects. In subjects who smoked cannabis, indomethacin decreased the elevation of prostaglandins induced by THC and attenuated the subjective "high" and the heart rate accelerating effects of THC.[15]
6. There was a slight increase in CBD exposure after 21 days of concomitant administration of clobazam (5 mg bid) with 750 mg of CBD bid, but no effect by stiripentol or valproate.[16]

It may be that even though cannabinoid pharmacokinetics are affected by other drugs, the interaction is more likely to be of clinical relevance in naive or occasional use subjects, in which aforementioned examples demonstrated 40–90% alterations in bioavailability. Chronic administration, as seen in example 6 resulted in little effect on cannabinoid levels, possibly reflecting that pharmacokinetic effects affecting cannabinoid bioavailability at high dose levels in subjects with tolerance are quite different than lower dose levels. Much more research is needed on this topic.

DDIS RELEVANT TO CANNABINOID EFFECTS ON EXOGENOUS DRUGS

Recalling the results on predicted effects of oral dosing of CBD and THC, where they found, unlike CBD, neither THC nor 11-OH-THC, showed inactivation of any of the CYPs tested, we would not expect to find the influence of oral THC to be involved in significant DDIs. THC has been studied primarily in smoked form at lower dose levels. The effects of CBD have been shown to be relevant at 70 mg/day. A review of the studies is given in the following.

Studies of Inhaled Cannabis

1. Smoked cannabis increases the clearance of theophylline by 40%, possibly by induction of CYP1A2-mediated theophylline metabolism. Whether it's the role of THC or the effect of smoke is in question.[17]
2. A case report of smoked cannabis (2.5 grams/week) and warfarin reported INR values increased to 11.55. That this effect is due to DDIs is in question. "An alternative theory is based on the fact that warfarin and Δ9-THC are both highly plasma protein-bound. Accordingly, Δ9-THC has the potential to displace plasma protein-bound warfarin, thus leading to an increase in warfarin concentrations and an increased INR."[18]
3. Smoked cannabis had no effect on indinavir or nelfinavir levels in HIV patients.[19]
4. Vaporized cannabis increased the analgesic effects of opioids without altering plasma opioid levels.[20]

Thus far, there is no clear determination of the effect of inhaled THC-rich cannabis on DDIs. As related earlier, no effect of oral THC occurred in all concentrations tested.

Studies of Cannabinoid Acids

The use of cannabis tea (200 ml herbal tea, 1 gram/l) for 15 days reported no interactions with docetaxel and irinotecan. We now know that cannabis tea contains primarily cannabinoid acids, so the actual THC level was likely to be small. Subjects' urine samples tested positive for cannabinoid metabolites (11-nor-THC-9-carboxylic acid).[21]

Studies of CBD, or CBD-rich Extract

1. A study of CBD for epilepsy required a 30% reduction in warfarin dose to maintain therapeutic INR values.[18]
2. CBD (2,000–2,900 mg/day) caused a threefold increase in tacrolimus. No effect of occasional use has been reported.[17]

3. Oral CBD (5–25 mg/kg/day) administered with clobazam led to a fivefold increase in plasma concentrations of the metabolite N-desmethylclobazam, which is metabolized by CYP2C19.[22] Administration of CBD (750 mg bid) with clobazam (5 mg bid) led to a 3.4- fold increase in N-desmethylclobazam, but non-significant changes in the level of clobazam.[16] Administration of high doses of CBD up to 50 mg/kg resulted in increases in topiramate, rufinamide, N-desmethylclobazam, zonisamide and eslicarbazepine.[23]

4. Oral administration of CBD (750 mg bid) with stiripentol (750 mg bid), a CYP2C19 substrate, led to a 1.6-fold increase in stiripentol.[16] Epidiolex at a dose of 20 mg/kg/day did not affect the pharmacokinetics of stiripentol and led to a small increase in stiripentol exposure (17% increase in C_{max}).[24]

5. Oral administration of CBD (750 mg bid) with valproate (500 mg bid) showed no effect on plasma levels.[12] Epidiolex at a dose of 20 mg/kg/day did not affect the pharmacokinetics of valproate or its metabolite.[21]

It should be noted that the doses of CBD or CBD extracted from cannabis that show DDI interactions are all high in these studies, ranging from perhaps 250 mg/day (5 mg/kg × 50 kg) to 1,500 mg/day up to 2,900 mg/day. Even at such high dosages, very few significant DDIs are noted. A side effect of overpowering hepatic enzymes with high doses of substrates can be extended to include high-dose CBD. Abnormal liver function test results were noted in participants taking concomitant CBD and antiepileptic drugs. Transaminase elevation occurred in 8% of participants taking Epidiolex at 10 mg/kg/day, as compared to 3% in placebo subjects. Caution is advised when high-dose CBD is used with medications with potential to cause hepatic injury or in people with hepatic impairment.[14]

CONCLUSION

Caution for the advent of DDIs continues to be promoted in cannabis risk literature. An example follows:

> Given the potential for drug interactions, it can be important to increase monitoring of medications that need to be within a specific therapeutic window, at least temporarily, if someone is starting medical cannabis for the first time, and to monitor patients much like they would if they were using herbal or dietary supplements.[25]

As aforementioned, there seems to be little indication that doses of THC or CBD normally used in medicinal cannabis pose any potential for DDIs. The exception would be when extremely high doses of cannabinoids are employed, at perhaps greater than 100 mg/day, as a conservative estimate. In these rare cases, caution should be employed, not only in measuring therapeutic levels of any drugs used but also in adjusting cannabinoid levels, especially in at-risk populations with reduced metabolism such as the elderly or those with impaired hepatic function. Much more research needs to be done on interactions between cannabis and other drugs at doses that patients are actually using, but human clinical trial research is scant.

> The widespread availability of these products highlights the urgent need for well-designed in vitro and clinical studies to investigate potential marijuana-drug

interactions ... with the end goal of informing health care providers and consumers about the safety of consuming marijuana products concomitantly with conventional medications.[26]

Contrary to what one may find in literature on the risk of DDIs as a contraindication to cannabis therapeutic use, its safety in most cases can easily be confirmed, or managed, if need be in high-dose cases.

REFERENCES

1. Bansal S, Maharao N, Paine MF, Unadkat JD. Predicting the potential for cannabinoids to precipitate pharmacokinetic drug interactions via reversible inhibition or inactivation of major cytochromes P450. *Drug Metabol Dispos.* 2020;48(10):DMD-AR-2020-000073.
2. Sulak D. A physician's perspective on optimal cannabis dosing. Leafly website. February 26, 2018. www.leafly.com/news/health/a-physicians-perspective-on-optimal-cannabis-dosing Assessed July 1, 2020.
3. American Society of Hospital Pharmacy. Lesson 1. Introduction to pharmacokinetics and pharmacodynamics. www.ashp.org/-/media/store%20files/p2418-sample-chapter-1.pdf Accessed July 1, 2020.
4. Watanabe K, Yamaori S, Funahashi T, et al. Cytochrome P450 enzymes involved in the metabolism of tetrahydrocannabinols and cannabinol by human hepatic microsomes. *Life Sci.* 2007;80:1415–1419.
5. Alsherbiny MA, Li CG. Medicinal cannabis-potential drug interactions. *Medicines (Basel).* 2018;6(1):3.
6. Jiang R, Yamaori S, Takeda S, Yamamoto I, Watanabe K. Identification of cytochrome P450 enzymes responsible for metabolism of cannabidiol by human liver microsomes. *Life Sci.* 2011;89(5–6):165–170.
7. Stout SM, Cimino NM. Exogenous cannabinoids as substrates, inhibitors, and inducers of human drug metabolizing enzymes: a systematic review. *Drug Metab Rev.* 2014;46(1):86–95.
8. Ujváry I, Hanuš L. Human metabolites of cannabidiol: a review on their formation, biological activity, and relevance in therapy. *Cannabis Cannabinoid Res.* 2016;1(1):90–101.
9. Stott C, White L, Wright S, et al. A phase I, open-label, randomized, crossover study in three parallel groups to evaluate the effect of rifampicin, ketoconazole, and omeprazole on the pharmacokinetics of THC/CBD oromucosal spray in healthy volunteers. *Springerplus.* 2013;2(1):236.
10. Horn JR, Hansten PD. 2014. Drug interactions with marijuana. *Pharmacy Times.* December 9, 2014. www.pharmacytimes.com/publications/issue/2014/December2014/Drug-Interactions-with-Marijuana Accessed June 20, 2020.
11. Mazur A, Lichti CF, Prather PL, et al. Characterization of human hepatic and extrahepatic UDP-glucuronosyltransferase enzymes involved in the metabolism of classic cannabinoids. *Drug Metab Dispos.* 2009;37(7):1496–1504.
12. Qian Y, Gurley BJ, Markowitz JS. The potential for pharmacokinetic interactions between cannabis products and conventional medications. *J Clin Psychopharmacol.* 2019;39(5):462–471.
13. Elmes MW, Kaczocha M, Berger WT, et al. Fatty acid-binding proteins (FABPs) are intracellular carriers for Δ9-tetrahydrocannabinol (THC) and cannabidiol (CBD). *J Biol Chem.* 2015;290(14):8711–8721.
14. Brown JD, Winterstein AG. Potential adverse drug events and drug-drug interactions with medical and consumer cannabidiol (CBD) use. *J Clin Med.* 2019;8(7):989.

15. Perez-Reyes M, Burstein SH, White WR, McDonald SA, Hicks RE. Antagonism of marihuana effects by indomethacin in humans. *Life Sci.* 1991;48(6):507–515.

16. Morrison G, Crockett J, Blakey G, and Sommerville K. A phase 1, open-label, pharmacokinetic trial to investigate possible drug-drug interactions between clobazam, stiripentol, or valproate and cannabidiol in healthy subjects. *Clin Pharmacol Drug Dev.* 2019;8:1009–1031.

17. Antoniou T, Bodkin J, Ho JM. Drug interactions with cannabinoids. *CMAJ.* 2020;192(9): E206.

18. Damkier P, Lassen D, Christensen MMH, et al. Interaction between warfarin and cannabis. *Basic Clin Pharmacol Toxicol.* 2019;124(1):28–31.

19. Abrams DI, Hilton JF, Leiser RJ, et al. Short-term effects of cannabinoids in patients with HIV-1 infection: a randomized, placebo-controlled clinical trial. *Ann Intern Med.* 2003;139(4):258–266.

20. Abrams DI, Couey P, Shade SB, Kelly ME, Benowitz NL. Cannabinoid opioid interaction in chronic pain. *Clin Pharmacol Ther.* 2011;90:844–851.

21. Engels FK, de Jong FA, Sparreboom A, et al. Medicinal cannabis does not influence the clinical pharmacokinetics of irinotecan and docetaxel. *Oncologist.* 2007;12(3):291–300.

22. Gaston TE, Szaflarski JP. Cannabis for the treatment of epilepsy: an update. *Curr Neurol Neurosci Rep.* 2018;18:73.

23. Gaston TE, Bebin EM, Cutter GR, Liu Y, Szaflarski JP. Interactions between cannabidiol and commonly used antiepileptic drugs. *Epilepsia.* 2017;58(9):1586–1592.

24. Ben-Menachem E, Gunning B, Arenas Cabrera CM, et al. A phase II randomized trial to explore the potential for pharmacokinetic drug-drug interactions with stiripentol or valproate when combined with cannabidiol in patients with epilepsy. *CNS Drugs.* 2020;34(6):661–672.

25. Slawek D, Meenrajan SR, Alois MR, et al. Medical cannabis for the primary care physician. *J Prim Care Community Health.* 2019;10:1–7.

26. Cox EJ, Maharao N, Patilea-Vrana G, et al. A marijuana-drug interaction primer: precipitants, pharmacology, and pharmacokinetics. *Pharmacol Ther.* 2019;201:25–38.

7 Delivery and Dosage of Cannabis Medicine

The choice of exactly which cannabis to take for each condition, for each individual, by what route, for how long, how much it will cost and how it may affect other medications one is taking are the ultimate questions that must be answered in order to use this or any medicine wisely. These are the questions for which patients seek professional advice. These are the answers that consultants are required to be able to provide in order to help patients achieve success. This chapter lays the foundation of knowledge in two basic arenas from which these answers will be solicited: delivery and dosage – no small task. We start with delivery, as the dosing variables are unique to each delivery method. There are actually seven categories of delivery methods: smoking, vaporizing, ingestion, oromucosal/sublingual, rectal/vaginal, topical/transdermal and a specific form of ingestion – raw (uncooked plant matter). About 10 years ago, a public health official made a statement that cannabis was unsafe as a medicine because it was smoked and it made people dangerously altered, that is, "stoned." At that time, I lamented that these official statements were being made by an appalling lack of current knowledge. In fact, there are six alternative modes of delivery to smoking, and of these, the topical and raw versions are inherently non-psychoactive, or more accurately, non-intoxicating. An educational poster about the different delivery methods that I created to address this lack of knowledge (with the exception of the rectal/vaginal methods, which were not widely available at that time) is displayed in Figure 7.1.

As you can see, smoking is but one among several options. It is true that recreational cannabis users have traditionally preferred to consume this plant by smoking or ingestion. However, accounts of ingestion, topical use and research on alternative delivery methods have been ongoing since the 1970s. It is only with the advent of cannabis therapeutic use that these dosage forms have become available to the general public in dispensaries. The challenge remains that those dispensing the medicine in dispensaries, "budtenders," are not clinicians and have no medical training. Based upon these shortfalls, budtenders are poorly equipped to help a patient decide which form and what dosage to use for medical applications. Worse, they often provide inaccurate and possibly damaging advice. To fill this breach, medical professionals must be educated on these matters.

DOI: 10.1201/9781003098201-17

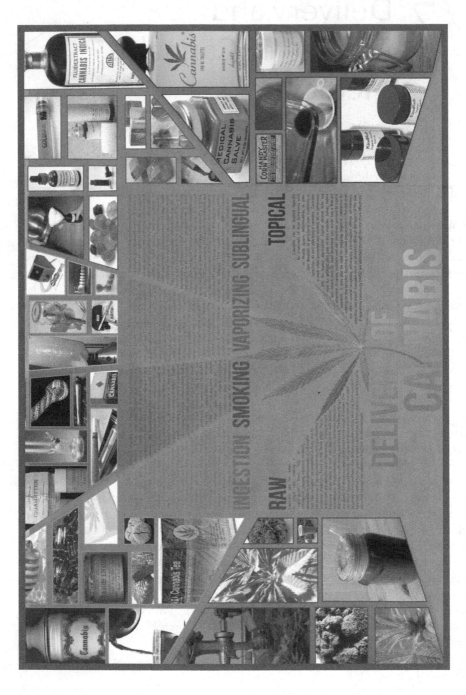

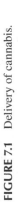

FIGURE 7.1   Delivery of cannabis.

DELIVERY METHODS

Different delivery methods yield their own bioavailability profile, not only for cannabinoids but for terpene constituents of the original plant matter. The pharmacokinetics and pharmacodynamics of cannabinoids vary by the route of administration with absorption exhibiting significant variability. "Absorption is affected both by intrinsic product lipophilicity and by inherent organ tissue differences (i.e., alveolar, dermal vs. gastric)."[1] Cannabinoids are highly lipophilic with very low aqueous solubility. Aqueous solubility is a key determinant of the rate and degree of absorption/bioavailability of any delivery format with increased aqueous solubility resulting in increased absorptivity. Cannabinoids are hydrophobic and are transported in the blood by lipoproteins and albumin.[2] These issues as well as convenience of use, availability, personal preference and cost, all factor into the delivery method chosen by the consumer. The type of extraction and formulation methods employed determine whether the resulting product will be full or partial spectrum. In general, full-spectrum products are more effective at lower doses than partial extracts due to the entourage effect that occurs among the various components of cannabis (see Chapter 2). A review of the common ways to consume cannabis has been compiled by the Canadian government as a resource.[3] An extensive review of pharmacokinetics (PKs) and absorption variables for various delivery methods has also been published.[1] Each of the seven delivery methods – smoking, vaporizing, ingestion, oromucosal/sublingual, rectal/vaginal, topical/transdermal and raw – is presented in the following sections.

SMOKING

Smoking cannabis is the classical method of cannabis delivery, used historically for centuries. Of course, smoking is not a preferred delivery method due to health concerns, such as inhalation of tar and hydrocarbons. Reducing the amount of plant matter by using cannabis with a high potency minimizes the amount of hydrocarbons inhaled. Cannabis flowers (aka buds) are now available in dispensaries with cannabinoid contents up to 25% by weight. Concentrates such as oils, kief, hash or wax can yield up to 80% of cannabinoids by weight. Cannabis is usually smoked, in a rolled cigarette (joint) or a pipe. Water pipes (bongs) reduce the level of inhaled smoke. Cannabis smoke is irritating to the throat and lungs and can cause bronchial inflammation and cough.[4] There are some pulmonary risks that may be associated with inhaling concentrated forms of cannabis, such as oils, wax, or hash due to petrochemical residue from an extraction process. Mold, pesticide and heavy metal contamination should be measured as well, although this is not yet standardized.[3] Numerous studies have evaluated the association between smoking cannabis and lung cancer. One large, early study found no association between cannabis inhalation and lung cancer.[5] Smoking by adding tobacco to cannabis is a preferred method for a minority of consumers in the United States, more so in European countries.[6] This not only exacerbates respiratory symptoms, but may also cause an increased dependence on use of this mix due to the addictive nature of tobacco.[7] Smoking delivery does avoid first-pass metabolism (see "Ingestion" section for more details), yielding less circulating 11-OH-THC as compared with oral ingestion.

TABLE 7.1
Smoking

Advantages	Disadvantages
Most well-known	Smoke may cause negative health effects
Rapid onset in 5–10 minutes	Can cause bronchial inflammation
Short acting, 2–4 hours	Can cause cough
No costly equipment needed	May be too short acting, 2–4 hours
Portable	
Simple method, easy to do	
Can select strain of cannabis desired	

Via inhalation, peak concentrations of cannabinoids are attained in 3–10 minutes. Maximum effects occur at 30–60 minutes and last for several hours.[8] From approximately 50% of the THC that survives pyrolysis (combustion), 16–53% is delivered to the smoker, while the rest is released into the air as sidestream smoke.[9] Total bioavailability has been estimated over a wide range, from 2% to 56%, due in part to intra- and intersubject variability in smoking dynamics.[10] The amount inhaled is determined by the depth and duration of inhalation with experienced users retaining more of the smoke. Given these dynamics, the final systemic bioavailability of THC has been measured at 23–27% for heavy users and 10–14% for occasional users.[11] Recovery of CBD by smoking is similar to THC, as well as having a similar PKs by inhalation.[1] Average bioavailability of CBD by smoking was measured to be 31%.[12] With smoking a single CBD containing cigarette, the average peak blood plasma level at 3 minutes resulted in a mean serum half-life of 31 hours and the average systemic availability ranged from 11% to 45%.[13] Upon inhalation, medicinal compounds pass through the lungs into the bloodstream. See Table 7.1 for a summary of the benefit/risk profile of the smoking delivery method.

VAPORIZING

Vaporizers are devices that heat cannabis to a specified temperature, below its ignition point. The temperature for vaporization of cannabis is 180–200°C (356–392°F). This process releases cannabinoids as a vapor without combustion and its toxic by-products, containing little or none of the carcinogenic tars and noxious gases found in smoke. Vaporized cannabis was found to be composed almost exclusively of cannabinoids with virtually no pyrolytic compounds. Furthermore, the vaporization does not raise exhaled CO levels.[14] Many vaporizer designs are available, including table-top, portable handheld models and vapor pens (vape pens). The choice of vaporizer is a major factor in determining extraction and delivery efficiency, as shown by the wide range of results from tests of different vaporizers. One study of the Volcano vaporizer (a table-top model) showed availability of 36–61% of the THC in the sample, similar to efficiencies reported by smoking cannabis.[15] Some studies have shown better efficiency than smoking, most likely because with traditional smoked preparations more THC is lost as a result of pyrolysis and sidestream smoke.[16]

Vaporized THC levels were similar over 6 hours when comparing smoking and vaporizing; however, vaporizing was associated with higher THC concentrations at 30 minutes and 1 hour compared with smoking, suggesting that absorption was faster with vaporizing.[17] THC showed 55% availability when 8 mg was vaporized alone or with low-dose (4 mg) CBD. The addition of high-dose CBD (200 mg) resulted in great variability in absorption rates.[18] This result may have more to do with saturation of cannabinoid levels in the subject from the high dose than inherent differences between CBD and THC. Vaporized cannabis may have differing concentrations and ratios of cannabinoids and terpenes compared with smoked cannabis. Terpenes vaporize at a lower temperature than cannabinoids, and often are not present in oils produced by high heat extraction processes. Hence, smoking or vaporizing full plant matter supplies a wider variety of entourage compounds than inhalation of vaporized concentrates (such as in vape pens). With newer extraction methods, the retention of a fuller spectrum of terpenes has been a major focus during optimal cannabis oil production.

There are clear advantages of vaporizing as compared with smoking. It was found that "Vaporizer users are only 40% as likely to report respiratory symptoms as users who do not vaporize, even when age, sex, cigarette use, and amount of cannabis consumed are controlled."[19] A study (having a pre-post design) reported a meaningful effect on patient symptoms in that switching to the vaporizer for 1 month improved self-reported respiratory symptoms by 73%, with statistically significant improvement in FVC in previous cannabis smokers (who did not use tobacco).[20] As with smoking, contaminants are a potential risk. In addition, there is a new lung injury risk linked to vape pens, termed e-cigarette or vaping product use-associated lung injury (EVALI). As of December 27, 2019, nearly 2,561 cases of EVALI were thought to be caused by inhalation of vitamin E acetate, an additive in some e-cigarettes and vaping products.[21] Other diluents found in electronic inhalant devices may include polypropylene glycol, propylene glycol, polyethylene glycol, vegetable glycerin and ethylene glycol. Complications seen with cannabis vaping products however have been rare, as these ordinarily do not include an array of diluents. As with all methods of consumption, it's best to use only lab-tested products, supplied with a Certificate of Analysis listing cannabinoid and terpene content, as well as contaminants such as additives, pesticides, mold and heavy metals. Upon inhalation, medicinal compounds pass through the lungs into the bloodstream. See Table 7.2 for a summary of the benefit/risk profile of the vaporizing delivery method.

TABLE 7.2
Vaporizing

Advantages	Disadvantages
Rapid onset in 5–10 minutes	Difficult to transport device
Short-acting, 2–4 hours	Portable device is not as efficient
No smoke, minimal health risk	Equipment is costly
No irritation to throat and lungs	May be too short-acting, 2–4 hours
Can select strain of cannabis desired	Concentrates may contain residual solvents

INGESTION

Ingestion of cannabis usually leads to a longer, stronger, and is reported to induce a more physical effect than smoking. Greater amounts must be used, up to three times as much per dose as compared with smoking. Oral preparations are a good choice if desiring long-acting effects. Preparations include edibles, capsules, oils and tea. Dosing is difficult and variable as absorption is dependent upon GI transit timing and the presence or absence of food in the gut. The onset of effects may be delayed by about an hour or more with peak concentrations and effects available for 1–6 hours. THC is subjected not only to degradation in gastric acid but also to first-pass metabolism in the liver that results in the production of 11-OH-THC, which is said to be more psychotropic than THC and causes sedation and disorientation. Oral bioavailability of THC, whether given in the pure form or in cannabis is low and variable, ranging from 6% to 20% with peak concentrations achieved between 60 and 120 minutes (and may take up to 6 hours). Duration of effects is 8–20 hours, with a serum half-life reported at 20–30 hours.[10] The oral bioavailability of CBD has been shown to be similarly low, 13–19%.[22] After chronic administration of high doses of CBD for 6 weeks, the half-life was 2–5 days.[13] The reported plasma half-life of oral CBD is 60 hours after administration of high doses for 7 days, according to Epidiolex® prescribing information.[23] These reports remind us that the clearance of cannabinoids including CBD and THC, with high-dose applications, takes longer than the acute one-time dosing utilized for most PK studies.

The PK profile of CBD has been reported to be similar to that of THC, whether it is administered orally, intravenously or inhaled.[1] On the other hand, in another report, when administered in concert with THC in comparing sublingual and oral doses of 16.2 mg THC and 15 mg CBD, the mean peak plasma concentration of THC was 11.2 µg/l and for CBD it was much lower, 3.7 µg/l. Mean maximum concentrations for THC, CBD and 11-OH-THC were <5, <2 and <7 ng/ml, respectively, across oral, sublingual or oromucosal and intravenous administration routes, with CBD having a lower C_{max}.[10] These results suggest that absorption of THC may be at least two times as efficient as CBD across multiple delivery systems. One explanation for this is that the PKs of mixed cannabinoids may produce differing results as compared to single cannabinoids. For example, cannabinoid acids may increase the absorption of neutral cannabinoids, demonstrating a type of entourage effect. Capsules filled with 10 mg total (THC + THCA) and 10–15 mg total (CBD + CBDA) showed mean peak plasma CBD concentrations four times higher in the unheated extract than in the heat-treated extract. The authors point out that "the use of unheated cannabis extract rich in acidic phytocannabinoids may beneficially affect the uptake and metabolism of CBD or other phytocannabinoids."[24] Cannabis is absorbed through the intestinal tract into the bloodstream. See Table 7.3 for a summary of the benefit/risk profile of the ingestion delivery method.

TABLE 7.3
Ingestion

Advantages	Disadvantages
Long-acting – average 8 hours	Slow onset 1 hour or more
Lasts through the night	May be too long-acting
Taste can be attractive – chocolates, cookies, candies	More product required
Easy to administer	Easy to overdose
Can achieve high doses	Dose is variable, affected by food
Can dose as other oral medicines, 2–3×/day especially in capsules	Unknown concentration in homemade edibles

OROMUCOSAL/SUBLINGUAL

Cannabis may be delivered via mucosal absorption in a rapid, dose-measured manner as a tincture, lozenge, mouthstrips or gum. Compared with ingestion, oromucosal absorption has a more rapid onset of action, less than half an hour, but can last 4–6 hours. Other terms that one may hear and are used interchangeably with oromucosal include sublingual and buccal. To provide this convenient delivery method, tinctures may be produced when an organic solvent is used to extract cannabinoids and other active components of cannabis. This is a classical method of herbal medicine delivery, used for centuries to prepare cannabis medicines. Extraction into an organic solvent such as alcohol or glycerin is a process that retains all the cannabinoids and terpenes, with alcohol retaining the chlorophyll as well. Alcohol-based products are fast-acting (15–45 minutes), lasting 2–6 hours. When alcohol-based products are ingested, they may be absorbed directly into the bloodstream through the pharynx and stomach lining, thus circumventing the first-pass metabolism. It is best taken sublingually (under the tongue) from a dropper bottle or delivered by an oral spray via an atomizer bottle. Tinctures may also be mixed with water and swallowed as well; however, this will delay the onset and extend the duration of effect. While both ethanol and oil extracts may be delivered as sublingual (oromucosal) products, oil is absorbed and delivered over a much longer period as compared with tincture products. Oil extraction is efficient as to yield and it retains all of the cannabinoids, only a little chlorophyll, but most terpenes are lost by evaporation if heat is used in the process.

Sativex® is an oromucosal spray containing 2.7 mg of THC and 2.5 mg of CBD in a 100 µl actuation dose whose PK profile has been studied in detail.[25] When comparing sublingual administration of CBD/THC (25 mg of each), lower plasma concentrations of CBD were observed.[10] As mentioned earlier, the absorption of THC may be at least two times as efficient as CBD across multiple delivery systems, including the oromucosal route when administered as mixed cannabinoids, with other

TABLE 7.4
Oromucosal/Sublingual

Advantages	Disadvantages
Rapid onset of action – 15 minutes	May have a harsh taste
Easily transportable	Difficult to hold in mouth for sublingual
No cannabis odor	May be too short acting, 4–6 hours
Measured dosing, good for low doses	Longer time to onset of action if swallowed
Moderately short-acting, 2–4 hours if sprayed, 4–6 hours if sublingual	

results showing that the PKs are comparable for CBD and THC.[1] Cannabinoid oral fluid concentrations and time course were evaluated for two routes of administration: oral THC and oromucosal Sativex, and compared to results after smoking and during monitoring abstinence in chronic daily cannabis smokers.[26] Each participant received oral synthetic THC, cannabis extract (Sativex) or oral THC placebo and Sativex placebo. Peak concentration of cannabinoids was reached in 15 minutes to 1 hour. Unlike oral THC, Sativex significantly increased oral fluid THC, CBD and CBN concentrations immediately following administration, implying that components of the extract (i.e., the terpenes) helped in cannabinoid absorption.[27] Much more work needs to be done to delineate the actual absorption of multiple cannabinoids at a range of doses from the full entourage of the cannabis plant as opposed to purified single cannabinoids. Cannabis is absorbed through oromucosal surfaces into the bloodstream. See Table 7.4 for a summary of the benefit/risk profile of the oromucosal/sublingual delivery method.

RECTAL/VAGINAL

Suppositories may be used rectally or vaginally. Oil preparations in a syringe (custom-made) have also been utilized. Rectal administration bypasses gastrointestinal metabolism in large part, to avoid first-pass metabolism and conversion to 11-OH-THC, resulting in less psychoactivity than ingestion. This method is good for delivery of low to high doses of cannabis to pelvic and lower abdominal areas. Rectal suppositories are most often made from cannabis infused into coconut oil or cannabis oil infused into cocoa butter. There exists a paucity of literature evaluating the absorption and bioavailability of rectal or vaginal delivery of cannabis formulations. Absorption of cannabinoids in suppository form is challenging due to their lipophilic nature. The exact formulation, method of extraction and solvent used are critical. In one study completed in monkeys, THC showed low to no bioavailability either rectally or vaginally from various suppository formulations.[28] Absorption was found to be improved with the hemisuccinate formulation (THC-HS).[29,30]

By employing the prodrug delivery of Δ9-THC via rectal administration of THC-HS in suppository formulation, it is hypothesized that it is possible to avoid potential acid lability of Δ9-THC in the stomach and the direct exposure via the portal circulation to the dominant hepatic extraction of Δ9-THC.[30]

A study of suppositories made in cocoa butter in which an unheated cannabis resin was used (perhaps containing mostly THCA) also showed little bioavailability.[31] Anecdotally, patients report feeling effects of rectally delivered THC-rich cannabis, so perhaps other entourage components besides cannabinoids are aiding absorption. A formulation containing cannabis delivered in flax-seed oil, introduced rectally via a syringe, was able to exhibit absorption that seemed to produce clinical effects (personal observation in clinical practice). The bioavailability of the rectal route once absorbed was found to be at least twice that of the oral route due to lower first-pass metabolism as compared with oral formulations.[30] Studies in the dog using rectal delivery of THC-hemisuccinate showed 67% bioavailability of THC.[32] In human subjects, rectal administration of 2.5–5 mg of THC (as a hemisuccinate) produced maximum plasma concentrations within 2–8 hours.[33] Another study analyzed the PK profile of THC delivered as THC-HS from 1.25 to 20 mg doses. Concentrations did not start to decline until 6–8 hours after dosing. Concentrations of 11-OH-THC were found to be generally very low, but highly variable. Cannabis once absorbed into the rectal veins is then distributed to the bloodstream.

Vaginal suppositories that are currently on the market are often formulated in medium-chain triglyceride (MCT) oil, coconut oil or cocoa butter. Little is known about the bioavailability of cannabis or cannabinoids delivered intravaginally, although transdermal absorption is most rapid with MCT oil. In an older study of rectal absorption in which vaginal suppository delivery was also tested, THC showed no absorption when delivered by vaginal suppository in various formulations.[28] The question of whether cannabis formulations show increased permeation by vaginal delivery as compared with pure cannabinoids has not been addressed. As it is likely to be a challenge here as for rectal delivery, vaginal delivery is not commonly used to achieve systemic effects. After passage through the vaginal membrane cannabinoids enter the bloodstream through the lamina propria layer into the exterior iliac vein to be distributed to the bloodstream. See Table 7.5 for a summary of the benefit/risk profile of the rectal/vaginal delivery method.

TABLE 7.5
Rectal/Vaginal

Advantages	Disadvantages
Rapid onset of action, 15 minutes	May be messy or uncomfortable
Moderately long-acting up to 8 hours	Hard to find
Allows for high concentrated doses	Variable absorption depending upon carrier
Minimizes first-pass effects	Limited dose range available, may need to be
Provides localized, pelvic distribution	custom-made

TOPICAL/TRANSDERMAL

Cannabis may be applied topically for treatment of local symptoms such as muscle spasm, inflammation or pain. Peripheral pain conditions respond to topical cannabis. Both THC and CBD as well as cannabinoid acids are therapeutic when applied topically. Cannabis is most often extracted into alcohol, oil or petroleum jelly for topical application. Cold alcohol extracts are a folk remedy for sore joints and are possibly the predecessor to modern topical alternatives. Cannabis oil is useful for massage, due to the muscle relaxant and anti-inflammatory properties of cannabis. Salves and balms may be used anywhere as a first-aid ointment. The inclusion of beeswax provides long duration of effect in the skin layer. Topical cannabis treatments typically do not have psychoactive effects, even if utilizing THC. Topicals primarily utilize CB2 receptors found in abundance in the skin, yet some effects on peripheral CB1 receptors have also been noted.[34]

> Cannabinoids act at peripheral sites and yield analgesia through the action on CB1 and CB2 receptors. Dorsal root ganglia cells contain mRNA for CB1 receptors. . . . Local analgesic actions of agonists for CB2 receptors include the inhibition of mast cell function and inflammatory pain.[35]

Newer evidence suggests that interaction with peripheral TRP receptors can modulate pain and inflammation effects as well.[36]

Because cannabis is lipophilic, it enters cell membranes of the skin; however, cannabinoids are highly hydrophobic, making transport across the aqueous layer of the skin the rate-limiting step in the diffusion process.[10,37] CBD was found to be about ten times more permeable than THC when used by dermal application – this phenomenon is thought to be due to the increased polarity of CBD as compared with THC.[37] Cannabinoid acids are likely also more permeable through the skin as they are more polar than neutral cannabinoids, but this has not been studied. The inclusion of solvents to aid passage through the dermis is important, such as dimethyl sulfoxide (DMSO), petroleum jelly, alcohol and even select terpenes are known to increase penetration. Ethanol concentrations of 30–33% significantly increased the transdermal flux of Δ8-THC and CBD.[1,37] The inclusion as terpenes, such as limonene, is known to increase transdermal permeation, highlighting the fact that full-spectrum cannabis products are likely to show increased efficacy as compared with pure cannabinoids.

The use of the term "transdermal" is a specific form of topical delivery that is ordinarily reserved for delivery and absorption methods that are designed to produce passage through the dermal layer into the systemic circulation for full body effects. Passage of cannabinoids through the various layers of the derma remain problematic, and several transdermal patch formulations have been developed to overcome this challenge.[38]

> Transdermal administration avoids the first-pass metabolism effect that is associated with the oral route and thus improves drug bioavailability. Furthermore, transdermal administration allows a steady infusion of a drug to be delivered over a prolonged period of time, while also minimizing the adverse effects of higher drug peak concentrations.[1]

TABLE 7.6
Topical/*Transdermal

Advantages	Disadvantages
Minimal psychoactive effect	Can be oily or messy
Helps peripheral, local symptoms	Range of potency due to solvent
Easily portable	Range of potency, concentration of products
Adjunct to internal use	May require large amounts, can be costly
*Transdermal – long-lasting, days and provides systemic effects	*Transdermal – limited products available

Another important effect of avoiding first-pass metabolism is reduced psycho-activity, even for THC-containing patches. The achievement of a significant steady-state plasma concentration of CBD at 15.5 ± 11.7 hours was demonstrated after transdermal gel application in animal studies. The authors conclude that CBD is useful for chronic pain treatment through this route of administration.[39] Various cannabis transdermal patches reportedly last from several hours up until 4 days. These are being used therapeutically for control of pain and inflammation. Cannabis must be absorbed through the layers of the skin to reach the bloodstream. See Table 7.6 for a summary of the benefit/risk profile of the topical/transdermal delivery method.

RAW

Raw cannabis has medicinal activity due to the presence of cannabinoid acids, the non-psychoactive precursors available in the live plant. Unheated edibles containing raw cannabis contain mostly cannabinoid acids. An evaluation of cannabis tea (raw cannabis heated in boiling water) contained seven times as much THCA as THC.[40] Cannabis may be eaten raw by eating tender young leaves right off the plant or juicing leaves and buds. It is usually juiced with other fresh vegetables, making a "super-green" food. A typical juiced regimen has been reported using THC-rich cannabis consisting of fresh juice daily divided into four to five doses, which was reported to be effective for chronic autoimmune disease.[41,42] The obvious problem with using raw fresh plant matter is access to it. Some dispensaries have available raw juiced cannabis sold in frozen form, but this is rare. It is mostly consumers that grow their own plants or have access to live plants that benefit from this delivery method. Cold extraction into rosin form or hash or an unheated tincture also provides cannabinoid acids. The therapeutic advantage of consumption of "live" plant matter as opposed to cannabinoid acids from full-spectrum extracts has not been studied. Cannabis is absorbed through the intestinal tract into the bloodstream. See Table 7.7 for a summary of the benefit/risk profile of the raw delivery method.

TABLE 7.7
Raw

Advantages	Disadvantages
Rapid onset of action, 15 minutes	May cause stomach irritation
Moderately long-acting, 6–8 hours	Cost for equipment if juicing
Non-psychoactive	Much daily preparation time, cannot store it
Success with chronic disease	Requires fresh plant supply, hard to find
Superfood, high in chlorophyll, vitamins and minerals	Can have contaminants – mold or pesticides

DOSAGE OF CANNABIS MEDICINE

The exact recommendations for dosage of cannabis will differ according to the delivery method. It's important to understand the principles underlying these choices. With medical cannabis, dosing is currently more an art than a science as there are rare few sources for evidence-based results published to help guide the clinician in determining dosing of medicinal cannabis. Most of the early dosing studies have been done only with smoking and apply to recreational users. Several general reviews of dosing cannabis have been published.[43–47] Dosing specific to CBD has also been reviewed.[48]

There are several inherent challenges regarding the dosing of cannabis. The first thing to recall is that cannabis is a botanical medicine, not a pharmaceutical drug. Single active ingredient pharmaceuticals, as most clinicians are accustomed to dosing, are far easier to standardize and regulate than a botanical medicine. Cannabis has many variables that do not fit well with the typical medical model for drug prescribing. Cultivars vary by their genetics and outwardly express their phenotypes, with differing cannabinoid profiles and terpene content. While many scientists comment on the problem, few present practical solutions – an example follows:

> Given the inherent variations in strain and phenotype of cannabis, the various routes of administration employed, and the multitude of debilitating or terminal conditions being treated in patients using medicinal cannabis, standards must be set that maximize the potential for symptomatic relief.[43]

Dosing remains highly individualized and relies to a great extent on titration (i.e., finding the right dose where potential therapeutic effects are maximized, while adverse or harmful effects are minimized). The most prudent approach to dosing in the absence of evidence-based guidelines is to "start low and go slow."[44] One of the great limitations encountered when using cannabis as a medicine occurs especially when patients use homegrown or black-market raw flower that may aptly be described as "non-standardized products." *If a product is not lab tested, accurate dosage is not possible.* Consumers who pursue these avenues should send a sample of their product to be lab tested to ensure freedom from pesticides, heavy metals and

other important contaminants as well as to understand the cannabinoid and terpenoid contents.

> Cannabis medicines, whether prescription or over-the-counter, should be ideally cul-
> tivated organically according to Mendelian selective breeding techniques without the
> necessity of genetic modification . . . and be made available to consumers with full
> information as to cannabinoid and terpenoid profiles, and certification that the material
> is free of pesticide microbial or heavy metal contamination.[46]

Fortunately, lab testing facilities are open to the public, although the accuracy of
results from many such facilities is still in question. A listing of testing facilities in
each state as of 2020 has been compiled.[49]

Another confounding variable to be mindful of is that there are likely to be different cannabis effects over a range of doses of cannabinoids. The biphasic dose
response of cannabinoids has been well documented, meaning differing responses
may occur at low versus high doses of cannabinoids, as well as a third response
at midrange. The familiar sine wave image as commonly used in pharmaceutical
dosing studies (as seen in Figure 7.2) for the action of cannabinoids is somewhat
simplistic as it implies the midrange to be an optimal dose. This depends upon the
desired effect.

In clinical applications, for example, saturated receptors such as may occur at
high doses may be required for antitumoral or anti-seizure effects. Also, low dose
may contribute an inhibitory effect, a plateau at midrange, while a stimulatory effect
may occur at high concentration, making the end ranges of the curve the desired
dose. Both stimulatory and inhibitory effects with CB1 receptor agonist administration have been reported in several neurobiological responses. In animal studies,
low doses of THC decreased locomotor activity, whereas higher doses stimulated
movement until catalepsy emerged.[50] The biphasic effect has been noted for non-CB

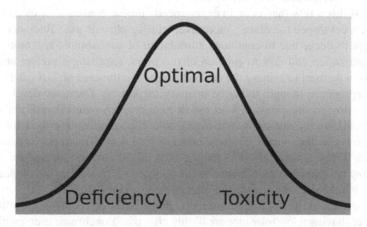

FIGURE 7.2   Biphasic dose–response curve.

Source: Häggström, M. 2014. Medical Gallery of Mikael Häggström 2014. *WikiJournal Med.* 1(2).
DOI:10.15347/wjm/2014.008. ISSN 2002–4436. Public Domain.

mechanisms exhibited by CBD as well. CBD at 150, 300 and 600 mg produced an inverted U-shaped (similar to a sine wave) dose–response curve for anxiety. Significant anxiolytic response was only achieved with an intermediate dose.[51] These results were confirmed in an experiment using CBD at 100, 300 and 900 mg. Subjective anxiety was reduced only with the CBD 300 mg dose.[52] Of course, these are all high doses utilizing purified CBD that has been reconstituted from crystalline powder, not cannabis. In animal studies, purified CBD showed a bell-shaped dose–response with a narrow therapeutic window. Upon testing a variety of CBD-rich cannabis extracts, it was found that CBD in the presence of other plant constituents, the dose-response occurred at a lower dose and over a wider range, indicating an entourage effect. The authors noted the following: "It is likely that other components in the extract synergize with CBD to achieve the desired anti-inflammatory action that may contribute to overcoming the bell-shaped dose-response of purified CBD."[53] Confirming the efficacy of cannabis versus a single cannabinoid, the dosing of cannabis for the treatment of pediatric epilepsy was found to be effective at a lower range than purified CBD.[54]

Thus, the chemical composition of the product and its source influence recommended dosage. In general, full flower or full-spectrum cannabis extracts are more efficient at lower doses than purified cannabinoid isolates. With cannabis-derived CBD containing a full complement of terpenes, botanical doses apply. Hemp-derived CBD may be sold with or without terpenes. If without, dosing should be treated as pure CBD derived from isolate, which may require ten times the dose as described earlier.

PRACTICAL CONSIDERATIONS

There are several points to consider when approaching how to determine effective dosing that are unique to each patient. These include the patient's tolerance, a consideration of endocannabinoid tone, any medications adjustments or interactions and the patient's preferences for delivery method.

First, is this a new (naive) or an experienced chronic consumer of cannabis? Has the patient developed tolerance – more likely during chronic use? Tolerance of THC is thought to occur due to continued stimulation of cannabinoid receptors leading to desensitization and downregulation of receptors, requiring a greater amount of cannabis to be used to achieve the desired effect.[55] In the case of THC, the CB1 and CB2 receptors are thought to be the primary targets.[56,57] Tolerance develops faster with high dosage situations, such as use of high-potency cannabinoids and chronic usage.[58] CBD-rich cultivars have different tolerance-producing effects than THC-rich cultivars as they target different primary receptors. Treatment in mice for 14 days with THC significantly reversed the increase in cerebral blood flow in mice, suggesting development of tolerance to the neuroprotective effect with repeated use of THC, but this was not seen with CBD at the doses employed.[59]

New users require and respond to much lower doses of cannabis. Low doses for naive users having a low tolerance are highly effective. For chronic users, with a high tolerance, doses need to be increased. In such cases, it is useful to consider tolerance-reducing strategies (discussed later in this chapter). The need for low doses, both in new users and to explore biphasic responses, has led to a caveat that has long been circulated for the dosing of cannabis, "start low and go slow." Recent years have brought the concept of "microdosing" into cannabis culture. Microdosing refers to using small amounts of a substance. It is not specific to cannabis or cannabinoids. Guidelines define a microdose to be at 1/100th of the expected pharmacological dose. A microdose or low dose of a cannabinoid is typically not in as low a range as 1/100th of a therapeutic dose, but higher, perhaps 1 mg of THC (approximately in the range of 1/10th the average dose). Many erroneously think microdosing applies to using low doses of THC to avoid the "high" effect.

The second point to consider: what is the patient's endocannabinoid tone? As previously discussed (see Chapter 3), the endocannabinoid tone refers to an individual's state of endocannabinoid balance, with accompanying descriptors such as excess or deficiency.[60] Unfortunately, there is no objective measure or laboratory test(s) to effectively categorize this state. Some conditions have been hypothesized to involve an endocannabinoid deficiency (i.e., low tone), such as migraine, irritable bowel syndrome or fibromyalgia, to name but a few.[61] In such an event, the patient would likely benefit from cannabinoid stimulation and may ultimately require higher doses of cannabis to achieve desired effects. Endocannabinoid excess or high tone might be reflected in higher plasma levels of endocannabinoids and/or activated cannabinoid receptors (CBrs). Such a condition may exist in chronic stress situations, such as in PTSD, in which CB1 receptors have shown increased availability.[62] This may explain the success of THCV as a therapy for PTSD, as it is a CB1 antagonist. Increased levels of eCBs have also been documented as a result of exercise, not a pathological situation, yet exercise may provide a mechanism other than cannabis for regulating endocannabinoid tone. Increased levels of AEA have been measured (but interestingly not of 2-AG) after 30–45 minutes and up to 5 hours of aerobic exercise.[63] A comprehensive review of the multitude of factors that modulate eCB levels, including pharmaceuticals, CAM (complementary and alternative medicine) therapies such as mind–body practices, the inclusion of other natural substances and lifestyle factors has been published.[64] Finding a level of homeostasis involves consideration of diet, lifestyle as well as a host of other factors. With cannabis, patients are able to self-regulate and self-titrate their dose while adjusting to other factors likely to affect their endocannabinoid tone.

Third, what other drugs/pharmaceuticals are coadministered? Is there a potential for cannabis/pharmaceutical interactions, which is rare (see Chapter 6)? An unusual instance in which DDIs (drug–drug interactions) may affect dosing is in the use of high dosages of CBD in pediatric seizure disorders. Or is there a potential for medication reduction and a decrease in polypharmacy (see Chapter 30)? Often, when decreasing the use of a pharmaceutical, the cannabis dosage may need to be increased during the weaning period of the drug. An example of this is cannabis use for sleep as sedative use is weaned.

Other considerations include the patient's preference and compliance for delivery method. Patients have favorite ways to use cannabis. Trying to bring in a new method often meets with resistance, sometimes due to the history of perceived benefit from previous usage. Some patients are entrained in using smoking as a delivery method, while other more cautious patients prefer topical use only, etc. Armed with the answers to these questions, we can proceed in determining the most likely effective dosage regimen(s) for each patient. The short answer to the question of how to dose cannabis is that it is a uniquely individualized process, dependent not only on the patient's condition but also on one's own endocannabinoid tone, chronicity of use and patient preferences.

Dosing recommendations for common delivery methods has largely been gleaned from anecdotal reports. Some information about oral use is provided by FDA-approved sources of cannabinoids. For example, the recommended dose for dronabinol is 10 mg twice daily. The recommended dose range for Epidiolex is 2.5–10 mg/kg twice daily, specifically for use in treatment of resistant childhood epilepsy.[23] With the development of Sativex (containing 2.7 mg of THC and 2.5 mg of CBD), much data has been collated about the pharmacokinetics and therapeutic dosing of this cannabis extract. It has been used at a dose of 1–6 sprays/dose = 5–31 mg of the cannabinoid mix, up to six times per day.[25]

DOSAGE SUMMARY

The dosage information summarized in the following sections is not empirical, but rather is practical, culled from anecdotal reports and clinical practice of cannabis medicinal use.

SMOKING DOSAGE

- 1 gram of cannabis flowers may contain 100–200 mg of cannabinoids (10–20%), concentrates provide higher doses (50–80% cannabinoids).
- Average amount in a joint (cannabis cigarette) = 0.5–1 gram of cannabis, at 20% cannabinoids, possibly 1/10th joint per puff, with 20% overall bio-availability, yields 2–4 mg cannabinoids inhaled/puff.
- Begin with one puff, wait 15 minutes, and then take another if needed.
- Effects last 2–4 hours.
- Smoking frequency may be 1–6 times/day.
- Amount used daily: from 1 to 7 grams (7 grams = 1/4 ounce)

VAPORIZING DOSAGE

- Tabletop and handheld vaporizers use cannabis flower, vapor pens generally use oil.
- For oil in a vaper pen containing 0.5 gram cannabinoids in an 80% oil, with 100 puffs, yields 4 mg cannabinoids inhaled/puff.
- Begin with one puff, wait 15 minutes, and then take another if needed.
- Effects last 2–4 hours.
- Vaporizing frequency can be 1–6 times/day.

INGESTION DOSAGE

- It is easy to overdose on edibles – start with small amounts!
- Effects come on slower and last longer if taken with food, up to 8 hours or more.

- Use depends on the potency of the substance, in general 5–20 mg are available in individual edibles.
- Capsules are easy to quantify, containing 10–50 mg cannabinoids.
- High doses in the hundreds of milligrams are available by use of concentrated oils
- Begin with only 1–2 mg of THC, 5–10 mg of CBD.
- Oral frequency is 2–3 times/day for 24-hour effects

OROMUCOSAL/SUBLINGUAL DOSAGE

- Typical tincture contains 10 mg cannabinoids/ml (one dropper is approx. = 1 ml).
- Lozenges, mints may range from 2.5 to 10 mg doses.
- Start with only 1–2 mg of THC, 5–10 mg of CBD.
- Begin with a few drops of tincture, wait 30 minutes and increase as needed.
- Lasts 2–4 hours as mouth spray or mouthstrips, 4–6 hours if sublingual with swallowing.
- Oromucosal frequency is 3–4 times/day for 24-hour effects

RECTAL/VAGINAL DOSAGE

- Suppositories typically in 5–50 mg doses.
- High-dose options can go up to hundreds of milligrams, such as for cancer treatment.
- Syringe delivery is typically custom-made.
- Start with 5 mg THC, 10 mg CBD (typically sold in higher doses of mixed cannabinoids).
- Suppository typically lasts 8 hours, frequency may be 2–3 times/day.

TOPICAL/TRANSDERMAL DOSAGE

- Higher dose may be required – a function of area to be covered.
- May apply 5–25 mg cannabinoids, in an appropriate base carrier.
- Check the concentration in the container, should be at least 200 mg cannabinoids in a 2-ounce jar
- Reapply every 4–6 hours as needed.
- Transdermal patches are designed for slow release over hours or one or more days, containing 30 mg cannabinoids on average.

DOSING DURATION

Clearly, it would seem that duration should be determined by duration of symptoms. There are several other factors to consider. For chronic users, tolerance will likely become an issue, and efficacy may be adversely affected by long-term cannabis therapy. In this case, it is useful to consider a tolerance break – using less of the substance. A tolerance break may be described as discontinuing cannabis consumption for as little as 3 days or up to 2 weeks if chronic high dosage has occurred. An additional strategy is to alternate cannabinoids. While taking a break from THC, one may use CBD or cannabinoid acids and vice versa. Reducing tolerance is a good reason to used mixed cannabinoid products in the first place, with lower dosages of the individual components. After a tolerance-reducing protocol, the goal is to have renewed sensitivity to the substance, thus limiting the need to use higher amounts. More is not better! The dose is reduced after a tolerance break, that is the point. A tolerance break is not a unique concept to cannabis or cannabinoids. In herbal medicinal practice, the procedure of an "herbal holiday" has been described.

> Always challenge a treatment: if after several weeks it is thought that the herb is useful, stop the herb for a period of time and see if it is still necessary. Take the herb for six days, then break a day. Or take it for four weeks and then break a week.[65]

A cannabis herbal holiday may be utilized regularly to mitigate long-term effects and to reduce tolerance. Suggested regimens include 1 day every week, 5–7 days every month and/or 1–3 weeks every season (3 months). If stopping the medicine is unadvisable, then change the cannabinoid content as advised earlier.

Indeed, a patient may and hopefully will arrive at a place with reduced symptoms when it is time to consider reduction or weaning of cannabis. The possibility of reduced dosage as condition(s) improve is a characteristic of herbal medicine, and cannabis is one of the most potent herbal medicines available. The user's own endocannabinoid system will determine how much medicine is required ongoing. As deficits become repaired, that is, nerve antioxidation, decreased joint inflammation, better mood or sleep, etc., the condition improves and reduction may not only be possible, but is advisable. Wean slowly off cannabis medicine over a series of weeks. For example, if oral use, from 10 to 5 mg the first week, then 2.5 mg, then off. If inhaled, reduce from 6 times/day to 5 times/day, etc. Stay at each level as needed if symptoms recur. Maintenance dosing is commonly required for chronic conditions.

CLINICAL PRACTICE PEARLS

In clinical practice, there are three overriding questions that a practitioner is tasked with answering: (1) What is the condition we are considering to treat with cannabis? That requires the knowledge not only of what diagnoses or complaints the patient has but also knowing the spectrum of what the therapeutic benefits of cannabis are. (2) What is the type or types of cannabis to use, its chemotype, suggested cultivars and ultimately what is available to the patients. (3) What is the delivery method and dosage to recommend? Exploring the cannabinoid and other secondary metabolite chemistry, physiological action and therapeutic potential has been addressed in the preceding chapters, and will be further elaborated in Part III under the heading of individual conditions. What is available to patients is locally determined and outside the control of the practitioner, yet a valuable consideration ultimately in making recommendations. In this case, clinicians are faced with constraints that may be likened to patients with a restricted pharmaceutical formulary, but with no central compilation of available inventory of products. It is a painstaking process to compile such information and is most often accomplished through patient feedback and online research of the stock carried by local dispensaries, something that physicians are unused to doing. The third consideration, that of delivery and dosage, is a much-asked question by those wishing to practice cannabis medicine with a woeful lack of guidance, nor a true understanding of the factors involved. The goal of this chapter was to address this pressing need.

REFERENCES

1. Bruni N, Della Pepa C, Oliaro-Bosso S, et al. Cannabinoid delivery systems for pain and inflammation treatment. *Molecules*. 2018;23(10):2478.
2. Elmes MW, Kaczocha M, Berger WT, et al. Fatty acid-binding proteins (FABPs) are intracellular carriers for Δ9-tetrahydrocannabinol (THC) and cannabidiol (CBD). *J Biol Chem*. 2015;290(14):8711–8721.
3. Gabrys R. Canadian Center on Substance Abuse 7th in Series. Clearing the smoke on cannabis: edible cannabis products, cannabis extracts and cannabis topicals. 2020. www.ccsa.ca/clearing-smoke-cannabis-edible-cannabis-cannabis-extracts-and-cannabis-topicals Accessed May 15, 2020.
4. Ribeiro LI, Ind PW. Effect of cannabis smoking on lung function and respiratory symptoms: a structured literature review. *NPJ Prim Care Respir Med*. 2016;26:16071.
5. Tashkin DP. Effects of marijuana smoking on the lung. *Ann Am Thorac Soc*. 2013;10(3):239–247.
6. Hazekamp A, Ware MA, Muller-Vahl KR, Abrams D, Grotenhermen F. The medicinal use of cannabis and cannabinoids: an international cross-sectional survey on administration forms. *J Psychoactive Drugs*. 2013;45(3):199–210.
7. Earleywine M, Barnwell SS. Decreased respiratory symptoms in cannabis users who vaporize. *Harm Reduct J*. 2007;4:11.
8. Carter GT, Weydt P, Kyashna-Tocha M, Abrams DI. Medicinal cannabis: rational guidelines for dosing. *IDrugs*. 2004;7(5):464–470.
9. Elzinga S, Ortiz O, Raber JC. The conversion and transfer of cannabinoids from cannabis to smoke stream in cigarettes. *Nat Prod Chem Res*. 2015;3:1.
10. Huestis MA. Human cannabinoid pharmacokinetics. *Chem Biodivers*. 2007;4(8):1770–1804.
11. Sharma P, Murthy P, Bharath MM. Chemistry, metabolism, and toxicology of cannabis: clinical implications. *Iran J Psychiatry*. 2012;7(4):149–156.
12. Millar SA, Stone NL, Yates AS, O'Sullivan SE. A systematic review on the pharmacokinetics of cannabidiol in humans. *Front Pharmacol*. 2018;9:1365.
13. Ujváry I, Hanuš L. Human metabolites of cannabidiol: a review on their formation, biological activity, and relevance in therapy. *Cannabis Cannabinoid Res*. 2016;1(1):90–101.
14. Loflin M, Earleywine M. No smoke, no fire: what the initial literature suggests regarding vapourized cannabis and respiratory risk. *Can J Respir Ther*. 2015;51(1):7–9.
15. Gieringer D, St. Lauren J, Goodrich S. Cannabis vaporizer combines efficient delivery of THC with effective suppression of pyrolytic compounds. *J Cannabis Ther*. 2004;4:7–27.
16. Spindle TR, Cone EJ, Schlienz NJ, et al. Acute effects of smoked and vaporized cannabis in healthy adults who infrequently use cannabis: a crossover trial. *JAMA Netw Open*. 2018;1(7):e184841.
17. Abrams DI, Vizoso HP, Shade SB, et al. Vaporization as a smokeless cannabis delivery system: a pilot study. *Clin Pharmacol Ther*. 2007;82(5):572–578.

18. Solowij N, Broyd SJ, van Hell HH, Hazekamp A. A protocol for the delivery of canna-bidiol (CBD) and combined CBD and Δ9-tetrahydrocannabinol (THC) by vaporisation. *BMC Pharmacol Toxicol.* 2014;15:58.

19. Earleywine M, Smucker Barnwell S. Decreased respiratory symptoms in cannabis users who vaporize. *Harm Reduct J.* 2007;4:11.

20. Van Dam NT, Earleywine M. Pulmonary function in cannabis users: support for a clini-cal trial of the vaporizer. *Int J Drug Policy.* 2010;21(6):511–513.

21. Centers for Disease Control. Outbreak of lung injury associated with the use of e-cigarette, or vaping, products. February 25, 2020. www.cdc.gov/tobacco/basic_information/e-cigarettes/severe-lung-disease.html Accessed November 8, 2020.

22. Mechoulam R, Parker LA, Gallily R. Cannabidiol: an overview of some pharmacologi-cal aspects. *J Clin Pharmacol.* 2002;42(S1):11S–19S.

23. Epidiolex® prescribing information Greenwich Biosciences Inc. Epidiolex website. 2018. www.epidiolex.com/sites/default/files/pdfs/1120/EPX-03645-1120_EPIDIOLEX_ (cannabidiol)_USPI.pdf Accessed May 15, 2020.

24. Eichler M, Spinedi L, Unfer-Grauwiler S, et al. Heat exposure of Cannabis sativa extracts affects the pharmacokinetic and metabolic profile in healthy male subjects. *Planta Med.* 2012;78:686–691.

25. Sativex oromucosal spray. Electronic Medicines Compendium (emc) website. www.medicines.org.uk/emc/product/602/smpc#gref Accessed May 15, 2020.

26. Karschner EL, Darwin WD, Goodwin RS, et al. Plasma cannabinoid pharmacokinet-ics following controlled oral D9-tetrahydrocannabinol and oromucosal cannabis extract administration. *Clin Chem.* 2011;57:166–175.

27. Lee D, Karschner EL, Milman G, et al. Can oral fluid cannabinoid testing monitor medi-cation compliance and/or cannabis smoking during oral THC and oromucosal Sativex administration? *Drug Alcohol Depend.* 2013;130(0):68–76.

28. Perlin E, Smith CG, Nichols AI, et al. Disposition and bioavailability of various formula-tions of tetrahydrocannabinol in the rhesus monkey. *J Pharm Sci.* 1985;74(2):171–174.

29. ElSohly MA, Stanford DF, Harland EC, et al. Rectal bioavailability of delta-9-tetrahydrocannabinol from the hemisuccinate ester in monkeys. *J Pharm Sci.* 1991;80(10): 942–945.

30. ElSohly MA, Gul W, Walker LA. Pharmacokinetics and tolerability of Δ9-THC-hemisuccinate in a suppository formulation as an alternative to capsules for the systemic delivery of Δ9-THC. *Med Cannabis Cannabinoids.* 2018;1:44–53.

31. Ofem OW, Ogechukwu OE, Okeke NC, et al. Some physical properties of novel Cannabis suppositories formulated with theobroma oil. *African J Pharm Pharmacol.* 2014;8(44):1127–1131.

32. ElSohly MA, Little TL Jr., Hikal A, et al. Rectal bioavailability of D9-tetrahydrocannabinol from various esters. *Pharmacol Biochem Behav.* 1991;40:497–502.

33. Brenneisen R, Egli A, Elsohly MA, Henn V, Spiess Y. The effect of orally and rectally administered delta 9-tetrahydrocannabinol on spasticity: a pilot study with 2 patients. *Int J Clin Pharmakol Ther.* 1996;34(10):446–452.

34. Richardson JD, Kilo S, Hargreaves KM. Cannabinoids reduce hyperalgesia and inflam-mation via interaction with peripheral CB1 receptors. *Pain.* 1998;75(1):111–119.

35. Jorge L, Feres C, Teles V. Topical preparations for pain relief: efficacy and patient adher-ence. *J Pain Res.* 2011;4:11–24.

36. Caterina MJ. TRP channel cannabinoid receptors in skin sensation, homeostasis, and inflammation. *ACS Chem Neurosci.* 2014;5(11):1107–1116.

37. Stinchcomb AL, Valiveti S, Hammell DC, Ramsey DR. Human skin permeation of D8-tetrahydrocannabinol, cannabidiol and cannabinol. *J Pharm Pharmacol.* 2004;56(3): 291–297.
38. Wallace W. Method of relieving analgesia and reducing inflammation using a cannabinoid delivery topical liniment. 2005. https://patents.google.com/patent/US6949582B1/en Accessed May 15, 2020.
39. Paudel KS, Hammell DC, Agu RU, Valiveti S, Stinchcomb AL. Cannabidiol bioavailability after nasal and transdermal application: effect of permeation enhancers. *Drug Dev Ind Pharm.* 2010;36(9):1088–1097.
40. Hazekamp A, Bastola K, Rashidi H, Bender J, Verpoorte R. Cannabis tea revisited: a systematic evaluation of the cannabinoid composition of cannabis tea. *J Ethnopharmacol.* 2007;113(1):85–90.
41. Dr. Courtney speaks on the Cannabis Issues Panel of experts and authors at the 18th Annual Southern Humboldt Hemp Fest. November 8, 2008. www.civilliberties.org/courtney.html Accessed May 15, 2020.
42. Lee M. Juicing raw cannabis. Beyond THC (O'Shaughnessy's) website. Winter/Spring 2013. www.beyondthc.com/wp-content/uploads/2013/03/Juicing-33.pdf Accessed May 15, 2020.
43. Aggarwal SK, Kyashna-Tocha M, Carter GT. Dosing medical marijuana: rational guidelines on trial in Washington State. *Med Gen Med.* 2007;9(3):52.
44. Government of Canada. Access to cannabis for medical purposes regulations: daily amount fact sheet (dosage). July 2016. www.canada.ca/en/health-canada/services/drugs-medication/cannabis/information-medical-practitioners/cannabis-medical-purposes-regulations-daily-amount-fact-sheet-dosage.html Accessed May 15, 2020.
45. Sulak D. A physician's perspective on optimal cannabis dosing. Leafly website. February 26, 2018. www.leafly.com/news/health/a-physicians-perspective-on-optimal-cannabis-dosing Accessed November 8, 2020.
46. MacCallum CA, Russo EB. Practical considerations in medical cannabis administration and dosing. *Eur J Intern Med.* 2018;49:12–19.
47. Lee, MA. CBD & cannabis dosing. Project CBD website. www.projectcbd.org/guidance/cbd-cannabis-dosing Accessed November 8, 2020.
48. Millar SA, Stone NL, Bellman ZD, Yates AS, England TJ, O'Sullivan SE. A systematic review of cannabidiol dosing in clinical populations. *Br J Clin Pharmacol.* 2019;85(9): 1888–1900.
49. Cannabis testing regulations: a state-by-state guide. Leafly website. February 24, 2020. www.leafly.com/news/health/leaflys-state-by-state-guide-to-cannabis-testing-regulations Accessed May 15, 2020.
50. Sañudo-Peña MC, Romero J, Seale GE, Fernandez-Ruiz JJ, Walker JM. Activational role of cannabinoids on movement. *Eur J Pharmacol.* 2000;391(3):269–274.
51. Linares IM, Zuardi AW, Pereira LC, et al. Cannabidiol presents an inverted U-shaped dose-response curve in a simulated public speaking test. *Braz J Psychiatry.* 2019;41(1):9–14.
52. Zuardi AW, Rodrigues NP, Silva AL, et al. Inverted U-shaped dose-response curve of the anxiolytic effect of cannabidiol during public speaking in real life. *Front Pharmacol.* 2017;8:259.
53. Gallily R, Yekhtin, Z, Hanuš. Overcoming the bell-shaped dose-response of cannabidiol by using cannabis extract enriched in cannabidiol. *Pharmacol Pharm.* 2015;6:75–85.
54. Sulak D, Sanneto R, Goldstein B. The current status of artisanal cannabis for the treatment of epilepsy in the United States, *Epilepsy Behav.* 2017;70(Pt B):328–333.

55. Gettman J. Marijuana and the brain. Part II: the tolerance factor. *High Times*. July 1995. www.marijuanalibrary.org/brain2.html Accessed May 15, 2020.
56. Hirvonen J, Goodwin RS, Li CT, et al. Reversible and regionally selective downregulation of brain cannabinoid CB1 receptors in chronic daily cannabis smokers. *Mol Psychiatry*. 2012;17(6):642–649.
57. González S, Cebeira M, Fernández-Ruiz J. Cannabinoid tolerance and dependence: a review of studies in laboratory animals. *Pharmacol Biochem Behav*. 2005;81(2):300–318.
58. Jones RT, Benowitz NL, Herning RI. Clinical relevance of cannabis tolerance and dependence. *J Clin Pharmacol*. 1981;21(S1):143S–152S.
59. Hayakawa K, Mishima K, Nozako M, et al. Repeated treatment with cannabidiol but not delta9-tetrahydrocannabinol has a neuroprotective effect without the development of tolerance. *Neuropharmacology*. 2007;52(4):1079–1087.
60. Howlett AC, Reggio PH, Childers SR, et al. Endocannabinoid tone versus constitutive activity of cannabinoid receptors. *Br J Pharmacol*. 2011;163(7):1329–1343.
61. Russo EB. Clinical endocannabinoid deficiency reconsidered: current research supports the theory in migraine, fibromyalgia, irritable bowel, and other treatment-resistant syndromes. *Cannabis Cannabinoid Res*. 2016;1(1):154–165.
62. Neumeister A, Normandin MD, Pietrzak RH, et al. Elevated brain cannabinoid CB1 receptor availability in posttraumatic stress disorder: a positron emission tomography study. *Mol Psychiatry*. 2013;18(9):1034–1040.
63. Tantimonaco M, Ceci R, Sabatini, S, et al. Physical activity and the endocannabinoid system: an overview. *Cell Mol Life Sci*. 2014;71:2681–2698.
64. McPartland JM, Guy GW, Di Marzo V. Care and feeding of the endocannabinoid system: a systematic review of potential clinical interventions that upregulate the endocannabinoid system. *PLoS One*. 2014;9(3):e89566.
65. Castleman M. *The New Healing Herbs: The Classic Guide to Nature's Medicine*. Emmaus, PA: Rodale Press Inc; 2001.

8 Adult Cannabis Practice

The adult population provides a basis for understanding theoretical and practical considerations needed as background for medical cannabis practice. Here we consider adults aged 26–60. Elements unique to younger and older age groups are presented in separate chapters. Multiple surveys indicate that adults comprise the majority of medical cannabis patients.[1-3] Information about medical and recreational cannabis users over the past 20 years and the differing characteristics that have become apparent between them is available from the results of several surveys.[4,5] A 2006 survey in California revealed that 50% of their medical cannabis patients were surprisingly older than expected, over age 35.[6] The most prevalent age for recreational users is younger adults, between ages 18 and 26 or 29.[5,7] In a 2013–2014 report comparing these two cohorts, 13% of US adults used cannabis in the past year, of which most (89%) were recreational, 10.5% were medical, with 36.1% reporting mixed use.[8] There were no significant differences found in race, education, past year depression and prevalence of cannabis use disorders between the two groups. Other reports seem to indicate recreational use is associated with a higher percentage of cannabis use disorder, but there are challenges with making this diagnosis (see "Cannabis Use Disorders" in Chapter 6). They also found medical cannabis users were more likely to have poorer health and lower levels of alcohol use disorders and non-cannabis drug use.[9] The distinguishing characteristic between recreational and medical cannabis users, one whose effect has not been explored in any studies I could find to date, is that *medical patients receive knowledgeable information about how to use cannabis therapeutically*! This may seem to be a given, but it is worth emphasizing, because that is the primary goal of this practice. While the number of medical cannabis patients has grown with the increase in medical cannabis state programs, there is no evidence that recreational use has decreased. Now that more states have approved non-medical decriminalized use, we are seeing an unfortunate trend, not yet measured, whereby previous medical cannabis patients have reverted to or moved on to the adult use category, and are no longer seeking medical advice.

There is an association between having pain as a motivator and seeking medical cannabis consultation.[10] In fact, pain is the number reason for seeking a medical cannabis recommendation. The percentage of medical cannabis patients carrying a diagnosis of pain across states range generally between 70% and 90%.[2,6,11] The variance in range of diagnostic prevalence is most likely a reflection of which diagnoses are approved in each state rather than actual incidence, with pain recorded as high as 97% in Hawaii and as low as 28% in New Mexico.[3,12] Other prominent diagnoses for medical cannabis approval include insomnia, mood disorders, muscle spasm, anorexia, relief of nausea and replacement of prescription medications.[1-3,5,6,12]

DOI: 10.1201/9781003098201-18

Estimates of common delivery methods vary between states and countries, but all seem to agree that smoking is the greatest preference by the adult age group whether medical or recreational. This is followed by vaporizing, then edibles, tinctures and lastly topicals.[1,2,3,5,12–14] These preferences apply only to average adult medical cannabis patients. Other demographic groups show altered preferences, that is, tinctures in pediatrics and increased topical use in elders. The choice of delivery method among adults has been presented in detail (see Chapter 7). But to recap, delivery choices reflect what a patient is familiar and comfortable with, what is available in their area and for some, hopefully, what is best for their condition. With this set of adults, we are seeing patients who actually have an interest in learning how to use cannabis medicinally. An important characteristic is that most, not all, adult medical patients have been exposed to cannabis before, and started with recreational use.[5] One of the most challenging aspects of working with many adult medical cannabis patients is how to decondition them from smoking THC-rich cultivars. Educating these patients about alternative delivery methods, the inclusion of other cannabinoids and how to determine the desired outcome in the absence of feeling "high" is a primary goal. With naive cannabis users, some adults, but more often found in the pediatric and elderly populations, there is a contrasting challenge, to decondition them from the stigma of using cannabis at all. Also challenging is a lack of follow-up, as previously discussed, pursuant to these visits not being covered by insurance.

RISKS

This category of patient is with minimal particular risks due to age. While tendency for overuse is greatest in the youth group, it is not gone entirely in the adult population. Knowledge of the general adverse effects and risks is required to assess a valuable benefit/risk ratio (see Chapter 6).

THERAPEUTIC EFFECTS

The adult population uses medicinal cannabis to treat a multitude of diagnoses, yet few are officially sanctioned. The National Academies of Sciences, Engineering, and Medicine (NASEM) published a review in 2017 that summarized available scientific research regarding the potential therapeutic effects and health risks of cannabis and cannabinoids. NASEM concluded that cannabis or cannabinoids are modestly effective for adults with (only) the following conditions when administered via specific routes: chronic pain, chemotherapy-induced nausea and vomiting and multiple sclerosis-related spasticity.[15] The report also concluded that there was inadequate information to assess the therapeutic effects of cannabis or cannabinoids for all the other conditions that were evaluated (a long list including most of the common diagnoses for which medical cannabis is approved). We are in early days of cannabis therapeutics being tested by clinical trials. A comprehensive listing of the therapeutic benefits of cannabis medicinal use seen in clinical practice is presented in Part III under individual condition sections. Often it is by patient feedback that we can learn how to most effectively use cannabis for a multitude of diagnoses. Yet, patients need to be guided as to what to use, how much and how often.

CONSULTATION PROTOCOL

Reviewing the mechanics of a typical consultation as applied to the adult population (given here as done in California) provides a template for how to manage medical cannabis patients. The adjustments made for other age groups will be listed in the following chapters. An in-depth questionnaire is completed by the patient prior to the visit, along with the directive to bring in or list any current medications (see Appendix for Patient History Questionnaire). Often the presenting complaint is not the only thing we address, as many patients are unaware of the benefits of cannabis for multiple functions, such as neuroprotection, especially if pain or dysfunction is not a current symptom. After a discussion of the benefits and risks, we discuss delivery and dosage with a mind toward what is available in the local area. Many, not all patients are discouraged by the cost, as cannabis is not covered by their insurance. Some prefer to grow their own plants, thereby reducing cost and participating in making their own medicine. After the initial visit, follow-up is encouraged in 3 months, or as needed, but few take advantage of that invitation, again a cost issue. Often, a patient will call to query for product advice if they can't find exactly what was suggested. Dosing strategies to cover an extended period of time must be proffered at this initial visit, as they may not return until the recommendation is expired. Directions for upward titration until a satisfactory dose is achieved should be provided. Tolerance is an issue with many chronic users and needs to be addressed at this first visit or in a follow-up. A medical cannabis recommendation is provided with the average length of duration being 1 year (see Appendix for Physician Statement form). Unfortunately, too many patients come in only once in a year, per legal requirement. This hinders our ability to properly adjust the dose or the product. Reducing or substituting for other medications is absolutely not something the patient should do on their own, and is best done at follow-ups and in collaboration with the patient's prescribing physician.

CLINICAL PRACTICE PEARLS

In my clinical cannabis practice, adults aged 26–60 comprised 43% of my patient population. They presented with a wide range of complaints. In fact, the presenting complaint of pain, while still most prevalent comprised only 55% of this group, followed by 25% with sleep issues, and 22% with various mood disorders. Other diagnoses covered the spectrum of medical conditions, as seen in Part III. Eighty percent had used cannabis previously. While many started out by smoking, most but not all of these medical cannabis patients did not remain as smokers. With appropriate guidance, they were directed to try vaporizing, tinctures, edibles and topicals. The important thing to note is that the patients needed to be educated and encouraged to try other methods. I worked in multiple diverse communities in California, including one in which most of the patients grew their own medicine. I had little success in disabusing this population of patients from smoking. Not only was it all that they knew, they were opposed to trying methods involving more cost. The simplest way to deal with patients who are comfortable with raw flower, that is, growers, is to encourage use of a vaporizer, at least part of the time. There are several easy recipes for making a cold alcohol extract from plant matter, which many patient growers appreciated. This, of course, makes a cannabinoid acid extract that could be taken internally or used topically for inflammation, among other uses.

Other than deconditioning from smoking, another challenge had to do with introducing CBD-rich products. This helps not only in reducing disorientation and counteracting several other adverse effects of THC but also in reducing tolerance. It can be difficult to find raw flower that has a mixed ratio of CBD/THC. For patients used to feeling the effects of THC, especially by inhalation, using a CBD-rich cultivar may hold little appeal. It was often more successful to introduce a CBD/THC 1:1 tincture for daytime use to treat pain, for example, with THC-rich cultivars reserved for use after work, in the evenings. This is not the case with all adults, especially those who were new to cannabis use. Here the reverse conditioning applies, starting with CBD-rich products, and slowly adding THC if indicated. Acclimating to the disorienting effects of THC is a necessary consideration for naive users.

Most adult cannabis patients had no problem with the concept and enactment of regular tolerance breaks. Some chronic, high-dose users were resistant though. Care must be taken in promoting a tolerance break for these chronic patients, who may actually have a cannabis dependence, as they may be wary of experiencing adverse symptoms during the withdrawal phase. For these clients, I usually advised a one-day/week tolerance break from the cultivar they were using to another type, most often with much less THC. This creates a tolerance break, while still offering something to take. Sometimes, just the act of smoking or vaporizing some form of cannabis brings relief, not least of which may be due to continuity of terpene benefits and/or a placebo effect.

When does the use of cannabis end for most adult medical cannabis patients? That is a question that we don't ordinarily ask in relation to chronic conditions being treated by pharmaceuticals. I bring it up here because, in my experience, the case with cannabis medicine is different. With short-lived symptoms, the question does not arise, medication is terminated, but with chronic use there may be some unusual consequences. For some of those adults who started with recreational use of smoked · THC-rich cannabis, and were successfully deconditioned to using products with a higher CBD content, possibly a 1:1 mix, cannabis use often declines, especially with my (the clinician's) encouragement. Symptoms relating to pain, sleep, mood disorders, inflammation, to name but a few, can effectively be treated by regimens leading to less impairment while bringing more inherent balance. It might be fair to speculate that a mixed CBD/THC protocol enhances endocannabinoid tone and brings homeostatic balance to individuals with dysfunction.

REFERENCES

1. Hazekamp A, Ware MA, Muller-Vahl KR, Abrams D, Grotenhermen F. The medicinal use of cannabis and cannabinoids: an international cross-sectional survey on administration forms. *J Psychoactive Drugs*. 2013;45(3):199–210.
2. Sexton M, Cuttler C, Finnell JS, Mischley LK. A cross-sectional survey of medical cannabis users: patterns of use and perceived efficacy. *Cannabis Cannabinoid Res.* 2016;1(1):131–138.

3. Webb CW, Webb SM. Therapeutic benefits of cannabis: a patient survey. *Hawaii J Med Public Health.* 2014;73(4):109–111.

4. Dai H, Richter KP. A national survey of marijuana use among us adults with medical conditions, 2016–2017. *JAMA Netw Open.* 2019;2(9):e1911936.

5. Walsh Z, Callaway R, Belle-Isle L, et al. Cannabis for therapeutic purposes: patient characteristics, access, and reasons for use. *Int J Drug Policy.* 2013;24(6):511–516.

6. Nunberg H, Kilmer B, Pacula RL, Burgdorf J. An analysis of applicants presenting to a medical marijuana specialty practice in California. *J Drug Policy Anal.* 2011;4(1):1.

7. Share of consumers in the United States who currently smoke marijuana as of July 2019, by age group. Statistica website. www.statista.com/statistics/737849/share-americans-age-group-smokes-marijuana/ Accessed November 19, 2020.

8. Compton WM, Han B, Hughes A, Jones CM, Blanco C. Use of marijuana for medical purposes among adults in the United States. *JAMA.* 2017;317(2):209–211.

9. Lin LA, Ilgen MA, Jannausch M, Bohnert KM. Comparing adults who use cannabis medically with those who use recreationally: results from a national sample. *Addict Behav.* 2016;61:99–103.

10. Hasin DS, Shmulewitz D, Cerdá M, et al. U.S. adults with pain, a group increasingly vulnerable to nonmedical cannabis use and cannabis use disorder: 2001–2002 and 2012–2013. *Am J Psychiatry.* 2020;177(7). appi.ajp.2019.1.

11. Kondrad E, Reid A. Colorado family physicians' attitudes toward medical marijuana. *J Am Board Fam Med.* 2013;26(1):52–60.

12. New Mexico Department of Health. Medical cannabis survey. 2013. www.nmhealth.org/publication/view/report/140/ Accessed November 19, 2020.

13. Schauer GL, King BA, Bunnell RE, Promoff G, McAfee TA. Toking, vaping, and eating for health or fun: marijuana use patterns in adults, U.S., 2014. *Am J Prev Med.* 2016;50(1):1–8.

14. Reinarman C, Nunberg H, Lanthier F, Heddleston T. Who are medical marijuana patients? Population characteristics from nine California assessment clinics. *J Psychoactive Drugs.* 2011;43(2):128–135.

15. National Academies of Sciences, Engineering, and Medicine. *The Health Effects of Cannabis and Cannabinoids: The Current State of Evidence and Recommendations for Research.* Washington, DC: The National Academies Press (US); 2017. www.ncbi.nlm.nih.gov/books/NBK423845/ Accessed November 19, 2020.

9 Pediatric Cannabis Practice

The thought of providing cannabis to a child is inherently disapproved of by most parents and health professionals. Stigma against cannabis is reflected in scientific literature and public opinion based upon its consideration as "marijuana" historically being a drug of abuse. Yet, there are valid therapeutic applications of cannabis use in children, as in adults, and arriving at that position entails overcoming this stigma and making informed choices.

> Many of the misconceptions regarding medical marijuana in the pediatric population stem from negative connotations associated with the term marijuana owing to its psychoactive effects. Therefore, it is important to define the various terms associated with products that are currently being used by the public as well as by pediatric researchers.[1]

Most professional opinions warn against cannabis use in children, in part due to ignorance about the range of potential therapeutic formulations that cannabis encompasses. The American Academy of Pediatrics (AAP), the American Medical Association, the American Society of Addiction Medicine and the American Academy of Child and Adolescent Psychiatry all have policy statements identifying marijuana use as a public health concern and opposing legalization.[2] The AAP published an updated policy statement on marijuana in youth in 2015 opposing the use of medical cannabis that was not FDA approved. (The FDA has approved one cannabis-derived formulation, Epidiolex, for the treatment of two forms of refractory childhood epilepsy in 2018.) The AAP cited the lack of evidence for cannabis use in children, as well as the potential long-term harms based on data derived from recreational use.[3] Indeed, there are valid risks in using THC-rich cannabis to developmental brain and neural function in children. "Such concerns are magnified when pediatric clinicians must consider MM [medical marijuana] use by children and adolescents, particularly because habitual marijuana use is associated with dependence, impaired neurocognitive development, and poor academic achievement in children."[4]

Currently, physicians are receiving increasing requests for advice regarding cannabis and/or CBD from parents. Little data about how health professionals are handling medical cannabis requests in minors is available as of yet. The prevalence of medical cannabis use or approvals in children in the United States has not been published. Data may be extracted from individual state registry statistics. In Colorado, for example, in May 2019, 330/5,817 minors (aged younger than 18 years) were registered medical cannabis patients, a prevalence of 5.6% of total medical cannabis patients. Seizures were listed as the main diagnosis for children aged younger than 10, while severe pain was primary for children aged 11–17 years.[3,5] Nevertheless, even if pediatric patients comprised as low as 1% of an estimated 3 million medical

DOI: 10.1201/9781003098201-19

cannabis patients in the United States, it is still a large number, 30,000 children. A 2017 survey reported that 50% of Canadian pediatricians had at least one patient who had used medical cannabis in the past year. Yet, only 4% of these pediatricians said they had actually authorized medical cannabis for one of their patients.[6] A discussion of pediatric medical cannabis use in Canada stresses careful evaluation of such a treatment course.

> Treatment plans that include cannabis should be constructed with careful attention to dose-finding, evaluation of efficacy and safety monitoring, and should only be conducted by clinicians or health teams with condition specific expertise and the ability to assess for, and evaluate, both efficacy and toxicity.[7]

The need for counsel to parents and their children is imperative, yet investigation of cannabis effects in minors is a greatly underresearched area and continues to be mostly shunned.

The dearth of knowledge about what cannabis products may be effective and safe to use in children is a limiting factor in pediatric cannabis therapeutics. Prior to CBD-rich cultivars and formulations becoming available, circa 2010 in some states, the choices for pediatric use were limited to THC-rich products, and to some extent, cannabis formulations containing cannabinoid acids – the non-psychoactive and non-impairing cannabinoids in unheated cannabis. Unfortunately, cannabinoid acid products are still less available than either THC-dominant or CBD-dominant products, but they do provide a safe alternative for some pediatric complaints. Even CBD use in minors is not yet adequately validated by clinical research.

> The pediatric literature lacks the same breadth owing to public stigma and restrictions on investigational use. This has resulted in retrospective and parentally reported data in epilepsy and behavioral conditions. Despite the overall lack of published data on CBD in pediatric patients, most of the literature is devoted to its use in epilepsy.[1]

A comprehensive review of studies done on cannabis or cannabinoid use for pediatric mental health conditions, epilepsy, spasticity for neurodegenerative diseases and neuropathic pain was compiled. The authors eliminated 18 of 20 potentially relevant studies noting challenges from small sample sizes, lack of publication bias assessment and lack of comparability due to differences between patients and the types and dosages of cannabinoids. They found CBD was associated with a reduction in seizure frequency in six primary studies, cannabis extracts or CBD-enriched cannabis extracts were associated with a reduction in seizure frequency in five studies and a CBD-rich cannabis extract resulted in significant improvement in spasticity in patients with severe complex motor disorders. They concluded, "The clinical effectiveness of medicinal or synthetical cannabinoids in children remains unclear."[8]

RISKS

General risks are outlined in Chapter 6 and reviewed for youth (aged 15 and older) in Chapter 10. We know little about specific risks that can be extrapolated to the pediatric population, focusing on children aged 14 or younger. There have been no clinical trials on long-term administration of cannabis or cannabinoids in pediatric populations.

> The current knowledge on the long-term side-effects of cannabinoids is based mainly on longitudinal follow-up of recreational cannabis users. . . . Notably, these studies contained very few participants under 10 years old and did not assess daily use of medical cannabis.[9]

The noted risks for minors center on THC-rich products with concerns about adverse cognitive effects. Neurological and brain function affecting cognition, intelligence, concentration and motor control undergoes active development during formative years, which may contribute to adverse long-term outcomes from THC-rich cannabis use in childhood.[10] It is predicted that an earlier age of onset of cannabis use may affect cognitive function.

> Age of onset, frequency and magnitude of MJ [marijuana] use were all shown to impact cognitive performance. Findings suggest that earlier MJ onset is related to poorer cognitive function and increased frequency and magnitude of MJ use relative to later MJ onset.[11]

There is no question that the adverse effects of memory impairment and poor executive functioning are of particular relevance in the developing brains of children. It is as yet unknown whether the benefit of low-dose THC especially in conjunction with coadministered CBD outweighs any potential risk in pediatric patients.

As with adults, there is the potential for adverse effects with CBD administered at high doses. As far as CBD in children at low to moderate doses (up to 0.5 mg/kg) is concerned, adverse effects may include mild sedation and dry mouth. At higher doses indicated to treat certain seizure disorders, adverse effects increase. A recent dosing trial for patients with Dravet syndrome compared safety and tolerability of 5, 10 and 20 mg/kg/day of purified CBD. There were some adverse effects, including pyrexia, somnolence, decreased appetite, sedation, vomiting, ataxia and abnormal behavior, all of which the authors say were well tolerated.[12] Of course, this was purified CBD administered at extremely high doses. The average dose of a CBD-rich cannabis extract for epilepsy is usually less than 5 mg/kg/day. As far as cannabinoid acids are concerned, any adverse effects from modest doses of THCA or CBDA whether in adult or pediatric populations have not been published, but are not predicted based upon their lack of activity at CB1 receptors.

THERAPEUTIC USE

Clinical cannabinoid use in a pediatric population was the subject of a literature review conducted in 2017, in which only 22 studies were identified. Benefit was strongest for chemotherapy-induced nausea and vomiting, with some benefit found for epilepsy. The conclusion was that there is insufficient evidence to support use for spasticity, neuropathic pain, post-traumatic stress disorder and Tourette syndrome.[10] There is scant documentation of what medicinal cannabis minor patients are actually using and for what purpose because this data hasn't been collected. Nevertheless, common conditions for which pediatric patients are approved for medical cannabis have been proposed to include cancer, epilepsy, nausea, pain, muscle spasm and palliative care.[3] The addition of behavioral and mood disorders, including autism spectrum disorder (ASD) and attention-deficit hyperactivity disorder (ADHD), should be added to this list to reflect what is clinically seen in states that allow these diagnoses to be approved for children. It is unfortunately true, that

> the literature on the prevalence and characteristics of medical cannabis use in children and youth continues to be scarce, with studies using widely different sampling methods and populations – making it challenging to draw any conclusions about the prevalence of and common indications for use.[13]

There is some data about cannabis treatment in seizure disorders, which appears to have some measure of success if used properly. One reviewer addresses why CBD and CBD-rich cannabis is being sought by parents of children with this condition. The reasons given are as follows: "1) prominent Internet and nation media attention; 2) reports of cases of children successfully treated with CBD products; and 3) the belief that treatments derived from natural products are safer or more effective."[1] One of the underreported complications of dosing in this population is the non-interchangeable use of full-spectrum CBD (containing the full entourage of the plant), broad-spectrum CBD (full spectrum with THC removed), CBD isolate (pure CBD) or Epidiolex – a CBD oral solution, which is the form used in most of the published research. The results of several studies and personal clinical experience show efficacy at doses of 2–5 mg/kg of CBD from a full-spectrum extract, while pure CBD is often tested up to 20 mg/kg, resulting in more side effects and potential for DDIs.[14] The efficacy of THCA containing cannabis extracts in treating pediatric seizure disorders has also been noted.[15] The use of medical cannabis shows promise for some cases of seizure disorder, but much more work needs to be done to delineate improved dosing protocols (see Chapter 46).

As with adults, cannabis is expected to alleviate pain in children. Medical cannabis effects on pain in children and youth have been reported in only two studies.[13] In one, dronabinol was effective in reducing neuropathic pain by 50%. The other study is the only one reporting on a cannabis oil extract for pain. The products tested had a CBD/THC 6:1 or 20:1 ratio. After 5 months, participants reported a very modest 1.41-point reduction in complex motor disorder pain on a 10-point scale, with improvements in dystonia, spasticity, motor function, quality of life, mood, appetite and sleep.[16] This study reminds us that when looking at improvement in chronic pain, improvement in other quality of life measures are significant contributing factors.

Cannabis use for pediatric behavioral disorders, including multiple mood disorders, ADHD and ASD, has been proposed and has some clinical relevance. In considering the scope of the problem, according to data collected as of 2016, 9.4% of children aged 2–17 years have received an ADHD diagnosis, 7.4% of children aged 3–17 had a diagnosed behavior problem, 7.1% had diagnosed anxiety, 3.2% had diagnosed depression while almost 2% of children have been diagnosed with ASD.[17–19] That is over one-quarter of all children who are challenged by behavioral or mood disorders. From speaking with parents, their primary objective in choosing to try medical cannabis for their children is the desire to avoid pharmaceuticals and/or that they haven't achieved adequate success by that route. In a few small studies in recent years, cannabis oil has been found to help some children with autism (see Chapter 19). Anecdotal reports of medical cannabis utility in treating ASD have arisen in popular media, while professional advice warns against its use. "The lack of high-quality evidence and the legal status of marijuana in the United States, which varies from state to state, puts parents of children with severe ASD in a difficult position, and one that is potentially outside the law."[20] Four uncontrolled case series of children with ASD and severe behavioral problems reported high tolerability and efficacy of artisanal CBD-rich cannabis strains. The treatment was reported to substantially decrease the irritability and anxiety in most of the participants and to improve the social deficits in about half of the subjects.[21] The observational study collected data on behavior via parental self-reporting before and after treatment to examine quality of life and mood changes in 188 teens diagnosed with ASD. After 6 months of treatment, 30% of patients reported significant improvement in symptoms, and more than 50% reported moderate improvement.[22] A protocol for a pilot study of CBD use in children with behavioral disorders and intellectual disabilities (ID) participants has been proposed in children aged 8–16 years with ID, with a maintenance dose of 20 mg/kg/day of pure CBD oil.[23]

There are no clinically relevant studies of cannabis use for ADHD in children within the context of this pediatric population (aged 0–14 years), although there are reports of its use in youth (older teens), with an orientation to adverse effects. One retrospective study of cannabis used in young adults who had a childhood diagnosis of ADHD found: "The extent to which cannabis use affects ADHD-related alterations in brain functional organization is unknown. . . . Our data suggest that cannabis use does not exacerbate ADHD-related alterations."[24] This suggests that the risks of using some THC-rich cannabis may be less than was imagined. A review of the few relevant studies on this subject concludes: "In sum, none of these studies provide sufficient, high-quality data to suggest that cannabis should be recommended for treatment of ASD or ADHD at this time."[2]

Yet as a clinician with multiple reports of benefit for autism and ADHD, and/or for other mental health diagnoses, what are we to tell the parents seeking advice? Perhaps the resolution is to consider the anecdotal reports of CBD-rich cannabis use for this population. There is scant literature on the use of CBD in the botanical dose range in children, as opposed to the higher dose range used for seizure disorders. Contrary to what would apply in most medical conditions, the doses these studies have been using are quite high, the range used for seizure control ranging from 5 to 20 mg/kg/day. In practice, I found a CBD-rich formula with anywhere from less than 1% up to 20% THC to be effective, especially for autism. Rigorous, large-scale, placebo-controlled trials are lacking, especially done at the more modest dose range.

CONSULTATION PROTOCOL

It is instructive at the outset to review the legal and ethical issues in recommending cannabis to a minor (the legal considerations may vary from state to state). First, a recommendation from a health care practitioner is required; in some states, two providers must certify for pediatric use. The list of approved conditions for minors varies among different states. In some states, approved forms of cannabis for minors are limited. The duration of approval is often still for 1 year, but frequent follow-ups are encouraged, if not required by approving practitioners. Physicians may be reluctant to provide these recommendations, as they are not well-informed about the risks and benefits of cannabis use in this population or likely in any population. A minor patient requires an adult willing to act as their caregiver/designated provider, usually a parent or guardian – who can enter a dispensary to purchase a product and supervise its use. In cases of pediatric cannabis consultations, the client(s) are not only the child, but one or more parents, sometimes a grandparent and or other legal guardians. Even after a minor has a medical cannabis approval, there might be other legal hurdles. In some states, parents who have provided medical cannabis to their children have been reported to the authorities, school officials or a state's Child Protective Services. There are also limitations upon when and where parents/providers/caregivers can administer this medicine to underage patients. Some states do not allow schools to authorize using or possessing medical cannabis on the premises, so children must leave school grounds to take their medicine. California, Illinois, Florida, Colorado and Washington are just a few states that have passed laws that allow parents to administer medical cannabis to their child at school.

CLINICAL PRACTICE PEARLS

This age group, which I present as a 0–14-year-old cohort, comprised only 2% of my private clinical practice, yet each child I have worked with has provided expertise about how to best use cannabis in children. This prevalence, while in alignment with that reported from medical cannabis program registries, is not expected to be representative of all clinical cannabis practices, as some physicians do not accept minors as patients citing a lack of familiarity with such cases. Pediatric patients in my practice ranged in age from 3 months upward, with the youngest ones (<5 years old) primarily presenting with a seizure disorder diagnosis. The primary diagnosis in this pediatric population overall was epilepsy, followed by autism, ADHD, anxiety, abdominal pain, anorexia, neurodegenerative disease and lastly pain. Surprisingly, in this group, pain was a relatively rare diagnosis, although traumatic injury pain such as joint pain was occasionally seen. The minors were almost all new users, or recently begun as some parents had already provided CBD-rich formulations, especially when it was available over the counter or supplied under the parents' own medical cannabis recommendation. Fortunately for these families, they came in for professional advice, as most were poorly informed. CBD-rich formulations were routinely advised for most diagnoses, with the addition of THC up to a maximum of 25%, that is, a CBD/THC 3:1 tincture, as needed for ADHD, pain or appetite. Often the addition of THCA- or CBDA-containing products were helpful for epilepsy and/or inflammation. One of the important things to keep in mind is that much benefit may be gained by specifying desirable terpene content, because the safety factor of terpenes is high even in children. For example, ADHD responds well to α-pinene, hence a tincture extracted from a cultivar rich in this terpene is useful, including

CBD-rich cultivars. In this case, such a "strain" would be most likely be known as a CBD-rich "sativa." Often this had to be homegrown and formulated as such distinctions are rarely available in commercially prepared cannabis tinctures. There was no instance in which I advised smoking cannabis to pediatric patients. Almost all were advised to use tincture as the delivery method, allowing precise measurement, by the drop, and ease of mixing THC-rich and CBD-rich formulations to reach the desired ratio. Often, they mixed the tincture with a small amount of juice, to improve the taste, and did the "swish and swallow" method. Other use included edibles or topicals for pain.

The question of advising use of cannabis in children is one where the risk/benefit ratio is of prime importance. In most cases, the negligible risk of employing a low to moderate dose of a CBD-rich product or a cannabinoid acid product produces measurably increased benefit over use of a pharmaceutical. It is long past time that medical professionals go beyond the stated risks associated with "marijuana," and deal in actual risks of the multitude of cannabis formulations that may be therapeutic in pediatric populations.

REFERENCES

1. Campbell CT, Phillips MS, Manasco K. Cannabinoids in pediatrics. *J Pediatr Pharmacol Ther.* 2017;22(3):176–185.
2. Hadland SE, Knight JR, Harris SK. Medical marijuana: review of the science and implications for developmental-behavioral pediatric practice. *J Dev Behav Pediatr.* 2015;36(2):115–123.
3. Nierengarten MB. Medical marijuana for children. *Contemp Pediatr.* 2019;36(7):32–36.
4. Adler JN, Colbert JA. Clinical decisions. Medicinal use of marijuana: polling results. *NEJM.* 2013;368(22):e30.
5. Colorado Department of Public Health and Environment. Medical marijuana statistics and data. https://cdphe.colorado.gov/medical-marijuana-registry-data Accessed November 20, 2020.
6. Ward M. Pediatricians seeing a growing demand for medical cannabis for kids. The Conversation website. May 10, 2020. https://theconversation.com/pediatricians-seeing-a-growing-demand-for-medical-cannabis-for-kids-132426 Accessed Nov 20, 2020.
7. Rieder MJ, Canadian Paediatric Society, Drug Therapy and Hazardous Substances Committee. Is the medical use of cannabis a therapeutic option for children? *Paediatr Child Health.* 2016;21(1):31–34.
8. Chao YS, McCormack S. Ottawa (ON): Canadian Agency for Drugs and Technologies in Health. Medicinal and synthetic cannabinoids for pediatric patients: a review of clinical effectiveness and guidelines. October 11, 2019. www.ncbi.nlm.nih.gov/books/NBK551866/ Accessed November 20, 2020.
9. Aran A, Cayam-Rand D. Medical cannabis in children. *Rambam Maimonides Med J.* 2020;11(1):e0003.
10. Wong SS, Wilens TE. Medical cannabinoids in children and adolescents: a systematic review. *Pediatrics.* 2017;140(5):e20171818.
11. Gruber SA, Sagar KA, Dahlgren MK, Racine M, Lukas SE. Age of onset of marijuana use and executive function. *Psychol Addict Behav.* 2012;26:496–506.
12. Devinsky O, Patel AD, Thiele EA, et al. Randomized, dose-ranging safety trial of cannabidiol in Dravet syndrome. *Neurology.* 2018;90:e1204–e1211.

13. Woo JJ, van Reekum EA, Rosic T, Samaan Z. Children and youth who use cannabis for pain relief: benefits, risks, and perceptions. *Adolesc Health Med Ther*. 2020;11:53–61.

14. Pamplona FA, da Silva LR, Coan AC. 2018. Potential clinical benefits of CBD-rich cannabis extracts over purified CBD in treatment-resistant epilepsy: observational data meta-analysis. *Front Neurol*. 9:759.

15. Sulak D, Sanneto R, Goldstein B. The current status of artisanal cannabis for the treatment of epilepsy in the United States. *Epilepsy Behav*. 2017;70(Pt B):328–333.

16. Libzon S, Schleider LB-L, Saban N, et al. Medical cannabis for pediatric moderate to severe complex motor disorders. *J Child Neurol*. 2018;33(9):565–571.

17. Centers for Disease Control and Prevention. Data and statistics on children's mental health. www.cdc.gov/childrensmentalhealth/data.html Accessed July 20, 2020.

18. Centers for Disease Control and Prevention. Data and statistics on autism spectrum disorder. www.cdc.gov/ncbddd/autism/data.html Accessed July 20, 2020.

19. Ghandour RM, Sherman LJ, Vladutiu CJ, et al. Prevalence and treatment of depression, anxiety, and conduct problems in US children. *J Pediatr*. 2019;206:256–267.e3.

20. Mamoser G. Here's what experts say about medical marijuana as treatment for autism. Healthline website. February 12, 2019. www.healthline.com/health-news/what-to-know-about-medical-marijuana-used-to-treat-autism Accessed November 20, 2020.

21. Aran A, Cassuto H, Lubotzky A, et al. Brief report: cannabidiol-rich cannabis in children with autism spectrum disorder and severe behavioral problems: a retrospective feasibility study. *J Autism Dev Disord*. 2019:49:1284–1288.

22. Bar-Lev Schleider L, Mechoulam R, Saban N, Meiri G, Novack V. Real life experience of medical cannabis treatment in autism: analysis of safety and efficacy. *Sci Rep*. 2019;9:200.

23. Efron D, Taylor K, Payne JM, et al. Does cannabidiol reduce severe behavioural problems in children with intellectual disability? Study protocol for a pilot single-site phase I/II randomised placebo controlled trial. *BMJ Open*. 2020;10(3):e034362.

24. Kelly C, Castellanos FX, Tomaselli O, et al. Distinct effects of childhood ADHD and cannabis use on brain functional architecture in young adults. *Neuroimage Clin*. 2016;13:188–200.

10 Youth Cannabis Practice

There is no absolute age cutoff when describing characteristics of older teens and young adults regarding cannabis use challenges and profiles. Here we look at patients aged 15–25, who can loosely be categorized as "youth." Notwithstanding legality issues, that some are minors and others are not, I present this age group as a unit because so many behaviors are similar in these young cannabis users. This is the age group where cannabis use traditionally begins, advances and patterns are set that are most often not therapeutic. Cannabis use recreationally by this age group has traditionally been high. The most prevalent age for recreational users is younger adults, between ages 18 and 26 or 29.[1] As reported in 2018, past year cannabis use in the 12–17-year age group was 12.5%, but increased to 45% by 21–22 years, declining mostly linearly with age to 14% by age 60.[2] The prevalence of cannabis users who apply for and receive medical approvals also show a considerable increase during this age range. In a 2016 study in Washington State, 8.6% of medical cannabis patients were in the 15- to 20-year-old age group, increasing to 35.2% for ages 21–30, reflecting the increase in registry once minor status is eliminated.[3]

This very diverse group of patients, constitutes the category of consumer who is most at risk for overusing cannabis, using it with poor discretion and not using it with a health goal in mind. This might be considered "recreational" use, but often these individuals are medicating something. If a young person wants to change their perspective, or alter their mood, there may be a problem, often reflecting an undiagnosed mood disorder. It appears that management of mood is a large factor in medical cannabis use in this population. This should come as no surprise, because one out of five teens are dealing with a mood disorder in any given year.[4] These include anxiety, depression, ADHD and others.[5] Consideration of physical, mental, social and emotional developmental issues are of importance here even more so than for pediatric patients.

> During adolescence, the brain undergoes significant developmental changes, establishing neural pathways and behavior patterns that will last into adulthood. . . . [B]ut adolescents' developing brains, coupled with hormonal changes, make them more prone to depression and more likely to engage in risky and thrill-seeking behaviors than either younger children or adults.[4]

Regular use of THC-rich cannabis in adolescence may interfere not only with cognitive functions but also with the development of important coping skills, including resilience, mastery and positive self-esteem, and in this way may contribute to dysfunction. Unless these younger patients receive professional advice about proper cannabis use, mood disorders or sleep can worsen, other overuse symptoms may ensue or tolerance-related adverse effects may occur. It is especially difficult with this age group to teach the concept that more is not necessarily better. Addressing

DOI: 10.1201/9781003098201-20

these complex issues is best handled by consultation with a qualified clinician. The American Academy of Child and Adolescent Psychiatry advises:

> Talking with your child about marijuana can help delay the age of first use and help protect their brain. If your child is already using marijuana, try asking questions in an open and curious way as your teen will talk more freely if not feeling judged. If you have concerns about your child's drug use, talk with your child's pediatrician or a qualified mental health professional.[6]

I would add that a qualified cannabis specialist may be as or more useful than a "drug" counselor. It is this category of patient, the young ones with mood disorders, perhaps not fully explored, diagnosed or treated, who turn to cannabis for relief, most often without professional advice, and do it wrongly, harmfully and potentially detrimentally, resulting in a worsening of their condition. It is this vulnerable young patient that we can best aid by providing instruction on best use practices. In my experience, the nature of these challenges, the type of presentation and, indeed, the way clients are able to handle cannabis evolve significantly for most in the mid-20s.

RISKS

This cohort comes with age-specific risks for effects to brain and neurological development, increased development of psychosis in vulnerable populations and/or for developing Cannabis Use Disorder if using THC-rich cannabis (see "Cognitive Function Risks," "Psychosis Risks" and "Cannabis Use Disorders" in Chapter 6). Again, risks are specific to THC-rich cannabis use, not CBD, cannabinoid acids, or CBD/THC mixed products with low THC content. Some of the studies upon which these conclusions are based show flaws in design and bias, and must be taken with discernment. Regarding cognitive function in adolescents, one study found the following:

> Those who had used cannabis ⩾50 times did not differ from never-users on either IQ or educational performance. Adjusting for group differences in cigarette smoking dramatically attenuated the associations between cannabis use and both outcomes. ... Teenage cannabis use alone does not appear to predict worse IQ outcomes in adolescents.[7]

Another study focused on adolescents with ADHD who used cannabis regularly. They found an association with impaired executive function and, potentially, for impaired cognitive function only when cannabis use began before age 16. When regular cannabis use was not started until after 16 years of age, there was no increase in cognitive deficits.[8] A study of 16–26-year-olds looked at the effect of regular cannabis use on neuropsychological performance, and whether aerobic fitness moderates these effects. While abstinence from prior cannabis use (i.e., the withdrawal period) was associated with decreased performance on working memory and psychomotor tasks, higher aerobic fitness level moderated this impact on visual memory, executive function and psychomotor speed.[9] Aerobic exercise is known to stimulate endocannabinoid tone, and may provide a good adjunct to cannabis use in youth.

Prevailing drug abuse literature cautions that adolescent substance abuse, including marijuana (they don't refer to this plant as cannabis), is a prevalent risk for which early intervention is indicated. There has been a hotly debated "gateway theory" especially applicable to youth, now largely debunked regarding the effects of cannabis use. The gateway hypothesis has been circulated since the 1970s suggesting that an adolescent's early experimentation with alcohol, tobacco or cannabis escalates to more addictive illicit drug use later in adulthood.[10] Finally, after years of promoting this theory in drug abuse literature, the National Institute of Drug Abuse has basically discredited it while not yet rejecting it. "These findings . . . are consistent with the idea of marijuana as a 'gateway drug.' However, the majority of people who use marijuana do not go on to use other, 'harder' substances."[11] In fact, it has been found that medical cannabis use decreases illicit drug use in young adults aged 18–26.

This is consistent with findings from the adult literature that those who use cannabis medically are less likely to use illicit substances, and that some medical cannabis patients are utilizing cannabis as a substitute for other substances such as alcohol, opioids, and illicit drugs.[12]

Some young adult patients have been described as subject to cannabis dependence or cannabis abuse disorder, which may or not be warranted. I've seen this diagnosis applied to medical cannabis patients smoking one joint/day, for several years, which is not normally excessive. At the other end of the spectrum, there are those patients who have smoked up to 4 grams/day of THC rich cannabis, that is, 4–8 joints/day, which clearly is indicative of tolerance if not dependence. Often these patients switch to the use of concentrates, as they have now developed a tolerance, are requiring high doses and their throat has discomfort. This excessive use is problematic. They might even be applying concentrates to a dabbing device, which aromatizes the contents that are then taken in by inhalation of the vapor (see "Cannabis Intoxication" in Chapter 6). Youth are more prone to inhale cannabis concentrates by means of dabbing than any other age group. According to a recent survey, 50% of the 18–24-year-olds polled have dabbed before or know someone who has, this prevalence decreasing with age.[13] An article on dabbing states, "Dabbing offers immediate physiological relief to patients in need but may also be more prone to abuse by recreational users seeking a more rapid and intense physiological effect." The author continues to say:

Our observations of patients who consume concentrates by dabbing are quite mixed and varied overall. Some individuals seem to be completely unaffected in terms of impairment, while others seem to be significantly incapacitated, sometimes to the point of vomiting or needing to sit down due to being overwhelmed.[14]

A recent study of cannabis use in adolescents in California found stronger associations of persistent cannabis use by those who had used combustible methods using concentrates (dabbing) than inhalation by more traditional smoked methods.

Youth may seek out and use cannabis concentrate products despite challenges with access to cannabis in this form either because they are interested in continued experiences with the sensory and pharmacological effects of cannabis concentrate specifically or because they have developed dependence owing to high levels of exposure to THC via use of cannabis concentrate.[15]

This persistence may indicate that withdrawal or discontinuance of high-dose use by youth is problematic. I have found that to be the case in clinical practice, occurring in the unwary young patient who develops a dependence without intending or wanting to.

THERAPEUTIC USE

There is little information from surveys or studies on the prevalence of diagnoses for which this specific age group seeks medical cannabis approval. There are numerous reports in the popular media by parents regarding the successful use of medical cannabis by adolescents for the treatment of a variety of health conditions. One might expect that as with adults, pain, sleep and mood disorders are common. It is worthwhile to look at the motives for cannabis use in this population. A survey in Canada of 20 adolescents aged 13–18 years of age revealed:

> [T]hey used cannabis to gain relief from difficult feelings (including depression, anxiety and stress), sleep difficulties, problems with concentration and physical pain. Most were not overly concerned about the risks associated with using marijuana, maintaining that their use of marijuana was not "in excess" and that their use fit into the realm of "normal."[16]

The authors summarized that 30% of teens self-report their recreational use of cannabis as therapeutic for mental health (anxiety, depression, ADHD, stress), insomnia and pain. Their reasons for use were listed as follows: no access to health care and prescriptions, prescriptions had side effects they didn't like, cannabis felt better, more socially acceptable and they got better relief from tension/stress. One author alluded to a potential placebo effect stating:

> As recreational cannabis use during youth is associated with serious adverse events and medical cannabis use is believed to have a relatively high placebo effect, decisions to use medical cannabis during childhood and adolescence should be made with caution and based on evidence.[17]

We cannot underestimate the motivation to pursue a "socially-accepted" practice, at least by one's peer group, as it affects this age group.

CONSULTATION PROTOCOL

Patients under the age of 18 require a parent or guardian to co-sign as a "caregiver" and be present at the cannabis consultation if a recommendation is to be approved in medical cannabis legalized states. Approvals are generally given for 1 year, but follow-up as needed is highly recommended. Those 18 and above can qualify in almost all medical cannabis states as patients without a caregiver and be allowed entry into a dispensary. In the nine states that have now passed adult use laws (see Figure 1.1), 18–20-year-olds still need to qualify as medical cannabis patients. In such states, many young adults aged 21 and above are now lost to medical surveillance, as they choose to not renew their medical cannabis status. These young adults often still need advice and will have much poorer outcomes without it.

Prospective patients who are not yet 18 and require an adult as caregiver must agree to supervised use. This does not always work out as intended. In fact, one of the biggest complaints I have heard from parents was that their teen children did not comply with restrictions, that is, no cannabis by smoking, or no THC use until after school or weekends. A frequent question from parents was how to make their teen accept conditions on cannabis use. My very inadequate answer was, "Well, other than my rescinding the recommendation in which case your child's use will be illegal, the problem remains, how to exert control over what your teenager does." We were sometimes able to extract a signed agreement from a teen, who was more amenable to making a bargain with me (the clinician) rather than with his/her parent. More often the issue of compliance was part of a larger challenge that existed in the family dynamic that was outside the scope of the clinical cannabis practice, yet this issue was often part of our discussion.

CLINICAL PRACTICE PEARLS

Patients aged 15–25 comprised about 20% of my cannabis medical practice. A good number of patients in this age group presented with a typical triad of complaints: anxiety, depression and insomnia. Is this a syndrome prevalent at this age? The most common diagnoses for this group in my practice included mood disorders – about half, including anxiety, depression, PTSD, ADHD, anger, stress, followed by insomnia. Other diagnoses included nausea, low appetite and headache. In contrast with the adult population, pain, other than headache, was not a common complaint. Of course, there were some traumatic injury complaints, including back pain, neck pain and various joint pains. This is reflective of the generally good physical health profile of most young people. Young women also came in complaining of premenstrual syndrome with symptoms of dysmenorrhea as well as low mood. Some young adult patients presented with autism with and without seizure disorder, but the percentage was not high, approximately 7% of the youth age group. What was truly rare were patients with diagnosed addiction disorders, that is, drugs, alcohol or tobacco. I did not see an association of these with cannabis use at all; in fact, the opposite was true. Many patients told me that cannabis was their preferred way of dealing with stress, of changing their perceptions, hence the desire to use it medicinally, safely and legally.

Patients in this age group often present with prior cannabis experience. Age of first use in my practice ranged from a few at ages 12–14, with most stating they started at ages 16–18, while some presented still totally new to the experience. Often those with a younger age of onset were using higher doses with accompanying tolerance, and almost all had been smoking it. Smoking was what this population was most familiar with, as is the case for recreational users. For those with prior use, at time of presentation the average amount of cannabis smoked was 0.5–2 mg/day. The only other avenue of delivery that was likely to be regularly used was vaporizing. This young population could be considered to be recreational users at the start, yet with medical advice their usage changed. What we are dealing with here is a population of recreationally habituated patients that need to unlearn bad habits. Not all, of course. Some new users displayed characteristics more reminiscent of the general adult population, with little to no bias toward specific use, or an expectation to get "high," and as such were easier to counsel.

As mentioned earlier, yet it bears repeating, often youth are conditioned to a certain level of cannabis use, and effecting change requires enforceable boundaries in the home. Refusal to comply with restrictions is not an uncommon adolescent trait. Requests from concerned parents about how to ensure enforcement were not uncommon. Surprisingly, in most cases, the teens followed the parents' caregiving instructions, but only after much work was expended to create a working partnership between the teen and the parent. Often counseling in the greater context of family dynamics by psychotherapy is helpful. Creating an environment where honesty and openness, as well as orienting toward positive therapeutic goals was the best recipe for success. In other words, don't expect compliance between teens and their parent caregivers at the outset. I imagine that as openness and therapeutic improvement occur, the teen begins to comply because he/she feels better. In the case that this does not occur, the cannabis clinician's primary reinforcement tool is to cancel the recommendation. This is a last resort, because then the teen would truly revert to recreational use, without benefit of advice.

There are further challenges in the youth group. These include dissuading smoking as a primary means of delivery, making the transition from recreational to medical use, appropriately dealing with underlying motivations, especially treating mood disorders. As far as deconditioning from smoking is concerned, vaporizing some or all of the time proved the most useful alternative. In the case of those youth patients who were free of parental interference in their decision-making, the caveat that had the most effect on behavior was the treatment of tolerance, thereby reducing cannabis use associated with reduced cost. This population often responds to cost considerations, and is in greatest need of tolerance intervention. Sometimes, just effecting a switch from THC-rich cultivars to a CBD/THC mix takes care of improved outcome, decreased dependency on the psychoactive THC effects and decreased tolerance. A true cannabis abuse disorder is a risk in this population. Helping the patient to recognize their dependency, offering alternative protocols as given previously, recommending counseling and being supportive as opposed to judgmental have brought the best results. How to advise patients in this youth age group about cannabis use is a uniquely individualized decision, as in all medicine.

REFERENCES

1. Share of consumers in the United States who currently smoke marijuana as of July 2019, by age group. Statistica website. www.statista.com/statistics/737849/share-americans-age-group-smokes-marijuana/ Accessed November 19, 2020.
2. Substance Abuse and Mental Health Services Administration. Key substance use and mental health indicators in the United States: results from the 2018 National Survey on

Drug Use and Health (HHS Publication No. PEP19–5068, NSDUH Series H-54). 2019. www.samhsa.gov/data/ Accessed July 23, 2020.

3. Sexton M, Cuttler C, Finnell JS, Mischley LK. A cross-sectional survey of medical cannabis users: patterns of use and perceived efficacy. *Cannabis Cannabinoid Res.* 2016;1(1):131–138.

4. Wile Schwarz S. National Center for Children in Poverty. Adolescent mental health in the United States: facts for policymakers. www.nccp.org/publications/pub_878.html#18 Accessed September 10, 2020.

5. National Alliance on Mental Illness. Mental health by the numbers. www.nami.org/mhstats Accessed September 10, 2020.

6. American Academy of Child and Adolescent Psychiatry. Marijuana and teens. No. 106. Updated October 2019. www.aacap.org/AACAP/Families_and_Youth/Facts_for_Families/FFF-Guide/Marijuana-and-Teens-106.aspx Accessed July 23, 2020.

7. Mokrysz C, Landy R, Gage SH, et al. Re IQ and educational outcomes in teenagers related to their cannabis use? A prospective cohort study. *J Psychopharmacol.* 2016:30(2):159–168.

8. Tamm L, Epstein JN, Lisdahl KM, et al. MTA Neuroimaging Group. Impact of ADHD and cannabis use on executive functioning in young adults. *Drug Alcohol Depend.* 2013;133(2):607–614.

9. Wade NE, Wallace AL, Swartz AM, Lisdahl KM. Aerobic fitness level moderates the association between cannabis use and executive functioning and psychomotor speed following abstinence in adolescents and young adults. *J Int Neuropsychol Soc.* 2019;25(2):134–145.

10. Lynskey MT, Agrawal A. Denise Kandel's classic work on the gateway sequence of drug acquisition. *Addiction.* 2018;113(10):1927–1932.

11. National Institute of Drug Abuse. Is marijuana a gateway drug? www.drugabuse.gov/publications/research-reports/marijuana/marijuana-gateway-drug Accessed November 19, 2020.

12. Woo JJ, van Reekum EA, Rosic T, Samaan Z. Children and youth who use cannabis for pain relief: benefits, risks, and perceptions. *Adolesc Health Med Ther.* 2020;11:53–61.

13. Gillespie C. 'Dabbing' pot is the new dangerous trend among teens: here's what to know. Health website. www.health.com/condition/smoking/dangers-of-dabbing-pot, Accessed November 19, 2020.

14. Raber JC, Elzinga S, Kaplan C. Understanding dabs: contamination concerns of cannabis concentrates and cannabinoid transfer during the act of dabbing. *J Toxicol Sci.* 2015;40(6):797–803.

15. Barrington-Trimis JL, Cho J, Ewusi-Boisvert E, et al. Risk of persistence and progression of use of 5 cannabis products after experimentation among adolescents. *JAMA Netw Open.* 2020;3(1):e1919792.

16. Bottorff JB, Johnson JL, Moffat BM, Mulvogue T. Relief oriented use of marijuana by teens. *Subst Abuse Treat Prev Policy.* 2009;4(7).

17. Aran A, Cayam-Rand D. Medical cannabis in children. *Rambam Maimonides Med J.* 2020;11(1):e0003.

11 Elderly Cannabis Practice

The elderly, also referred to as "seniors," aged 60 and above, represent a unique population due to the specific health challenges of aging. The elderly are more at risk for falls, psychomotor disturbances, memory or cognitive deficits and have a slower metabolism, all contributing to increased risk (from THC-rich products) and heightened sensitivity to cannabis as compared with younger adults.[1] A review of cannabis use in older populations points out:

> Older adults are a vulnerable group because of age-related physiological changes and a high prevalence of comorbidity and polypharmacy, which increase the likelihood of adverse drug events. Thus, the data on safety and efficacy of cannabis reported in trials with young adults cannot be extrapolated to frail older adults.[2]

There is also the likelihood that many in this group have held a considerable stigma against cannabis, having long been taught that cannabis is a drug of abuse. Yet with medical cannabis becoming more widespread, and with the advent of non-impairing (non-psychoactive) forms of cannabis, an increasing number of seniors have now expressed an interest in trying cannabis or CBD. As we will see, trying this therapy is not the same as sticking with it. Repeated encouragement and direction are necessary with older patients. An excellent patient-friendly review of cannabis and CBD for seniors is published by the National Council for Aging Care.[3]

Seniors' use of cannabis has been increasing over the past 25 years that medical cannabis has been available, with older adults comprising the fastest growing user group. The proportion of adults aged 65 and over with past year cannabis use increased tenfold from 2002 to 2014, from 0.2% to 2.1%.[4] A continued rise is ongoing, doubling yet again to 4.2% by 2018.[5] Among older adults, 75% consider cannabis use to have no or only slight health risks if used once or twice a week.[6,7] At least 30% of medical cannabis users are 50 years or older, both in the United States as of 2016, and in an international population surveyed in 2013. Some states report even higher percentages.[6,8] It is the over 60-year age group that we wish to focus on in this elderly section. We can estimate that perhaps 5% of these may use cannabis, and most of these, medicinally.

RISKS

There is little actual research investigating cannabis use regarding specific risks attributed to this population (see Chapter 6 for general population risks). A recent

DOI: 10.1201/9781003098201-21

literature review concluded that risks of cannabinoid use in older patients appear to be moderate, and their frequency is comparable to other analgesic drug classes.

> Despite numerous small studies describing a modest side effect profile of cannabinoids, we are aware of only one systematic review evaluating the safety profile of cannabis and cannabis products in the elderly. This systematic review found that cannabinoids were associated with a higher rate of adverse events than the control [as is found for adults in general].[9]

Of the general risks, the ones including psychomotor impairment, possibly affecting gait, and cognitive impairment are postulated to loom the largest for this population. The most common side effects reported in the review included drowsiness, dry mouth, coordination disturbance and headache. A prospective study addressed the safety and efficacy of cannabis in older subjects. In this population, the most common side effect was dizziness (9.7%). Contrary to expectations, the rate of falls was not elevated.[10] Adverse effects on coordination and cognition arise specifically from THC-rich cannabis, while the adverse effects of dry mouth and possible sedation may arise from both CBD and THC use.

In a study of the pharmacokinetics and pharmacodynamics of THC dosed from 3 to 6 mg in older subjects, they found the pharmacodynamic effects of THC were smaller than effects previously reported in young adults (most likely due to the lower dose range tested in this population). At this low dose, they concluded that "THC appeared to be safe and well tolerated by healthy older individuals."[11] The potential for increasing drug–drug interactions (DDIs), with cannabis as one of the drugs, has been touted as a risk for the elderly. The opposite is in fact the case. Cannabis at therapeutic doses does not cause DDIs in general (see "Drug Interactions" in Chapter 6), but it can reduce the effects of polypharmacy that in itself is a risk in seniors.

> In the United States, 35.8% of older adults take five or more prescription medicines. This increases to 67.1% when we throw in over-the-counter medication and supplements. Seniors at long term care facilities are at great risk, up to 91% take at least 5 meds daily.[12]

Cannabis can and does reduce polypharmacy in older adults, thereby substituting a botanical medicine for a pharmaceutical one, decreasing the likelihood of DDIs. It is well-documented that cannabis can often reduce or eliminate one or more prescription medicines (see Chapter 30). To best do this requires collaboration between the prescribing physician and the cannabis specialist, both of whom have little knowledge of each other's expertise. One of the changes that must occur if cannabis is to be used therapeutically is greater communication between providers. "Patients are more likely to consider deprescribing if the physician recommends it. . . . Deprescribing must occur with clear interphysician communication to formulate a comprehensive patient care plan."[12] Physicians knowledgeable about the adverse and therapeutic effects of cannabis must become part of the patient's greater health care plan, especially in the elderly.

In clinical practice, patients must be advised of potential risks. For a long time, these were solely based upon the effects of using THC-rich products. I noticed that many of my older patients had a fear of using cannabis due to the long list of potential adverse effects of which they were informed, especially disorientation, and the fear of being "high." As of about 2015, I was providing my patients with separate categorization of risk for the effects of THC and the effects of CBD because, clearly, they are not the same (see Appendix for Acknowledgement of Disclosure). There was, to my knowledge, no accepted or even published list of CBD side effects utilized in clinical cannabis practice at that time, so I constructed my own list based upon patient feedback. This advisement form that all patients signed resulted in less fear of cannabis use, especially for CBD-rich cultivars and products. Based upon an evaluation of potential risk, it is advised that CBD-rich products, topicals and/or cannabinoid acids might make preferred choices of cannabis medicine for this cohort.

THERAPEUTIC EFFECTS

There is little specific information about the therapeutic effects of cannabis in this population. Clinical trials are scarce. A 2014 review of the effects of cannabis and cannabinoids in patients aged 65 and older found only five studies reporting specifically on older subjects. They concluded that cannabinoids might be useful in treatment of anorexia and behavioral symptoms in dementia.[13] A 2017 review went a bit further, referring to efficacy of cannabis for Parkinson's disease, dementia, sleep disturbance and malnutrition in the elderly. The authors conclude: "Lastly, the medical literature suggests that cannabinoids have a relatively safe profile for use in geriatrics, with drowsiness being the most common complaint."[14] In fact, neither of these reviews reflect the primary reason that older patients use cannabis, and that is for control of pain. A prospective study of medical cannabis patients above 65 years of age found that the most common indications for cannabis in the elderly were, in fact, pain and cancer. They reported that after 6 months of treatment, 93.7% reported improvement in their condition, and the use of prescription medicines, including opioids, decreased.[10] A survey of medical cannabis patients aged 50 and older in Florida was reported in 2020. Here it was reported that 45% of patients utilized cannabidiol (CBD)-only preparations, 33.1%, used mixed THC and CBD products and 21.7% used all of the above. The main diagnoses were musculoskeletal disorders and spasms (48.4%) and chronic pain (45.4%).[7] These reports indicate that older medical cannabis patients are receiving benefit for the most common complaints, including pain and muscle spasms. Palliative care may also be required in this population. The types of pain I saw in my elderly patients were largely arthritic and/or neuropathic. One prospective observational study of 184 geriatric medical cannabis patients in Israel followed their progress for 6 months from 2017 to 2018. Most were 75 years of age or older.[15] Most suffered from chronic pain (77%) and other age-related conditions, such as sleep disturbances, cancer-related symptoms, mood disorders and Parkinson's disease. The majority of the subjects (66%) utilized cannabis oil sublingually as the sole method of administration. This study employed relatively low doses of cannabis with 5 mg of THC and 5 mg of CBD, a day divided into three doses with an upward titration of 5 mg every 3 days. After 6 months of treatment, 58.1% were still using cannabis.

Clinical information about cannabis use in the elderly is as yet an underresearched area, especially in a time when this is the fastest growing population of cannabis users. More studies need to be done, especially using CBD-rich medicines, which is what many of the senior population are using. Surprisingly, no studies on topical use in this population have been done, which is an omission, as many of the elderly make use of this non-impairing delivery method.

CLINICAL PRACTICE PEARLS

As a clinician in a cannabis specialty practice, seniors aged 60 and above made up a large percentage of my practice, originally at 30% but increasing to 40% of all my medical cannabis patients. My practice on the Central Coast of California included a community with a large number of retirees, well endowed with funds, so cost for their visit or their cannabis medicine was not as great a limiting factor as one may encounter with many of the elderly. My patient population included those in their 60s, 70s, 80s and 90s, even up to age 104! The high number of seniors comprising my patient population was due to several factors: referrals from other patients, referrals from other physicians and the advent of greater availability of CBD-rich products, which became a boon to recommending cannabis with less potential for adverse effects. About half of these older adults were new to cannabis use, thus half had used it before. In contrast to younger adults, rarely did these seniors choose to smoke cannabis, most preferred tincture and topicals, followed by vaporization and edibles. Typical requests from my senior patients were to experience less pain, reduce pharmaceutical medications and to have better sleep. The top three presenting complaints were pain (59%), insomnia (27%) and mood disorders (16%). The range of complaints were as expected for their age: joint pain and osteoarthritis, back pain, insomnia, peripheral neuropathy and following these, mood disorders, including depression and/or anxiety. Cardiovascular disease other than hypertension was not common. Neurological disease, including Parkinson's disease, Alzheimer's disease and multiple sclerosis, as well as various cancers were also conditions we treated with cannabis. The few cases of dementia I saw were mild, while the patient could still attend a doctor's visit. Unfortunately, a good portion of the visits by the elderly were one-time events. Over half did not choose to follow up with me or most likely continue with cannabis therapy. There are many reasons for this low level of participation, not least of which is little support at home, in their living environment or from their other physicians.

A survey we did at a local assisted living facility (ALF) showed remarkably good compliance and follow-up, likely due to a cannabis nurse being present on-site facilitating this.[16] The use of cannabis medicine in this senior retirement community spread to more than half the residents. Fourteen of 24 residents used some form of cannabis, mostly CBD-rich tinctures and topicals. We administered a simple ten-question survey to 12 patients aged 78–97 who had been using cannabis in whatever form they chose for at least 6 months prior (see Appendix for the survey). Most chose to use a tincture, and self-titrated to an average dose of 10 mg of a CBD-rich cultivar.

Some used THC-rich edibles before bed to help with sleep, and two used cannabis in tea, claiming benefit from the resulting cannabinoid acid brew. The most common diagnoses were neuropathic pain and insomnia. Most not only claimed benefit but also recommended cannabis use to their friends. The THC-containing edibles were suggested by the delivery service that brought products directly to the center. A common problem especially with the elderly who seek much direction are suggestions made by product sales agents whether by delivery service or in a dispensary. No matter how hard we tried to minimize THC-rich products in this group, some unwittingly chose it anyway, and stayed with it. Some patients achieved a considerable reduction in their other prescription medication use. The most notable was the reduction of four tablets of Vicodin per day to half tablet, and with better pain control on the cannabis regimen. The most influential factor in compliance and ease of use was the presence of the on-site nurse who helped with questions and offered reassurance. Follow-up almost 2 years later showed ten patients still taking cannabis medicine, with two having moved to skilled nursing where continuance was not permitted. Some patients discontinued use, but resumed upon follow-up. The stated reasons for stopping included lack of education about the benefits, not knowing how to use the product, and inadequate follow-up. An extension of this may include those who chose not to participate in cannabis therapy at all, stating they were afraid of the side effects. Patients' comments included: "We feel good about taking it. We wish we knew about this sooner"; "Few suppliers carry high CBD or grow it. High CBD/THC needs to be grown for the many people who need neuropathic pain relief." Challenges we encountered frequently were the desire to use as little cannabis medicine as possible, perhaps due to some stigma yet attached to its use and fear of use during the day. A patient who was using cannabis only at night due to fear of daytime use, unsurprisingly related: "Use of cannabis so far has not reduced neuropathic pain or otherwise had apparent effects during daytime." Most were totally at a loss as to what to take, requiring explicit advice from a professional. Remarks included, "Not sure how to quantify dosage"; "Not using cannabis, quit because it was ineffective and I didn't know who to turn to for help." That would have been me, the cannabis specialist, or the on-site nurse, yet our communication was not adequate. The model of having an on-site cannabis facilitator is an excellent means of ensuring compliance of proper use of cannabis medicine. Without this reinforcement, mistakes happen, the elderly may use the wrong product in the wrong dosage and are at risk for discontinuance.

My oldest patient first came to see me at age 103 for chronic nausea. We settled upon CBD-rich lozenges or mouth spray, which she said helped, at our follow-up at age 104. Patients show us that cannabis can be safe and effective in the elderly, but the products used must be carefully inspected, dosage must be slowly titrated and ongoing reassurance and guidance is imperative. Instructing a caregiver, relative, attendant or even a friend in what the older patient needs to take and what not to take is crucial. Senior patients need to have more supervision, more direction and more frequent follow-ups than the average adult patient. Coordination with their primary care provider is always a good idea. Patient education is so important with this age group who may have less internet searching skills, and really value a trusted opinion.

REFERENCES

1. Minerbi A, Häuser W, Fitzcharles MA. Medical cannabis for older patients. *Drugs Aging*. 2019;36(1):39–51.
2. Ahmed AI, Van den Elsen GA, Van der Marck MA, Olde Rikkert MG, Medicinal use of cannabis and cannabinoids in older adults. Where is the evidence? *J Am Geriatr Soc*. 2014;62(2):410–411.
3. National Council for Aging Care. The complete guide to medical marijuana and CBD. October 24, 2017. https://aging.com/the-complete-guide-to-medical-marijuana-for-seniors/ Accessed November 28, 2020.
4. Substance Abuse and Mental Health Services Administration (SAMHSA). Results from the 2012 National Survey on Drug Use and Health: summary of national findings. 2013. NSDUH Series H-46, HHS Publication no. (SMA) 13–4795. www.samhsa.gov/data/sites/default/files/NSDUHnationalfindingresults2012//NSDUHresults2012.htm Accessed September 12, 2020.
5. Han BH, Palamar JJ. Trends in cannabis use among older adults in the United States, 2015–2018. *JAMA Intern Med*. 2020;180(4):609–611.
6. Lloyd SL, Striley CW. Marijuana use among adults 50 years or older in the 21st century. *Gerontol Geriatr Med*. 2018;4:1–14.
7. Brown JD, Costales B, van Boemmel-Wegmann S, et al. Characteristics of older adults who were early adopters of medical cannabis in the Florida medical marijuana use registry. *J Clin Med*. 2020;9(4):1166.
8. Han BH, Sherman S, Mauro PM, et al. Demographic trends among older cannabis users in the United States, 2006–13. *Addiction*. 2017;112(3):516–525.
9. Beedham W, Sbai M, Allison I, Coary R, Shipway D. Cannabinoids in the older person: a literature review. *Geriatrics (Basel)*. 2020;5(1):2.
10. Abuhasira R, Schleider LB, Mechoulam R, Novack V. Epidemiological characteristics, safety and efficacy of medical cannabis in the elderly. *Eur J Intern Med*. 2018;49:44–50.
11. Ahmed AIA, van den Elsen GAH, Colbers A, et al. Safety and pharmacokinetics of oral delta-9-tetrahydrocannabinol in healthy older subjects: a randomized controlled trial. *Eur Neuropsychopharmacol*. 2014;24(9):1475–1482.
12. Halli-Tierney AD, Scarbrough C, Carroll D. Polypharmacy: evaluating risks and deprescribing. *Am Fam Physician*. 2019;100:32–38.
13. Van den Elsen GAH, Ahmed AIA, Lammers M, et al. Efficacy and safety of medical cannabinoids in older subjects: a systematic review. *Ageing Res Rev*. 2014;14(1):56–64.
14. Katz I, Katz D, Shoenfeld Y, Porat-Katz BS. Clinical evidence for utilizing cannabinoids in the elderly. *Isr Med Assoc J*. 2017;19(2):71–75.
15. Abuhasira R, Ron A, Sikorin I, Novack V. Medical cannabis for older patients-treatment protocol and initial results. *J Clin Med*. 2019;8(11):1819.
16. Malka D. Cannabis therapeutic use in the elderly. Presented at CannMed 2017 Premier Medical Marijuana Conference. April 10, 2017. Reviewed in Brown, K. *Cannabis Business Times*. A small-scale study with big results. November 18, 2015. www.cannabisbusinesstimes.com/article/a-small-scale-study-with--big-results/ Accessed November 19, 2020.

12 Pet Cannabis Practice

Cannabis has been used historically in animals dating back to the 1800s. "Patent medicines containing cannabis, usually in an alcohol tincture, were sold to horse owners for colic and other equine ailments, and topical liniments were used externally for joint and lameness problems."[1] In modern times, much of the research on the effects of cannabis and cannabinoids have been gleaned from laboratory animal experiments, verifying the safety of cannabinoids at extremely high doses and the therapeutic potential for numerous conditions. A review of many of these animal experiments has been published.[2] Cannabis acts on the endocannabinoid system (ECS) in animals not identically, but similarly to humans. Much of the therapeutic effects of cannabis in humans has been not only learned from animal studies but is applicable to animals, including our pets. Pet owners have shown great interest in using cannabis products, especially CBD preparations. "The use and demand for cannabis products in veterinary medicine is growing rapidly, mainly by pet owner demand. Unfortunately, it is growing faster than most practitioners have the time to educate themselves about it."[3] A study found that 82.2% of veterinarians agreed or strongly agreed that there are medicinal uses of CBD products for dogs. Many veterinarians with clinical experience using cannabis products (79%) said CBD was somewhat or very helpful for chronic pain in animals; over 62% said it was helpful for managing anxiety. Over 80% of those vets said there were no reports of adverse effects aside from sedation.[4]

The problem is that veterinarians still can't legally "prescribe" or even recommend cannabis for their patients, although they are able to discuss risks and benefits with their clients in a few states, not all. Veterinarians have not been protected federally from even speaking with pet owners about medical benefits. Federally, cannabis is a Schedule I drug for pets as well as humans. Furthermore, the FDA has not approved the use of cannabis or hemp in any form in animals. There is no FDA approval process for animal supplements, including cannabis products marketed as nutritional supplements. Laws and their enforcement vary between the states. This has led some states to practice more lenient policies, especially those that have approved adult use, notably Colorado, Washington, Oregon and most recently California, the first to pass legislative action to protect veterinarians. California has a statute signed into law in 2018 that affords veterinarians the opportunity to discuss cannabis with their clients, although they may not prescribe or recommend its use. The Veterinary Medical Association of California has published guidelines that advise a documented physical examination and collection of relevant clinical history, including prior medical records. It also provides that discussion of the indication and safety of the use of cannabis be documented. Yet it stipulates that, "Reminder to the client that cannabis is not being recommended or prescribed by the veterinarian."[5] The Colorado Veterinary Medical Association has a similar view. Its position statement says, "Veterinarians have an obligation to provide companion animal owners

DOI: 10.1201/9781003098201-22

with complete education in regard to the potential risks and benefits of marijuana products in animals." They also stipulate that, "It is illegal in the State of Colorado for a veterinarian to prescribe marijuana for animal use."[6] The resulting lack of freedom to discuss cannabis therapeutic use in pets by veterinarians has led pet owners to make their own unmedically supervised decisions.

A survey of hemp product (99.7% CBD or greater by definition) consumers in 2015 found that in the past year, 59% of respondents used hemp products for their dogs and 12% gave them to their cats, in the form of pet treats, tinctures and topical preparations. Reasons cited for giving CBD to companion animals included caring for aging pets and treating conditions such as anxiety, pain and seizures.[7] According to a 2018 nationwide survey of 1,068 dog owners nearly 80% of respondents said they had ever given hemp or cannabis products for their dogs.[8] This somewhat greater percentage may reflect differences in the demographic sampled and/or the inclusion of cannabis as well as hemp products. These are extremely high numbers and likely reflect a bias from sampling hemp product consumers. The type of hemp or cannabis product most commonly used were capsules or pills marketed for animals (57%), as compared to capsules or pills marketed for humans (3.9%). It is more common for pet products to be offered as tinctures if actually prepared from extracts of cannabis than from pure hemp-derived CBD; therefore, it is likely that most respondents were using CBD only products. Topical or transdermal use is rare. Cannabinoid receptors have been shown to be activated in the skin of dogs with atopic dermatitis, suggesting the efficacy of topical applications for skin disorders, but there is the challenge that they may lick it off.[3,9] Other forms of cannabis such as cannabinoid acid containing products have been suggested for pets and are now just becoming available.

How do pet owners know what to use for their animals? In the days prior to CBD becoming available over the counter, pet owners have consulted their cannabis specialist physician for advice on what to give their pets. That happened in my practice multiple times. Currently, some veterinarians are gaining knowledge and, in some states can talk with their clients. Now that CBD is more widely available. many pet owners are just relying on the internet for information on what and how much to give. There is little information on that subject from scientific studies, but there is a growing accepted dosing format, presented later in this chapter.

TOXICITY

The American Veterinary Medical Association (AVMA) has expressed concern about the safety of cannabis products for use in animals. In a letter on this subject, it is opined:

> We continue to receive reports from our members indicating that animal owners are actively purchasing these products and administering them to their pets and horses to treat medical conditions, often in the absence of veterinary consultation, and without the assurance that comes with FDA review and approval of therapeutic claims.[10]

In humans, we have much information about the risks of using cannabis. In pets, there has been emphasis placed on accidental ingestion of large amounts of cannabis reported as toxicity, with delta-9-THC listed by the American Society for the Prevention of Cruelty to Animals (ASPCA) Poison Control Division as being the intoxicant in *Cannabis sativa*. The most common route of exposure to THC in companion animals is via ingestion. Approximately 66% of exposures involve pets accidentally ingesting edible goods. The second most common source of cannabis exposures involves ingestion of plant material, followed by cannabis oils or tinctures.[11] A study of 250 cases of cannabis toxicity in pets showed 96% to be in dogs, with cats rarely at 3%.[12] The ASPCA lists possible intoxication symptoms as prolonged depression, vomiting, incoordination, sleepiness or excitation, hypersalivation, dilated pupils, low blood pressure, low body temperature, seizure, coma and death (rare).[13] Death due to cannabis ingestion is not actually a potential outcome, as the suspected lethal dose of THC in dogs is >9 grams/kg.[3] The AVMA lists the symptoms of THC toxicity as lethargy, central nervous system depression, ataxia, vomiting, urinary incontinence or dribbling, increased sensitivity to motion or sound, dilated pupils, hypersalivation and bradycardia. THC absorption in animals is similar to that of humans, with clinical signs evident within 30–60 minutes of ingestion or up to several hours. Toxicity may last from hours to days depending on the dose, elimination being complete in 5 days. Treatment is largely supportive, with hydration and/or sedation as needed. Rarely treatment with activated charcoal or gastric lavage is indicated.[11]

CBD does not show signs of toxicity even when used at relatively high doses. A 2016 study was designed to test the safety, toxicity and pharmacokinetics of CBD use in dogs. The canine test subjects received CBD via three different routes: a transdermal cream applied to the ears, capsules with a powder form of CBD or oil tinctures. For each delivery method, 10 mg/kg/day or 20 mg/kg/day doses were tested for 6 weeks. The most notable effect was elevation in serum alkaline phosphatase (ALP) that occurred in some dogs. All of the dogs in the study experienced diarrhea, while the dogs that received the transdermal formula had reddened skin after application that was not of clinical concern. The study concluded that this particular CBD-dominant product (at very high doses), with no terpenes, appeared to be well tolerated in dogs. The study revealed that of the three delivery methods, oil tinctures had the highest and most stable bloodstream absorption rates.[14,15] The therapeutic dose level of CBD in animals is much lower that what was tested here, determined to be less than 2 mg/kg, but in actuality it is likely even lower for most applications.

THERAPEUTIC EFFECTS

There is some information about the therapeutic effects of CBD and hemp-derived products for pets, gleaned from research studies and consumer surveys. There is little other than anecdotal reports of the therapeutic effects of THC-containing products in pets aside from animal study research. We know from consumer surveys that hemp products have been used in pets to treat pain, arthritis, inflammation, seizures, anxiety and sleep.[7] A survey of hemp and/or cannabis use in dogs reported essentially the same reasons for use. Less than 5% reported any side effects, mostly sedation, followed by decreased salivation and polydipsia. We know from human studies that CBD can reduce inflammation, anxiety and seizures and may help neuropathic and inflammatory pain. It is generally not useful for sleep unless combined with THC or with sedating terpenes (such as β-myrcene). This reminds us that hemp extracts with full terpene content are not only more effective than pure CBD but can also aid in specifying which effects to expect from the product.

Thus far, two research studies on osteoarthritis (OA) and epilepsy have provided information on cannabis use in dogs. In the osteoarthritis study, dogs with radiographically confirmed OA were treated with a hemp strain extracted by ethanol and heat containing 10 mg/ml of CBD as an equal mix of CBD and CBDA, with "a robust terpene profile." Preliminary testing was of 2 or 8 mg/kg dosage of the formulation in oil. The half-life of elimination of CBD was 4.2 hours for both doses. The clinical trial settled upon 2 mg/kg every 12 hours for 4 weeks. Decreased pain was evident at 2 weeks of treatment. The authors concluded "that 2 mg/kg of CBD twice daily can help increase comfort and activity in dogs with OA."[16] This statement seems to be somewhat misleading, as the product used according to the article actually contained 1 mg/kg of CBD and 1 mg/kg of CBDA (a cannabinoid acid) as well as terpenes, a vastly different product than pure CBD! For the epilepsy study, a CBD hemp extract was used, containing CBD 100 mg/ml with trace amounts of other cannabinoids. Dogs with intractable idiopathic epilepsy were given 2.5 mg/kg of the oil twice daily for 12 weeks in addition to existing antiepileptic treatments. Dogs in the CBD group had a significant reduction in seizure frequency (median change, 33%). Since a responder was defined as ≥50% decrease in seizure activity, the clinical relevance of the results has not been promoted. The authors suggest future studies at higher doses of CBD.[17]

In an unpublished study, a veterinarian gave 30 horses doses of 25–50 mg of CBD in a hemp extract once or twice daily to address complaints of anxiety, gait abnormalities, mild to severe laminitis and metabolic syndrome. The horses weighed an average of 1,000 pounds. It was found that for anxiety and mild cases of lameness or gait abnormalities, 25 mg once or twice/day was effective at reducing symptoms.[1] The efficacy of this low dose of hemp extract (25 mg/455 kg = 0.05 mg/kg) may show that "microdoses" in animals, as in people, may be therapeutic (see the next section – "Dosing"). There is also a report of tumor remission in dogs with less than 1.0 mg/kg of THC given twice daily. Positive effects of 100% CBD with no THC were reported as well. The authors saw a reduction in the size of the mass in about 6 weeks. They conclude, "The dose used in these successful cases was 0.5–1.0 mg/kg BID of CBD. Not all tumors respond to this dosage, but in those that do respond it is remarkable to watch."[18]

DOSING

The optimum dosing for animals has not been determined, although there are several opinions and projections from veterinarians that have some experience with cannabis and/or CBD use in pets as well as anecdotal reports from pet owners. We can attempt to extrapolate from human oral dosage estimates. For example, THC starting at 1 mg/50 kg person translates to a starting point of 0.02 mg/kg of THC from a cannabis extract. For CBD starting at 5 mg/50 kg translates to 0.1 mg/kg of CBD from a cannabis or hemp extract. Again, from humans, this dose may escalate slowly to a likely maximum that is increased tenfold or greater for seizure control, to 1 mg/kg of CBD from a hemp extract. An opinion often quoted at multiple pet CBD sites on the internet is similar, suggesting the CBD range to be 0.05–1 mg/kg/day with the THC range somewhat higher than projected previously, at 0.1–0.25 mg/kg/day.[1] No scientific citation is given for this much quoted opinion. Unfortunately, the OA study done with dogs using a 2 mg/kg dose of CBD/CBDA has likely not established the minimum effective dose. In an extensive review of all aspects of veterinary cannabis including dosing, it is concluded as follows:

> The data from veterinarians who have been recommending phytocannabinoids for their patients shows that veterinary species have a "biphasic response" to cannabis dosages in the same way that humans do. Microdoses are considered to be less than 0.5 mg/kg BID [twice/day] of cannabinoids. Macrodoses would be greater than 2.0 mg/kg BID.[1]

Clearly, the authors are not making a distinction as to which cannabinoid, CBD or THC, to which they are referring, although likely it is CBD. They also recommend a CBD/THC mixed ratio tincture for slowly bringing THC into the picture stating, "In rare situations in veterinary species, it may be necessary to provide a high THC formulation for improved pain management or to better address the needs of the oncology patient. THC:CBD/4:1 is typically the ratio that is being used clinically."[1] That is quite similar to clinical practice in human patients, in which the introduction of 20% THC in a CBD/THC mix (to produce a 4:1 mix) does not ordinarily cause psychoactive or adverse effects. Early studies in the 1970s showed that dogs have a high density of CB1 receptors in their hind brain that govern balance and cardiovascular function. Tolerance to THC developed in about a week with gradual upward titration. As is the case for humans, the author suggests, "Once tolerance has been developed, the canine patient can then tolerate larger doses if their condition warrants dose escalation."[18]

CLINICAL PRACTICE PEARLS

My experience with pet clients is gleaned from several pet owners who came in for advice on what to give their pets, a dog and a cat. Really, they considered these pets as family members, and were quite earnest in seeking care with cannabis, but I didn't know what to tell them, other than to extrapolate from human data as expressed previously in the "Dosing" section. One of my patients used cannabis for pain in her cat stating, "My 18-year-old cat, Sammy, continues to live free of pain, thanks to cannabis. In the beginning, I thought I could keep him comfortable for a few months. He's been using this magical medicine for 30 months."

Being accustomed to the therapeutic benefits of cannabis for people, and knowing of several tinctures already available on the market for pets, I tried some with my own pets, in ways not reflected in published anecdotes. First, with my aged dog who had significant knee as well as general osteoarthritis, I gave him a tincture with a formula that I found to work well for pain, inflammation and mobility. It contained about 40% CBD, 35% THCA and 25% THC. The dose was 15 mg by tincture directly into his mouth twice daily. That translates to a combined cannabinoid dose of 0.65 mg/kg, with 0.18 mg/kg being THC. The THC was maximized to treat pain, the THCA is a strong anti-inflammatory without being sedating, and CBD is relaxing and anti-inflammatory. In this 25% THC combination, none of the unpleasant side effects of THC were evident. Cannabinoid acids are now finally being marketed for humans, yet rarely for pet populations. In fact, THCA is still considered a Schedule I drug, because it is extracted from a "marijuana" source. My dog took this daily tincture for the last 3 years of his life, to age 14. Without it, he found it too painful to get up from his bed other than for essential functions. With it, he was able to walk miles and had a much improved quality of life. My other experience was with my cat who developed squamous cell carcinoma of the ear. After surgical resection of the affected portion of the ear, followed by cryotherapy when it came back, the vet said he estimated the cancer would be extensive within 6 months, and I should prepare for then putting the cat out of his discomfort. I tried a concentrated topical cannabis oil with a CBD/THC ratio of 1:1 on the ear, but it was not effective in halting the spread, likely poorly penetrating to the subdermal tissues. There is anecdotal evidence for concentrated oil applied topically being effective in humans for basal cell carcinoma, but his squamous cell carcinoma had spread to underlying tissues. I began to give the cat oral medicine, CBD mixed with CBDA or THCA in tincture form mixed into some wet food. It was a larger dose, approximately 8 mg twice daily, close to 2 mg/kg twice daily of this mix. The progression of the cancer slowed. We had 3 more years together.

To review what we know about what to expect when we give pets cannabis therapeutically, I offer the following summary:

1) Their endocannabinoid system interacts with cannabis. CBD and THC bind to receptor sites as in humans. In fact, whatever effects one expects to see in humans can likely be extrapolated to pets, at least it may be beneficial to try. As found earlier, people are using cannabis to treat pain, arthritis, sleep and anxiety in their pets, with success.
2) The best form of delivery is by tincture, as compared to powder in capsules. Oil tinctures were tested, but we would expect similar if not better results with alcohol tinctures. The effects may last 4–8 hours.
3) We know a 2 mg/kg dose of CBD can help arthritis pain. The recommended dose of CBD products on the market is much lower, from 0.02 mg/kg to a maximum of 1 mg/kg, although this is for hemp extracts, not for purified CBD. The best bet is to start low and increase slowly, just as with people.
4) Small doses of THC-rich cannabis, especially when given in concert with CBD, can be helpful for pets in pain or in some cancers. The research on how much to use in this regard has not been adequately studied.
5) As far as how much help veterinarians can be, that not only depends on what the state laws are and whether they'll even be able to participate in discussing the topic but also upon how much will they know. Will their advice be informed, biased or no opinion? As in most alternative therapies, the consumer is the pioneer. Consumers will likely scour the internet for poorly researched claims. This is a problem that needs to be addressed. For

more information on what to expect, your best bet is to talk to an informed veterinarian or a cannabis consultant such as health care practitioners who have been advising human clients.

REFERENCES

1. Hartsel JA, Boyar K, Pham A, Silver RJ, Makriyannis A. Cannabis in veterinary medicine: cannabinoid therapies for animals. In: Gupta RC, Srivastava A, Lall R, eds. *Nutraceuticals in Veterinary Medicine*. Swizerland: Springer, Nature; 2019:121–155.
2. Landa L, A. Sulcova A, Gbelec P. The use of cannabinoids in animals and therapeutic implications for veterinary medicine: a review. *Veterinarni Medicina*. 2016;61:111–122.
3. Cital S. Cannabis for animals: a look into cannabis as medicine for pets. *Cannabis Science Tech*. 2019;2(2):56–60.
4. Kogan L, Schoenfeld-Tacher R, Hellyer P, Rishniw M. US veterinarians' knowledge, experience, and perception regarding the use of cannabidiol for canine medical conditions. *Front Vet Sci*. 2019;5:338.
5. Veterinary Medical Board of California. Guidelines for veterinarian discussion of cannabis within the veterinarian client-patient relationship. January 1, 2020. www.vmb.ca.gov/forms_pubs/cannabis_discussion.pdf Accessed November 10, 2020.
6. Colorado Veterinary Medical Association Position Statement on Marijuana and Marijuana-Derived Products in Companion Animals. *CVMA Voice*. 2017;1. www.vin.com/apputil/image/handler.ashx?docid=8700488 Accessed November 10, 2020.
7. Kogan LR, Hellyer PW, Robinson NG. Consumers' perceptions of hemp products for animals. *J Am Holistic Vet Med Assoc*. 2016;42(Spring Issue).
8. Kogan LR. Dog owners' use and perceptions of cannabis products. *J Am Holistic Vet Med Assoc*. 2018;51(Summer Issue).
9. Campora L, Miragliotta V, Ricci E, et al. Cannabinoid receptor type 1 and 2 expression in the skin of healthy dogs and dogs with atopic dermatitis. *Am J Vet Res*. 2012;73:988–995.
10. Donlin JD. American Veterinary Medical Association letter. Re: Docket No. FDA-2019-N-1482 for scientific data and information about products containing cannabis or cannabis-derived compounds; Public Hearing; Request for Comments. www.avma.org/sites/default/files/2020-01/FDA_2019_07_16_2019-N-1482.pdf Accessed July 1, 2020.
11. American Veterinary Medical Association Council on Biologic and Therapeutic Agents. Cannabis: what veterinarians need to know. January 2018. https://news.vin.com/apputil/image/handler.ashx?docid=8473679 Accessed November 10. 2020.
12. Janczyk P, Donaldson CW, Gualtney S. Two hundred and thirteen cases of marijuana toxicoses in dogs. *Vet Hum Toxicol*. 2004;46:19–21.
13. American Society for the Prevention of Cruelty to Animals. Marijuana. www.aspca.org/pet-care/animal-poison-control/toxic-and-non-toxic-plants/marijuana Accessed July 1, 2020.
14. Bartner LR, McGrath S, Rao S, et al. Pharmacokinetics of cannabidiol administered by 3 delivery methods at 2 different dosages to healthy dogs. *Canadian J Vet Res*. 2018;82:178–183.
15. McGrath S, Bartner L, Rao S, et al. A report of adverse effects associated with the administration of cannabidiol in healthy dogs. *J Am Holistic Vet Med Assoc*. 2018:34–38(Fall Issue).
16. Gamble LJ, Boesch JM, Frye CW, et al. Pharmacokinetics, safety, and clinical efficacy of cannabidiol treatment in osteoarthritic dogs. *Front Vet Sci*. 2018;5:165.
17. McGrath S, Bartner LR, Rao S, Packer RA, Gustafson DL. Randomized blinded controlled clinical trial to assess the effect of oral cannabidiol administration in addition

to conventional antiepileptic treatment on seizure frequency in dogs with intractable idiopathic epilepsy. *J Am Vet Med Assoc.* 2019:254(11):1301–1308.

18. Silver RJ. Veterinary cannabis: regulatory, pharmacology, safety, applications (pain & cancer). www.isvma.org/wp-content/uploads/2019/10/SilverVeterinaryCannabis-1.pdf Accessed July 1, 2020.

Part III

Clinical Case Examples for Medical Conditions

13 Alzheimer's Disease, Dementia

ALZHEIMER'S DISEASE, DEMENTIA AND CANNABIS

It has been the hope that the neuroprotective properties of cannabinoids might offer promise in treating brain degenerative disorders such as dementia. As yet, the much-acclaimed success of these compounds in animal studies has not been tested in humans. The mechanism involved in causing Alzheimer's disease (AD) is not known, but there are some theories. The nervous tissue of the brain in people with AD shows an increase in abnormal structures such as plaques and tangles. Plaques build up between nerve cells. They contain deposits of a protein fragment called beta-amyloid. Tangles are twisted fibers of another protein called tau. Tangles form inside dying cells. In addition, levels of acetylcholine are abnormally low in the brains of Alzheimer's patients.

The effect of cannabinoids on AD has been studied in several laboratories globally in animal models and cell studies in the past few years. We know that CB1 receptors regulate neurotransmitters involved in excitotoxic neurodegenerative processes. It was shown that CB1 agonism is able to prevent tau hyperphosphorylation in cultured neurons. Microglial activation induced in vivo by beta amyloid peptide was prevented by cannabinoid administration. THC, specifically, competitively inhibits the enzyme acetylcholinesterase (AChE) as well as prevents AChE-induced amyloid β-peptide aggregation.[1] In an animal model of AD, treatment with 3 mg/kg of THC, once daily for 4 weeks with addition of a cyclooxygenase inhibitor reduced the number of beta-amyloid plaques and degenerated neurons. The results suggest that modulation of the endocannabinoid system in AD patients by cannabinoids could provide a mechanism to delay the progression of the disease.[2–5] A study comparing brain tissue from people who had AD before they died with age-matched controls found a dramatically reduced functioning of cannabinoid receptors in the diseased brain tissue, suggesting that patients had lost the capacity to experience cannabinoids' protective effects. They concluded that "Alterations in the localization, expression, and function of cannabinoid receptors occur in AD and may play a role in its physiopathology."[6]

CBD is also neuroprotective, although it does not primarily act at CB receptors. CBD makes an ideal candidate for treatment of neurodegenerative disease. CBD has multiple routes of action affecting brain chemistry that are CB receptor independent. Some of these include interacting with neurotransmitter systems, including glutamate receptors, serotonin receptors, vanilloid receptors, TRPV channels, cytokines, among others, to produce decreased psychosis, anti-inflammatory and antioxidant effects. However, the dosage and chronicity of use needed to impact the pathogenesis of AD or to reverse it has not been determined. What do we know about the effect of CBD on AD? In vitro studies showed CBD suppression of tau protein

DOI: 10.1201/9781003098201-24

hyperphosphorylation and the production of nitric oxide.[7] In transgenic animal models for AD, CBD reduced reactive gliosis and the neuroinflammatory response as well as promoted neurogenesis.[8] In a study of AD mice treated with a high dose of purified CBD (20 mg/kg) by daily oral administration for 8 months beginning at 2.5 months of age, they found that long-term CBD treatment can prevent the development of a social recognition deficit.[9] Many studies have been done with combinations of THC and CBD, the CBD potentially acting as an antithesis to THC psychoactivity. A study in mice was done using a THC-enriched botanical extract, a CBD-enriched botanical extract or a mix injected during 5 weeks at the early stages of the symptomatic phase. They found that THC and CBD, as well as the combination of both natural cannabinoids, reduce memory impairment, but only the combination prevented learning deficiency.[10]

It has also been suggested that CBD can be helpful for agitation and mood effects with AD, specifically for Sundowner's syndrome. Sundowner's syndrome, also known as "late-day confusion," is seen in some cases of AD and dementia in which labile mood behaviors escalate, such as anger, crying, fear and wandering. Before CBD became more prominent, studies focused on the effects of THC on dementia, which were inconclusive.[11] For example, treatment with 2.5 mg dronabinol daily for 2 weeks significantly improved the neuropsychiatric inventory total score for agitation and aberrant motor and nighttime behaviors.[12] In another report, THC 1.5 mg given 2×/day did not help neuropsychiatric symptoms in dementia.[13] In one recent small study of ten patients given medical cannabis, significant decrease was found in delusions, agitation, aggression, irritability, apathy, sleep and caregiver distress.[14] There are no published studies about the effect of CBD in those with dementia or for agitation in AD, although it has been proven effective in patients with Parkinson's disease psychosis.[15] There is one clinical trial now underway, testing an oral solution of CBD up to 60 mg/day with AD participants.[16] A recent pilot study conducted with elderly patients with dementia, treated with approximately a 2:1 CBD/THC extract, showed a decreased need for psychotropic medications, and neuropsychiatric and behavior scores decreased by 40% and a rigidity score by 50%.[17]

One systematic review of 12 primary studies of the use of cannabinoids for dementia concluded, "Overall, limited evidence from the studies included this report suggested that medical cannabis may be effective for treating neuropsychiatric symptoms associated with dementia (i.e., agitation, disinhibition, irritability, aberrant motor behaviour, nocturnal behavior disorders, and aberrant vocalization and resting care)."[18] Alzheimer's disease patients are thought to make up a small percentage of those seeking help with medical cannabis. In the five states where information was available regarding qualifying conditions for certification, dementia was the indication for <0.5% of medical cannabis certifications.[19]

PATIENT REPORTS

To move on to patient results from my practice, I did see several patients with Alzheimer's disease or dementia in my practice, or consulted with family members about their care, but few actually followed up with me after the first visit to provide sufficient information for case reports. These patients aged in range from their 60s to their 80s, and most only came in once. Several soon became restricted to care facilities that required a physician's order for cannabis dispensation, which is problematic, especially in facilities that receive federal approval or funding. As cannabis remains a Schedule I drug, it is not able to be dispensed in most skilled nursing facilities. Now that hemp-derived CBD products are available, access in care facilities should be changing. Anecdotal reports from family members who privately dispensed CBD-rich cannabis to their relative said it helped a lot for agitation and Sundowner's syndrome. Here are some illustrative case reports.

Patient 1: This is an 87-year-old male with a diagnosis of AD for 5 years. He came in with his wife who had already tried giving him a CBD-rich edible. She didn't know the dose. His dementia was not severe. He was able to fill out his own questionnaire, answer questions and was relatively well-functioning. His medications included memantine and galantamine. The couple thought cannabis might be useful to slow the progression of the disease, as symptom control was not a current issue. I did not encourage the use of cannabis as a disease-modifying agent, but advised a CBD-rich product might be useful for anxiety or agitation. At our next visit, he reported using a half of a CBD/THC 3:1 edible, only two to three times/week. He was now ambulating with a cane to help with balance. When asked how the cannabis affected him, he reported, "I remember to dot the i(s) in my name, and helps with attention to detail." He continued to take a small dose of an edible daily, and even progressed to a CBD/THC 1:1 product. The dosage was never clear to me as he got the product from a private delivery service. He said he thinks cannabis was helping his cognitive function. At the time of our last visit, he was 90 years old.

Pearls: Dementia encompasses a wide range of function. This patient was relatively high functioning, even though he was diagnosed with AD. For those who can handle a small amount of THC, such as in a small dose of a 1:1 product, it is conceivable that improved alertness or a positive shift in perception might result. I advised the patient to take no more than 5 mg of his edible product, providing less than 3 mg each of THC and CBD. This low dose strategy may be useful for patients with mild to moderate dementia.

Patient 2: This is an 83-year-old female who presented for pain management due to osteoporosis and compression fractures as well as multiple joint pains. She also had mild dementia, accompanied by paranoia and memory loss. She had a caregiver and lived with her daughter. She was new to cannabis use. Her daughter was interested in using cannabis for pain management, although she was on no current pain medications. Her dementia was being treated by memantine. She also had poor sleep, being treated by Trazodone. Over the next few years, her dementia progressed, but her mood was helped by a CBD/THC 20:1 tincture given daily. I did recommend its use twice daily if needed, but that did not happen.

Pearls: For a patient complaining of pain, one might think a higher proportion of THC might have been useful, but not at the outset in an elderly patient with dementia and paranoia. Many elderly patients will have pain complaints, but one must be careful introducing THC into those with dementia and paranoia. In contrast to the previous well-functioning patient, who on his own increased his THC use, I am cautious with most dementia patients. The 20:1 mix is typical to use for most dementia patients.

CANNABIS THERAPY SUMMARY

The question of whether cannabis can be used as preventive for the onset of dementia is a subject widely debated in the literature. It is possible that an ongoing dose of CBD-rich cannabis, or even THC-rich cannabis (possibly taken earlier in life), can be neuroprotective. How much and how long to take it has yet to be studied. We do know that CBD-rich cannabis has been used effectively for agitation and is useful in AD patients, especially if they are "sundowning." In this case, 5–10 mg of a tincture given at 5 p.m. is a good strategy. For patients with agitation or anxiety throughout the day, a 3×/day dosing schedule may be useful. An example is a patient with Lewy body dementia who had agitation throughout the day began on a dose of CBD/THC 20:1 tincture approximately 2 mg 3×/day, increased to twice that over the next few weeks, and ultimately took 10 mg 3×/day. The agitation remained stable or may have slightly improved over the next 2 years. Tinctures can range from hemp-CBD that has less than 0.3% THC to CBD/THC in a ratio of 20:1, which has 5% THC. In rare cases, in patients with fatigue or inertia, we can try to increase the THC content by 10–20% carefully. The assistance of family members in providing daily medicine to a patient in a restricted facility is often required.

REFERENCES

1. Eubanks LM, Rogers CJ, Beuscher IV AE, et al. A molecular link between the active component of marijuana and Alzheimer's disease pathology. *Mol Pharm.* 2006;3:773–777.
2. Di Iorio G, Lupi M, Sarchione F, et al. The endocannabinoid system: a putative role in neurodegenerative diseases. *Int J High Risk Behav Addict.* 2013;2(3):100–106.
3. Bilkei-Gorzo A. The endocannabinoid system in normal and pathological brain ageing. *Philos Trans R Soc Lond B Biol Sci.* 2012;367(1607):3326–3341.
4. Maroon J, Bost J. Review of the neurological benefits of phytocannabinoids. *Surg Neurol Int.* 2018;9:91.
5. Campbell VA, Gowran A. Alzheimer's disease: taking the edge off with cannabinoids? *Br J Pharmacol.* 2007;152(5):655–662.
6. Ramirez BG, Blázquez C, Gómez del Pulgar T, Guzmán M, de Ceballos ML. Prevention of Alzheimer's disease pathology by cannabinoids: neuroprotection mediated by blockade of microglial activation. *J Neurosci.* 2005;25:1904–1913.
7. Walther S, Halpern M. 2010. Cannabinoids and dementia: a review of clinical and preclinical data. *Pharmaceuticals.* 2010;3(8):2689–2708.
8. Watt G, Karl T. In vivo evidence for therapeutic properties of cannabidiol (CBD) for Alzheimer's disease. *Front Pharmacol.* 2017;8:20.
9. Cheng D, Spiro AS, Jenner AM, Garner B, Karla T. Long-term cannabidiol treatment prevents the development of social recognition memory deficits in Alzheimer's disease transgenic mice. *J Alzheimer's Dis.* 2014;42:1383–1396.
10. Aso E, Sánchez-Pla A, Vegas-Lozano E, Maldonado R, and Ferrer I. Cannabis-based medicine reduces multiple pathological processes in AβPP/PS1 mice. *J Alzheimer's Dis.* 2015;43:977–991.
11. Liu CS, Chau SA, Ruthirakuhan M, Lancot KL, Herrmann N. Cannabinoids for the treatment of agitation and aggression in Alzheimer's disease. *CNS Drugs.* 2015;29(8):615–623.
12. Walther S, Mahlberg R, Eichmann U, Kunz D. Delta-9-tetrahydrocannabinol for night-time agitation in severe dementia. *Psychopharmacology.* 2006;185:524–528.

13. Van den Elsen GA, Ahmed AI, Verkes RJ, et al. Tetrahydrocannabinol in behavioral disturbances in dementia: a crossover randomized controlled trial. *Am J Geriatr Psychiatry.* 2015;23:1214–1224.

14. Shelef A, Barak Y, Berger U, et al. Safety and efficacy of medical cannabis oil for behavioral and psychological symptoms of dementia: an-open label, add-on, pilot study. *J Alzheimer's Dis.* 2016;51(1):15–19.

15. Zuardi AW, et al. Cannabidiol for the treatment of psychosis in Parkinson's disease. *J Psychopharmacol.* 2009;23(8):979–983.

16. Forester B, Mclean Hospital. Open-label trial of a cannabidiol solution for the treatment of behavioral symptoms in older adults with Alzheimer's dementia. https://clinicaltrials.gov/ct2/show/NCT04075435 Accessed March 13, 2020.

17. Broers B, Patà Z, Mina A, Wampfler J, de Saussure C, Pautex S. Prescription of a THC/CBD-based medication to patients with dementia: a pilot study in Geneva. *Med Cannabis Cannabinoids.* 2019;2:56–59.

18. Peprah K, McCormack S. Ottawa (ON): Canadian Agency for Drugs and Technologies in Health; CADTH Rapid Response Report: Summary with Critical Appraisal. Medical cannabis for the treatment of dementia: a review of clinical effectiveness and guidelines [Internet]. July 17, 2019. https://pubmed.ncbi.nlm.nih.gov/31525011/ Accessed March 13, 2020.

19. Maust DT, Bonar EE, Ilgen MA, et al. Agitation in Alzheimer disease as a qualifying condition for medical marijuana in the United States. *Am J Geriatr Psychiatry.* 2016;24(11):1000–1003.

14 Anorexia, Low Appetite

ANOREXIA, LOW APPETITE AND CANNABIS

Anorexia is a term that refers to lack of appetite. The role of cannabis in appetite stimulation has received notoriety in the case of cachexia, malnutrition and weight loss associated with cancer, chemotherapy or HIV/AIDS. Marinol (dronabinol) is FDA approved for the treatment of anorexia associated with weight loss in patients with HIV/AIDS.[1-3] But many patients use cannabis to stimulate appetite in a greater context, such as disinterest in food, the effect of stimulants on appetite, stress or as a side effect of some medications. In the extreme case of anorexia nervosa, which has psychological components, cannabis can offer appetite stimulation as well as anxiety reduction.

Cannabinoids appear to regulate eating behavior at several levels within the brain and the intestinal system. One of the humoral factors evoking hunger is ghrelin, a peptide hormone that is released in both the gastrointestinal tract and the brain. Leptin, another hormone, is the main signal in which the hypothalamus senses and modulates food intake. Intravenous leptin injection into rats reduces hypothalamic levels of the endocannabinoids, anandamide and 2-arachidonyl-glycerol. The endocannabinoid system (ECS) is intricately involved in the regulation of these hormonal levels.[4] Activation of endocannabinoids drives the release of leptin and ghrelin. THC is thought to exert these effects as well by binding to CB1 receptors. A dose relationship was shown between THC levels and ghrelin, less directly for leptin, in the plasma of HIV subjects.[5] The stimulating effect of THC is more pronounced at lower as compared to higher doses, implying a biphasic response curve. In mice, lower doses of THC increased feeding, while higher doses decreased feeding. It is thought that activation of CB1 induces appetite, promotes food consumption and reduces energy expenditure.[4]

Early studies of dronabinol in HIV/AIDS patients showed promising increases in caloric intake and stabilization or gains in weight. The effects of dronabinol 2.5 mg 2x/day or cannabis in HIV patients showed modest or no effect on weight gain, although subjects receiving placebo lost weight.[3,6] In patients with advanced cancer, 2.5 mg THC and 1 mg CBD or THC alone were compared with placebo. Increase in appetite between the three groups was not different, but these results may be different for a full-spectrum cannabis product.[2] Enhanced chemosensory perception of food was noted with dronabinol at low doses, 2.5 mg 2–3x/day. While the food tasted better and appetite and caloric intake increased, there was no weight gain.[7] Few studies have looked at the effect of cannabis on the weight of healthy subjects, and the results are conflicting. Early studies did confirm increased eating when volunteers smoked cannabis, several cigarettes per day. Overeating was matched by a body weight increase, averaging 2.3 kg in the 3-week study.[8] According to a study in normal volunteers, low doses of smoked cannabis had no effect on food intake,

DOI: 10.1201/9781003098201-25

but higher doses did increase daily calorie intake.[9] One factor that most studies do not take into effect is the tolerance that chronic use may generate, with decreasing effects over time. In fact, one adverse effect of chronic cannabis use is the development of lack of appetite unless it is stimulated by exogenous cannabinoids, such as THC. People who experience withdrawal after chronic use often report a lack of appetite during the withdrawal period.

In contrast, CBD does not acutely stimulate appetite, but may antagonize weight gain. In animals, the induction of hyperphagia by CB1 and 5HT1A agonists could be decreased with a high dose of CBD (20 mg/kg), while more modest doses, 2.5 and 5 mg/kg/day for 14 days reduced the weight gain in rats.[10,11] In a human study, it was suggested that CBD might actually attenuate the appetite-stimulating effect of THC. They found that CBD/THC cultivars with a high ratio showed reduced attentional bias to drug and food stimuli compared with low CBD/THC ratios.[12] A testing of the effect of CBD on appetite in the absence of THC-induced hyperphagia has not been done in humans.

The situation with patients with anorexia nervosa is more complex. A pilot study of nine outpatients with anorexia nervosa treated with THC showed a significant improvement in depression and perfectionism scores with a minimal weight gain, 0.95 kg over 4 weeks. THC was given, 1 mg/day for 1 week, then 2 mg/day sublingual for 3 weeks.[13] Similar modest results were obtained with dronabinol. The participants received dronabinol 2.5 mg 2×/day for 4 weeks and gained 0.73 kg.[14] It is unclear whether the physiological response to cannabinoids differs in anorexia nervosa patients from the normal response, or whether the effect of cannabinoids is insufficient to overcome the strong drive for weight loss that these patients have. A study of the effect of CBD on anorexia nervosa patients has yet to be reported. A pilot study is underway.[15] As CBD can reduce anxiety, which is a formative psychological component in anorexia nervosa, it may help this eating disorder.

PATIENT REPORTS

To move on to patient results from my practice, most of the patients I saw with appetite complaints also had concomitant digestive and/or anxiety disorders. They ranged in age from 15 to 60 years. There were also some patients claiming poor appetite as a condition for which they were seeking cannabis approval, in part as a consequence of chronic cannabis use, by which their appetite-stimulating mechanism was linked to being habituated to cannabis as a trigger. Most of these were youth (aged 18–25). This is an unintended side effect that is transient, as appetite returns to normal after a 2–4-week abstinence from cannabis. Here are some illustrative case reports.

Patient 1: This is a 23-year-old female with complaint of nausea, low appetite, anxiety and depression. She was a prior medical cannabis patient from another state. She had a history of chronic loose stools episodically for 3 years. She had previously taken Prozac, which she said made her feel flat, and was now off medications. She had been using a significant amount of cannabis, up to 6×/day of large bong hits, now using it only once in the evening. The weaning off cannabis was difficult for her, leaving her with morning nausea and vomiting for 9 months after she stopped. Now she had residual nausea and loss of appetite, with continued anxiety. She really didn't know that chronic, heavy cannabis use may have contributed to her symptoms, yet she claimed: "Nothing has helped my stomach in 2+ years except cannabis." I explained that she had been overusing it and could continue at the new lower rate, THC only in the evening, preferably before dinner to help appetite, and that she should try a CBD-rich mouth spray for daytime anxiety and nausea. After a year, the nausea and anxiety were much reduced, she was using a bong or vaporizer 2×/day, yet had not tried a CBD-rich product. All was well until the next year when anxiety and intestinal bloating with queasiness resurfaced, likely stress-induced. I again advised adding CBD, this time a CBD/THC 1:1 mix for daytime use, to add to her nightly use of THC. She clearly did not appreciate the efficacy of CBD because it did not produce a "high," so had been slow to utilize it. This strategy of a 1:1 mix was helpful.

Pearls: This is a case of chronic cannabis use causing nausea, vomiting and low appetite upon withdrawal, compounded by underlying digestive disorder and anxiety issues. Having said earlier that the withdrawal syndrome usually manifests for less than a month, clearly the patient's underlying pathology contributed to extended symptoms. This underscores the need for individualized dosing to find the specific place where cannabinoid homeostasis can occur.

Patient 2: This is a 19-year-old female with a diagnosis of anorexia nervosa, anxiety and depression. She was here with her mother who was acting as a caregiver for anorexia treatment. She had a history of being treated for eating disorder since age 14, including inpatient over the past year due to dehydration. Her weight fluctuated from 70 to 100 lb, currently 79 lb. Her medications included Lexapro and Effexor, with prior use of Lamictal and other SSRIs. She was new to cannabis use. Her participation in psychological counseling was inconsistent. I advised a CBD-rich tincture for anxiety as well as smoking a THC-rich strain for appetite. I also recommended a local eating disorders outpatient treatment program. Over the next year, she experimented with various strains, settling on rare use of cannabis, 2×/week, for appetite, and sometimes before bed. She had been hospitalized again, down to 70 lb, with a current weight of 93 lb. She was off all medications. She had not tried counseling. She said her mood was good. I again advised using the cannabis at least daily for appetite.

Pearls: Unfortunately, patients with anorexia nervosa are often resistant to treatment suggestions. She allowed cannabis use up to several times per week, which was not enough to be fully therapeutic. Yet, she was happier to be on cannabis, such as it were, rather than her other medications. The fact that her mood did not deteriorate off psychiatric medications may have been facilitated by cannabis, but it's hard to know at such a low dose.

Patient 3: This is a 60-year-old female with anorexia with binge-purging, anxiety, PTSD and insomnia. She reported a history of multiple SSRI medications, but was off these currently, saying "they made her feel dead." She was doing ongoing counseling. Her experience with cannabis was rare, but she thought CBD-rich helped. I advised CBD-rich capsules or tincture daily, as well as an indica strain before bed. She tried a CBD/THC 2:1 tincture, but preferred a capsule daily with 14 mg of CBD and 5 mg of THC. She said her eating disorder was improved, anxiety decreased and she felt "less dissociated." She did not like the THC-rich indica. Her eating disorder symptoms improved on this regimen.

Pearls: Here is a case of an eating disorder, although not specifically "anorexia nervosa." In this instance, cannabis was effective in treating her mood disorder, which was beneficial in maintaining her appetite. We had no need of THC-rich cannabis to stimulate appetite, as her underlying psychological issues were what responded to therapy. A CBD/THC 2:1 mix has proven effective in other cases not only for anxiety but for mood stabilization and PTSD.

Patient 4: This is a 47-year-old male with sequelae from gastric cancer, post total gastrectomy and chemoradiation treatment 10 years prior. He had difficulty swallowing, with chronic nausea, low appetite and radiation enteritis with abdominal pain and diarrhea. He has been using cannabis for his whole adult life, more consistently since these events. He smoked 2–3×/day as well as having edibles made with cannabis butter. His weight had gone down 30 lb post-surgery, now he maintains at around 160 lb. His medications include Paregoric and Lomotil daily. In the 5 years we worked together, his cannabis use did not vary much, nor was I able to offer him any useful advice, other than to support his use of a strain that worked well for his appetite, pain and nausea. He states that without cannabis, his appetite is decreased and eating is more difficult.

Pearls: Where to begin? This patient is post-chemotherapy, has painful swallowing and constant nausea, all contributing to low appetite. I don't know of any substance that can address all these issues as well as cannabis. This is a rare case where my knowledge was not required, because the patient already found an optimum cannabis therapy. Being supportive as a medical professional was helpful in itself.

CANNABIS THERAPY SUMMARY

The case of low appetite often has multifactorial causes, which fortunately cannabis in the right formulation can address in one therapy as opposed to separate medicines for appetite stimulation, anxiety reduction and nausea. The challenging part is that while THC is an appetite stimulant, CBD is not, and can at times, decrease appetite. So, if we are treating anxiety as well as trying to minimize psychoactivity, a CBD/THC mix is a good choice. Individual cultivar selection may prove useful, especially for concurrent mood disorders, such as the inclusion of D-linalool for anxiety and D-limonene for depression. Some varieties high in α-humulene may actually suppress appetite. Also, dosage and tolerance are crucial issues. The emotional and physiological components of lack of appetite need to be addressed as well. An example is a patient with anorexia and bipolar disorder who benefitted from a mild dose of vaporized THC-rich cannabis 2×/day for appetite stimulation and mood stabilization. More challenging are those cases in which low appetite is actually caused by chronic cannabis use. The treatment here is a slow weaning process of the THC component in the cannabis, so the downregulated CB receptors can rebalance. Appetite invariably returns to a more natural state when tolerance is reduced. It is imperative to teach patients that they may be causing the very symptoms they wish to avoid by improper use of this medicine. There are of course cases where appetite is decreased during or post-chemotherapy, and ongoing stimulation by THC-containing cannabis is best achieved by regular low doses, such as vaporizing 4×/day.

REFERENCES

1. Abrams DI. Integrating cannabis into clinical cancer. *Curr Oncol.* 2006;23(Suppl 2):S8–S14.
2. Strasser F, Luftner D, Possinger K, et al. Cannabis-In-Cachexia-Study-Group. Comparison of orally administered cannabis extract and delta-9-tetrahydrocannabinol in treating patients with cancer-related anorexia-cachexia syndrome: a multicenter, phase iii, randomized, double-blind, placebo-controlled clinical trial from the Cannabis-In-Cachexia-Study-Group. *J Clin Oncol.* 2006;24:3394–3400.
3. Badowski ME, Perez SE. Clinical utility of dronabinol in the treatment of weight loss associated with HIV and AIDS. *HIV AIDS – (Auckl).* 2016;8:37–45.
4. Horn H, Böhme B, Dietrich L, Koch M. Endocannabinoids in body weight control. *Pharmaceuticals (Basel).* 2018;11(2):55.
5. Riggs PK, Vaidaa F, Rossib SS, et al. A pilot study of the effects of cannabis on appetite hormones in HIV-infected adult men. *Brain Res.* 2012;431:46–52.
6. Lutge EE, Gray A, Siegfried N. The medical use of cannabis for reducing morbidity and mortality in patients with HIV/aids. *Cochrane Database Syst Rev.* 2013;4:CD005175.
7. Brisbois TD, de Kock IH, Watanabe SM, et al. Delta-9-tetrahydrocannabinol may palliate altered chemosensory perception in cancer patients: results of a randomized, double-blind, placebo-controlled pilot trial. *Ann Oncol.* 2011;22:2086–2093.
8. Kirkham TC, Williams CM. Endogenous cannabinoids and appetite. Nutr Res Rev. 2001;14:65–86.
9. Sansone RA, Sansone LA. 2014. Marijuana and body weight. *Innov Clin Neurosci.* 2014;11(7–8):50–54.
10. Scopinho AA, Guimarães FS, Corrêa FM, Resstel LB. Cannabidiol inhibits the hyperphagia induced by cannabinoid-1 or serotonin-1A receptor agonists. *Pharmacol Biochem Behav.* 2011;98(2):268–272.
11. Bergamaschi MM, Queiroz RH, Zuardi AW, et al. Safety and side effects of cannabidiol, a Cannabis sativa constituent. *Curr Drug Saf.* 2011;6:237–249.
12. Morgan CJA, Freeman TP, Schafer GL, Curran HV. Cannabidiol attenuates the appetitive effects of Δ9-tetrahydrocannabinol in humans smoking their chosen cannabis. *Neuropsychopharmacology.* 2010;35(9):1879–1885.
13. Avraham Y, Latzer Y, Hasid D, Berry EM. The impact of Δ9-THC on the psychological symptoms of anorexia nervosa: a pilot study. *Isr J Psychiatry Relat Sci.* 2017;54(3):44–51.
14. Andries A, Frystyk J, Flyvbjerg A, Støving RK. Dronabinol in severe, enduring anorexia nervosa: a randomized controlled trial. *Int J Eat Disord.* 2014;47(1):18–23.
15. Guido F. Center for Medicinal Cannabis Research. The role of cannabidiol (CBD) in regulating meal time anxiety in anorexia nervosa. 2019. www.cmcr.ucsd.edu/index.php/background/studies/active-studies/228-gray-anorexia-nervosa Accessed November 20, 2020.

15 Anxiety

ANXIETY AND CANNABIS

The studies on the psychological effects of cannabis and its effect on anxiety have been many, contradictory and most often done with THC-rich cannabis. As with all mood disorders, the potential benefits and harms of cannabis have been debated at great length without appropriate understanding of the components of the plant and confounding factors. A longitudinal study of 8,598 cannabis users showed no increased risk of anxiety at follow-up. They also found no associations between anxiety and cannabis use at onset. Adjusted for all confounders (alcohol and illicit drug use, education, family tension, place of upbringing), the associations that might have been attributed were no longer statistically significant.[1] A 2012 review of cannabis and anxiety concluded that there were no studies that directly addressed the key questions. They found

> some benefit of non-THC cannabinoids (nabilone and cannabidiol) among a small number of study participants. THC, the most prominent medicinal compound in cannabis, is known to cause an anxiety reaction in high doses in some patients. CBD, the second most common compound in cannabis, appears to ease anxiety even if taken in high doses.[2]

Use of THC and THC-rich cannabis has shown contradictory effects on anxiety. To review the effects of THC on the endocannabinoid system, we recall that it is a CB agonist, and its stimulation of CB receptors shows a bidirectional dose–response curve. It is generally thought that low doses of CB1 receptor agonists elicit anxiolytic effects, while high concentrations are anxiogenic.[3,4] Pharmacological blockade of CB1 receptors induces anxiety in rats, and inhibition of anandamide metabolism produces anxiolytic-like effects.[3] In a study in mice, they found that in contrast to other CB1 agonists, THC at high doses of 0.25–10 mg/kg did not show anxiolytic responses.[5] In contrast, another animal study showed that the administration of a low dose of THC (0.3 mg/kg) produced clear anxiolytic-like responses. Further, in a study of health volunteers, a 7.5 mg dose of THC reduced negative emotional responses to stress, while 12.5 mg of THC produced small increases in anxiety.[6] It may be that the therapeutic range needed for THC to be anxiolytic in an average person would be less than 10 mg. Of course, this is not directly translatable to cannabis with the added effect of terpenes making lower doses more effective, with specificity of action determined by the terpene profile. The mechanisms of the effects of cannabinoids on anxiety-related responses also appear to involve CB1 and non-CB1 receptors, including the 5HT1A receptor.[7] In an animal study using cannabinoid agonists, low doses elicited antidepressant-like behavior and enhanced 5-HT neurotransmission,

DOI: 10.1201/9781003098201-26

while high doses opposed those effects.[8] It has also been suggested that "Effects of THC and CBD to increase tryptophan concentrations in unstimulated peripheral blood cells in the nanomolar concentration range, may give some explanation for the observed well-being after smoking marijuana."[9]

This brings us to the effects of CBD. As the anxiolytic effects of CBD have become more well-known, interest in the therapeutic use of cannabis for anxiety has grown. CBD is an allosteric modulator at CB receptors, and does have activity at the 5HT1A receptor among others.[10] In human studies of the brain, it was found that CBD increased blood flow to the areas of the brain that are known to control anxiety.[11] A 300-mg dose of CBD was found to be as effective as the two known antianxiety medicines and was significantly more effective than the placebo.[12] Patients with social anxiety disorder who received a single dose of CBD (600 mg) significantly reduced anxiety, cognitive impairment and discomfort in their speech performance.[13] This was confirmed with CBD 400 mg causing reduced anxiety in social anxiety subjects.[14] A dose-dependent response has been shown for CBD. CBD (100, 300 and 900 mg) induced anxiolytic effects with a dose-dependent inverted U-shaped curve. Anxiety measures were reduced with CBD 300 mg, but not with CBD 100 and 900 mg.[15] As with pure THC, these numbers are not expected to extrapolate directly to effective cannabis doses, which are much lower. Finally, CBD has been shown to attenuate the anxiogenic effect of THC. Volunteer subjects received CBD (1 mg/kg), THC (0.5 mg/kg) or both. Results showed that the increased anxiety following the administration of THC was significantly attenuated with the simultaneous administration of CBD. In another study, anxiety was reduced with administration of 15, 30 or 60 mg of CBD concurrent with 30 mg of THC.[16]

Anxiety is a common complaint for which people seek to use cannabis. In a recent survey, medical cannabis users perceived a 58% reduction in anxiety. Two puffs were sufficient. CBD (>11%)/THC (>26.5%) cannabis produced the largest perceived changes in "stress." It is useful to recall that CBD works well for anxiety, but a significant THC component is indicated for stress management. In this survey, no difference between efficacy of CBD versus THC was found, possibly because of low dose, that is, two puffs.[17] Although stress and anxiety are not equivalent, we might expect that a CBD/THC 2:1 mix (as was used earlier) would be effective for stress, whereas the inverse would be preferred for anxiety. In a Canadian survey, 60% of participants reported anxiety as a symptom, while 15% were actually diagnosed with an anxiety-related disorder. This study sought to differentiate efficacy based upon strain profile. All of the cultivars chosen were grouped into three categories by their terpene profile. Three of the four most effective strains for anxiety were Kush varieties, which all shared a similar chemotype with high levels of trans-nerolidol, β-caryophyllene and D-limonene.[18] It is thought that the terpene profile, which determines many cultivar characteristics, is most important in specifying mood effects allowing some THC-rich strains to actually be relaxing. In the earlier study, it could be the D-limonene content that was contributing to a feeling of well-being. D-Linalool is the terpene most associated with effectiveness for anxiety. It induces a sedative and calming effect and is used for the treatment of nervousness and anxiety.

PATIENT REPORTS

To move on to patient results from my practice, anxiety was a common complaint, often confused with or codiagnosed with depression. In fact, it is important to distinguish between the two, as the cannabis therapeutic options differ with each. The patients presented in all ages, from the teens to the 80s. Included in this category were patients with significant anxiety disorders such as panic disorders and obsessive-compulsive disorder (OCD). Often, we had to consider a multimodal approach for coexisting diagnoses, such as low appetite or insomnia. Here are a few illustrative case reports.

Patient 1: This is a 52-year-old female diagnosed with anxiety and depression, previously suffering from agoraphobia that was now improved. She was using cannabis by pipe 2–3× daily for the past 12 years. Her medications were decreasing at the time of this visit, Effexor from 225 mg/day to 75 mg/day and Trazodone from 100 mg to 50 mg at night. She credited cannabis and counseling for her improvement. Over the next year, she continued to smoke a sativa strain for her depression, but decreased it to 2×/week as needed, and was able to cut the Trazodone in half. She did not like indicas as they gave her a "hangover." Around this time, a sedating strain of CBD, Cannatonic, became available and she used it before bed. This had a CBD/THC ratio of 2:1 and was somewhat sedating. She added CBD oil by vaporization, yet her condition actually worsened over the next year, to include recurrent nightmares and rare agoraphobia. Ongoing counseling may have induced these latent symptoms, possibly resulting from PTSD. Over the next 2 years, she tried Buspar, then got off of it. She had ongoing improvement that she attributed in part to meditation and her new cannabis regimen. This consisted of a CBD-rich tincture, 20 mg, plus a raw cannabis smoothie every morning. At our last visit, she said she was "doing well" for the first time in the 6 years she had been seeing me.

Pearls: So many factors are involved here, outlining the need for perseverance through a mental health healing process. Symptoms may get worse before they get better. Of note is the non-escalation of pharmaceuticals during this process, potentially due to cannabis as a medicine. The utilization of a sedating strain of a CBD/THC hybrid was a superior sleep medicine for her than a THC-rich strain Also, we don't have much information about raw cannabis for mood disorders, but we do know it can promote vitality and well-being.

Patient 2: This is a 68-year-old male who had been treated successfully in the past year for prostate cancer. He came in for help with anxiety and headaches, which he thought were due to sinus congestion. He was on blood pressure medicine and Sudafed daily. He also was dealing with urethral inflammation. He thought his anxiety might be related to stress over the cancer diagnosis. While he was considered to be in cancer remission, he was worried about recurrence. He was new to cannabis use. On review of his history, I discovered he was an excessive coffee drinker, having 5 cups/day for many years. Interestingly, many of his symptoms could also be addressed by limiting caffeine, including anxiety, headaches and hypertension. I advised a caffeine wean down to 2 cups/day and a CBD-rich tincture 2×/day for anxiety and inflammation. By our next visit, his blood pressure medicine was reduced, anxiety was improved, by vaporizing a few times a week. Headaches were also improved, and his coffee was down to 3 cups/day. He never used the tincture, but was satisfied with reduced anxiety. I again advised him to wean to 2 cups/day of caffeine.

Pearls: Anxiety associated with a cancer diagnosis is common and may need short-term help until the patient becomes accustomed to his/her change in health status. The main point about this case is the benefit of taking a good history, especially from an "alternative" health perspective. Lifestyle adjustments, such as with caffeine, or other nutritional advice are often part of what the patient needs. Having a cannabis consultation practice that is wide in scope can provide individualized patient advice for cannabis therapy to be more successful.

Patient 3: This is a 56-year-old male with long-standing complaints of anxiety. He had a history of cannabis use in the past, but recently was experimenting, trying to find the right strain or product. He was on several supplements such as St. John's wort and SAMe. He had previously used Buspar and Ambien or Lunesta, but was now off medications. He also was doing psychotherapy. His cannabis use was 2–3 puffs/day of a CBD-rich strain, which was hard to find. We agreed he would continue with this type of strain, or go to a tincture if he couldn't find it. By the next year, he was growing his own CBD-rich strain, still sleeping poorly due to anxiety, and had been prescribed lorazepam as needed for sleep. Subsequently, he was prescribed gabapentin 300 mg at night, presumably for anxiety and a flare of low back pain. At our last visit, he was about the same, with ongoing anxiety, but he was still using very little cannabis, only 2–3 puffs per day.

Pearls: This patient did not use enough cannabis to be therapeutic. I think there was still somewhat of a stigma about needing it, or depending upon it that he was leery of. This is common with patients with anxiety, worry about the effects of a new medication. Our visits, once a year were not sufficient to overcome his reluctance to utilizing CBD-rich medicine appropriately. There needs to be more support from the patient's entire health care team.

Patient 4: This is a 26-year-old male with anxiety, depression and insomnia. His medications at our first visit were Lexapro 20 mg/day, Ambien 10 mg at night and Xanax 2 mg in the afternoon, down from 3×/day. He had recently started cannabis by smoking in the evenings to replace Ambien for sleep. He was also doing counseling 2×/month. He was smoking tobacco 10 cigarettes/day. He went on to smoke cannabis in the evenings, and spent the next year getting off tobacco and reduced Xanax to 1/4 mg/day. He also had a flare of asthma and was started on Singulair. I advised him to switch to a tincture or edible and discontinue smoking cannabis. He did not follow that advice, continued to smoke it, but switched to a CBD-rich strain, Harlequin, with a CBD/THC ratio of 2:1. This continued for another year, with the addition of an indica chocolate for sleep. At this time his anxiety was much reduced, he was sleeping better and he continued on Lexapro for depression. His asthma improved as he switched to a bong and he was able to stop Singulair.

Pearls: There's something about smoking cannabis that fills an emotional need in some patients, especially in those who give up tobacco. Switching to a water pipe was the best he could do and still effectively treat his anxiety with a CBD-rich strain. There are terpenes in the full flower that can be effective for anxiety. In his case, Harlequin is not a typical antianxiety strain but is known to have β-myrcene and α-pinene. The α-pinene may have been beneficial for his asthma, while the β-myrcene is sedating, as well as relaxing. I always tell my patients to stick with a strain that truly works for them, as often the patient knows best.

Patient 5: This is a 16-year-old male presenting with multiple psychological issues, including anxiety, depression, obsessive compulsive disorder (OCD) and racing thoughts. He also reported poor appetite, having previously been hospitalized for anorexia and anxiety. Currently, he was doing counseling and eating better. He had already experimented with cannabis, smoking a few times a week for the past 3 years, which he claimed made him feel better. I advised a CBD-rich tincture. Over the next year, he continued to smoke that became daily, and added the tincture. He got better on this regimen, stating it helped him manage his emotions instead of being paralyzed by them. His appetite improved as well. He continued on this regimen for the next few years, saying that cannabis kept him balanced.

Pearls: Anxiety in teens often presents challenges that are not as prevalent in adults. Teens gravitate more often to smoking for delivery than other methods. It's more socially acceptable in this age group. The challenge is to ensure that it doesn't become excessive. Even with parental supervision, teens often escalate their cannabis use, especially by smoking, and unwary parents are kept in the dark. This teen increased to daily smoked cannabis, while under parental supervision. I would have preferred greater use of tincture, but accepted his choice. It is a judgement call. Is smoking one joint/day worse than being hospitalized for mental health dysfunction? Perhaps being responsible for reporting to me his physician, and his parents kept his usage at this modest level.

CANNABIS THERAPY SUMMARY

There are as many varied responses to using cannabis for anxiety as there are solutions. A successful treatment seems to be more dependent on the individual than the therapy. Important to consider are the levels of THC and CBD and/or the cultivar of the cannabis plant that is used. Also, the dose that the patient takes, the patient's emotional condition and their endocannabinoid "tone." As you can see, cannabis choices to treat anxiety range across the whole spectrum of plant chemotypes and delivery options, from THC-rich to CBD-rich, from smoked to tincture to raw, encompassing many different strains. What's important to remember is that there really are stimulating THC-rich strains that can exacerbate anxiety, and these must be avoided. Also, the higher the THC dosages in cannabis therapy, the more likely it is to be anxiogenic. In patients with significant anxiety, such as in OCD or panic episodes, it has been my experience that patients respond best to low THC content such as found in CBD/THC 20:1 mixed products. A good starting dose might be 5 mg of a CBD-rich product, and increase from there as needed until you reach a desired result. Another aspect of treating anxiety with cannabis is the need to manage coexisting conditions. For example, for a mixed anxiety/depression presentation, it's often best to choose a CBD/THC mix, preferably with appropriate terpenes such as D-linalool and D-limonene, both relaxing and uplifting. This is the art of working with cannabis for individualized solutions. Or, for anxiety accompanied by insomnia, a THC-rich product, while sedating, may be too agitating, A CBD-rich strain with some THC and with β-myrcene will be both relaxing and sedating. Remain aware of the need to adjust cannabis dosages and/or frequency as pharmaceuticals are withdrawn. Effective cannabis dosing may need to be increased as the medication is withdrawn. Anxiety is a condition for which cannabis is extremely effective, especially with CBD-rich products. In my experience, the benefit/risk profile is high, and cannabis is a smart choice.

REFERENCES

1. Danielsson AK, Lundin A, Agardh E, Allebeck P, Forsell Y. Cannabis use, depression and anxiety: a 3-year prospective population-based study. *J Affect Disord.* 2016;193:103–108.
2. Campos-Outcalt D, Hamilton P, Rosales C. Arizona Department of Health Services Medical Marijuana Advisory Committee Report. Medical marijuana for the treatment of generalized anxiety disorder. An evidence review. 2012. www.azdhs.gov/documents/licensing/medical-marijuana/debilitating/Debilitating-Conditions-Anxiety.pdf Accessed June 10, 2020.
3. Viveros MP, Marco EM, File SE. Endocannabinoid system and stress and anxiety responses. *Pharmacol Biochem Behav.* 2005;81(2):331–342.
4. Tambaro S, Bortolato M. Cannabinoid-related agents in the treatment of anxiety disorders: current knowledge and future perspectives. *Recent Pat CNS Drug Discov.* 2012;7:25–40.
5. Patel S, Hilliard C. Pharmacological evaluation of cannabinoid receptor ligands in a mouse model of anxiety: further evidence for an anxiolytic role for endogenous cannabinoid signaling. *J Pharmacol Exp Ther.* 2006;318(1):304–311.
6. Childs E, Lutz JA, de Wit H. Dose-related effects of delta-9-THC on emotional responses to acute psychosocial stress. *Drug Alcohol Depend.* 2017;177:136–144.
7. Schier AR, Ribeiro NP, Silva AC, et al. Cannabidiol, a cannabis sativa constituent, as an anxiolytic drug. *Rev Bras Psiquiatr.* 2012;4(supl.1):S104–S117.
8. Bambico FR, Katz N, Debonnel G, Gobbi G. Cannabinoids elicit antidepressant-like behavior and activate serotonergic neurons through the medial prefrontal cortex. *J Neurosci.* 2007;27(43):11700–11711.
9. Jenny M, Schröcksnadel S, Überall F, Fuchs D.The po tential role of cannabinoids in modulating serotonergic signaling by their influence on tryptophan metabolism. *Pharmaceuticals (Basel).* 2010;(8):2647–2660.
10. Blessing EM, Steenkamp MM, Manzanares J, Marmar CR. Cannabidiol as a potential treatment for anxiety disorders. *Neurotherapeutics.* 2015;12(4):825–836.
11. Crippa JA, Zuardi AW, Garrido GEJ, et al. Effects of cannabidiol (CBD) on regional blood flow. *Neuropsychopharmacology.* 2004;29:417–426.
12. Zuardi AW, Cosme RA, Graeff FG, Guimarães FS. Effects of ipsapirone and cannabidiol on human experimental anxiety. *J Psychopharmacol.* 1993;7(1 Suppl):82–88.
13. Bergamashi MM, Queiroz RH, Chagas MH, et al. Cannabidiol reduces the anxiety induced by simulated public speaking in treatment-naïve social phobia patients. *Neuropsychopharmacology.* 2011;36(6):1219–1226.
14. Crippa JA, Derenusson GN, Ferrari TB, et al. Neural basis of anxiolytic effects of cannabidiol (CBD) in generalized social anxiety disorder: a preliminary report. *J Psychopharmacol.* 2011;25(1):121–130.
15. Zuardi AW, Rodrigues NP, Silva AL, et al. Inverted U-shaped dose-response curve of the anxiolytic effect of cannabidiol during public speaking in real life. *Front Pharmacol.* 2017;8:259.

16. Zuardi AW, Shirakawa I, Finkelfarb E, Karniol IG. Action of cannabidiol on the anxiety and other effects produced by delta-9-THC in normal subjects. *Psychopharmacology.* 1982;76:245–250.
17. Cuttler C, Spradlin A, McLaughlin RJ. Naturalistic examination of the perceived effects of cannabis on negative affect. *J Affect Disord.* 2018;235:198–205.
18. Kamal BS, Kamal F, Lantela DE. Cannabis and the anxiety of fragmentation: a systems approach for finding an anxiolytic cannabis chemotype. *Front Neurosci.* 2018;12:730.

16 Arthritis (Immune-Mediated)

ARTHRITIS (IMMUNE-MEDIATED) AND CANNABIS

Immune-mediated arthritis is distinguished from the more commonly found arthritis of aging, such as osteoarthritis (OA) (see Chapter 41), due to their differing pathophysiology. In research presented at the 2019 Annual European Congress of Rheumatology (EULAR) meeting, it was reported that of the 1,059 arthritis patients (OA and non-OA types), 37% have tried cannabis, and of those, 97% said it helped their symptoms.[1] Many immune-mediated arthritis patients find cannabis useful in treating the pain and stiffness caused by their disease. What is less commonly understood is that cannabis is a promising therapy to halt the progression of the disease due to its anti-inflammatory and immune-modulating effects.

As for all immune-mediated diseases, the endocannabinoid system has an important role in the modulation of immune-mediated arthritis.[2,3] The endocannabinoid system is activated in arthritis patients as shown by analysis of their synovial fluid. Not only are cannabinoid receptors found in joint tissue, but AEA and 2-AG were also identified in the synovial fluid of OA and rheumatoid arthritis (RA) patients, but not detected in synovial fluid from normal volunteers.[4] This report also notes that non-steroidal anti-inflammatory drugs (NSAIDs), which act via the inhibition of cyclooxygenase, have been shown to inhibit FAAH, suggesting that current treatment of inflammatory pain using NSAIDs may interact with endocannabinoid metabolism in addition to arachidonic acid metabolism. In RA, the main function of T-cells is to activate macrophages and fibroblasts transforming them into cells causing joint destruction. The endocannabinoid system and. by extension, cannabinoid agonists such as THC have a host of immunomodulatory effects, particularly on immune cells, including T cells, B cells and macrophages, generally causing a reduction in pro-inflammatory cytokines and an increase in anti-inflammatory cytokines.[5]

Immunomodulatory effects attributed to THC have been linked to activation of CB2 receptors.[2] Other pathways are involved in modulation of RA as well. Preclinical studies indicate that the effects of peripherally administered cannabinoids occurred via TRPV-1 ion channels, as well as cannabinoid receptors.[6] Less is known about CBD involvement in immune modulation, but it acts by alternative mechanisms, still being elucidated.[7] CBD has anti-inflammatory and anti-oxidative properties, both useful for RA. In a mouse study of collagen-induced arthritis, a model of arthritis that resembles RA, CBD administered after onset of clinical symptoms effectively blocked the progression of arthritis, by reducing cell-mediated joint destruction.[7] CBD effects included a dose-dependent suppression of lymphocyte proliferation. The doses used here were high, with optimal results found at 25 mg/kg per day orally. Such a dose would not be reached clinically in humans. Rheumatoid arthritis was one of the first conditions studied in a human clinical trial with a cannabis-based medicine (CBM), done in Great Britain in 2005. It employed a nabiximol extract with approximately a CBD/THC 1:1 ratio. Dosage was graduated until a mean of about 28 mg of cannabinoids/day. After a 5-week trial, they found that the CBM group showed a significant effect on easing pain, improving the quality of sleep, and on suppressing the disease as measured by the 28 joint disease activity score.[8] This study remains the only randomized, controlled trial of cannabis effects on RA to date. Several recent reviews show we have not made much progress with research, mainly due to lack of further human trials.[9,10] With regard to rheumatic disease, they conclude that there is limited evidence to support the therapeutic use of cannabinoids and question long-term risk. A later review states, "With only pharmaceutical preparations studied to date, and without any formal study of herbal cannabis preparations, no comment can be made regarding effects for herbal cannabis preparations in patients with rheumatic diseases."[11] Of course, that is not entirely correct, as the cannabis-based medicine used earlier is actually a plant extract. Cannabinoid acids (such as found in the raw plant) have also shown promise in in vitro studies of immune-mediated joint inflammation.[12] Although cannabis therapy has not yet been reported to effectively treat inflammatory/immune-mediated arthritis such as psoriatic arthritis, a new clinical trial is being conducted to study its effects on psoriatic arthritis subjects.[13] The study involves a very low dose of pure CBD, 10–30 mg/day, so any results have to be interpreted loosely, as therapeutic levels may not be reached. The conclusions reached for cannabis and rheumatoid arthritis may be applicable to all forms of immune-mediated arthritis.

Physicians are unclear about what to say to patients who want to use cannabis to treat RA. Results from a survey of Canadian rheumatologists published in 2017, most reported at least 1 query per week from patients seeking advice on the use of medical cannabis.[6] One review of the topic concluded that, "Cannabinoid therapy of RA could provide symptomatic relief to joint pain and swelling as well as suppressing joint destruction and disease progression."[14] it is clear that more research needs to be done on the use of cannabis in rheumatic diseases. That is why our experience with patients using all forms of cannabis, THC-rich, CBD-rich, vaporized or ingested often is the best current way to find answers.

PATIENT REPORTS

To move on to patient results from my practice, most of my patients with inflammatory arthritis were aged from their 30s to 70s at the time of presentation, with varying levels of pain. There was a wide range of products used for this condition. Some patients chose to use mostly THC, some mostly CBD, some topical primarily and all combinations thereof. The patients with psoriatic arthritis often continued the use of topicals begun earlier when their disease showed psoriasis only. Here are a few illustrative case reports.

RHEUMATOID ARTHRITIS (RA)

Patient 1: This is a 67-year-old female with a 15-year history of RA. Some joints were significantly affected with swelling and pain. She was taking Norco for the pain, five 10 mg tablets per day. She also had a long history of disease-modifying anti-rheumatic drug (DMARD) use, including Plaquenil, Methotrexate, Enbrel, Orencia and Remicade, all of which had stopped being helpful. Currently, she was using a prednisone regimen from 5 to 25 mg depending on the severity of her symptoms. She was new to cannabis use. She wanted to get off the Norco but had no alternative. I strongly advised her to start on a CBD/THC 1:1 tincture dosed at 10 mg 3x/day. She was leery of the THC and got a CBD/THC 20:1 tincture instead used at a dose of 5 mg/day. During the following year, she developed Bell's palsy and was started on gabapentin. Fortunately, she followed my weaning instructions and was off the Norco in a year. After this time, she was lost to follow-up.

Pearls: Is this an example of placebo effect or microdosing success? This is a rare case where a small dose of CBD was sufficient to manage her pain during an opiate wean. Or perhaps the addition of gabapentin contributed to her pain management. It taught me to never undermine a patient's belief in anticipating a positive outcome, even when the expectation of a result based on statistically significant dosing would be low.

Patient 2: This is a 57-year-old male with a 25-year history of RA in some daily pain. He described it as 3 on a scale of 10. It was being treated with methotrexate and naproxen 2x/day. He had knee, shoulder and big toe joint replacements. He was new to cannabis use. We started him on a CBD/THC 2:1 tincture with a dose of 15 mg 2x/day. After 1 year, his naproxen was cut in half, he stated he had less pain especially in his feet and ankles, and more importantly, he could stand longer, for up to 5 hours and be more active. This regimen continued throughout the following year with the same results.

Pearls: Pay attention to quality of life. Cannabis may not be able to cause a significant reduction in medication, but may be an adjunct to improved outcome. Being able to be more active was a great bonus for this gentleman.

Patient 3: This is a 52-year-old female with an 8-year history of RA. She also had a whiplash injury in the past resulting in chronic neck pain. She has been taking Humira since her diagnosis. At time of presentation, she was already using cannabis by vaporizing 3–5x/week. She was happy with this regimen. I advised her to add topical for her stiff neck and add a CBD-rich tincture. The next visit she reported relief with the topical and continued to vaporize, but methotrexate had been added to her medications. She now wanted to try CBD and switched to a CBD/THC 20:1 tincture at a dose of 10 mg daily. She was also using an indica tincture 10 mg 3x/week. She was able to discontinue methotrexate on this regimen. Her head and neck pain were improved as well.

Pearls: It's often difficult to get patients to try something new. In this case, it wasn't until our third visit that she increased her cannabis dose to a more therapeutic level. It may have been the fact of adding another medication that prompted her to use cannabis to try and replace it, and not just as an add-on.

Patient 4: This is a 70-year-old male with joint pain and swelling in the left first toe. His diagnosis was presumed arthritis, which was determined to be rheumatoid by subsequent testing. He had been smoking cannabis for 45 years. I advised the addition of topical cannabis for his toe. After the new diagnosis came in, I advised a CBD/THC 1:1 tincture 2–3×/day. The patient chose to use concentrated CBD-rich oil 3×/day instead, and continued to smoke cannabis. Over the 4 years we worked together, he did not take any prescription medicines, and managed his RA with cannabis only.

Pearls: This is an unusual presentation for an RA patient, not to be taking DMARDs, biologics or even NSAIDs as the majority of patients with this condition. It is most likely a milder case than ordinary, not presenting until older age, but it is indicative that long-term cannabis use might delay the progression of RA and that both THC-rich and CBD-rich cannabis can be an effective therapy.

REACTIVE ARTHRITIS

Patient 1: This is a 43-year-old male with reactive arthritis. He already had a hip replacement that failed and needed to be redone. He reported that the current reactive arthritis may have been related to high cobalt and chromium levels from the failed hip arthroplasty. He was already using cannabis as a medical marijuana patient at our first meeting, but not regularly, only smoking it occasionally. He was on prednisone, 20 mg/day for the past 2 months. By our next visit, the prednisone was down to 2.5 mg, but he was taking methotrexate and Remicade. He was also using an indica tincture before bed. I advised adding a CBD-rich tincture during the day. He continued to smoke cannabis in the evenings, sometimes used a tincture, yet had to resume a higher prednisone dose, 5 mg/day and went off methotrexate. This continued for the next few years as his arthritis moved into new joints.

Pearls: I don't think I was able to influence this patient. That happens a lot. Especially in adults in their 20s, 30s and 40s, smoking cannabis is their preferred route of administration. He thought he was doing well to keep his cannabis usage low, only in the evenings, and I wanted him to use more to help decrease inflammation. Now that the benefits of CBD are becoming more well-known, more patients will use it.

PSORIATIC ARTHRITIS

Patient 1: This is a 36-year-old female who came in complaining of arthritis for 5 years, for which she had been using cannabis medicinally. She was smoking rarely, using a CBD-rich edible daily and topical on her hands. The psoriatic arthritis diagnosis was still in question. Her only medication was Aleve or Tylenol. By the next year, she had graduated to THC-rich edibles 5 mg 2×/day, was smoking every night, and continued using a topical. By the next year, the diagnosis was confirmed, and her hand pain was worse. She was now using THC edibles and CBD edibles, smoking and topical. She said if she misses a dose, her pain is worse. She continued on this cannabis regimen with no other medications for the next few years.

Pearls: With this patient as with others with psoriatic arthritis, topical and internal cannabis seem to be additive. She was also significantly younger than most patients with psoriatic arthritis, and unusual in that she took no biologic medicine. Also unusual was the absence of psoriasis. It could be that topicals are more important in psoriatic arthritis as preventive for psoriasis.

Patient 2: This is a 57-year-old male with psoriasis and arthritis likely psoriatic. He had a 35-year history of cannabis use. He was using topical for psoriasis, vaporizing during the day and using an indica tincture at night. He also did ultraviolet light skin treatments. He basically continued on this regimen for years, adding a daytime CBD-rich tincture as well. He said the twice daily tincture kept his joints deinflamed. He was on no medications. His cannabis dosage was consistent and sufficient, approximately 10 mg by tincture 2×/day, plus additional 3×/day vaporizing, plus topical. Psoriasis remained mild on the cannabis plus UV regimen. The psoriatic arthritis did not seem to be progressing, nor was his joint pain increasing.

Pearls: This is again an example of cannabis likely replacing an immunosuppressive medication. It is rare for patients with psoriatic arthritis to remain stable and able to treat their pain without a pharmaceutical. It is tempting to postulate that the long history of cannabis use may have contributed to the expression of a milder disease than otherwise would have manifested.

CANNABIS THERAPY SUMMARY

I have found the need to educate my patients with immune-involved arthritis about the difference between pain relief with cannabis, which they all come in wanting, and therapeutic protocols needed to treat their disease. There are three levels of intervention here. Pain relief can be achieved with relatively low doses of CBD or THC, maybe 5–10 mg, or a few puffs by smoking or vaporizing. The next level is as an anti-inflammatory, which in itself reduces pain, but also can replace an anti-inflammatory medication. This may require a higher dose of CBD or THC or a mix, but it should be taken daily, not just after the pain has onset. And the deepest level may be its action as an immunomodulator, possibly acting as a DMARD. It is unclear what dose to suggest for this effect, but possibly this was achieved in some of the earlier patients. The results with the mouse model tested a high dose of pure CBD, 25 mg/kg, yet no evaluation of the minimum effective dose for disease modification has been done. In these patient reports I did not relate the use of topical for RA, but it should also be considered in these cases as well as for psoriatic arthritis. It does help for flare-ups, but it does not replace an internal dose in achieving the more intrinsic actions on the joints.

REFERENCES

1. Gelman L. 57% of arthritis patients have tried marijuana or CBD for medical reasons (and more than 90% say it helped). https://creakyjoints.org/eular-2019/medical-marijuana-cbd-usage-arthritis-patients-study/ Accessed March 5, 2020.
2. Gui H, Tong Q, Qu W, Mao CM, Dai SM. The endocannabinoid system and its therapeutic implications in rheumatoid arthritis. *Int Immunopharmacol.* 2015;26(1):86–91.
3. Barrie N, Manolios N. The endocannabinoid system in pain and inflammation: its relevance to rheumatic disease. *Eur J Rheumatol.* 2017;4(3):210–218.

4. Richardson D, Pearson RG, Kurian N, et al. Characterisation of the cannabinoid receptor system in synovial tissue and fluid in patients with osteoarthritis and rheumatoid arthritis. *Arthritis Res Ther.* 2008;10:43–57.
5. Nagarkatti P, Pandey R, Rieder SA, Hegde VL, Nagarkatti M. Cannabinoids as novel anti-inflammatory drugs. *Future Med Chem.* 2009;1(7):1333–1349.
6. Lampner, C. Cannabinoids in the treatment of RA: current status and future prospects. *Rheumatoid Arthritis Advisor.* May 20, 2019. www.rheumatologyadvisor.com/home/rheumatoid-arthritis-advisor/cannabinoids-in-the-treatment-of-ra-current-status-and-future-prospects/ Accessed May 30, 2020.
7. Malfait AM, Gallily R, Sumariwalla PF, et al. The nonpsychoactive cannabis constituent cannabidiol is an oral anti-arthritic therapeutic in murine collagen-induced arthritis. *Proc Natl Acad Sci.* 2000;97(17):9561–9566.
8. Blake DR, Robson P, Ho M, Jubb RW, McCabe CS. Preliminary assessment of the efficacy, tolerability and safety of a cannabis-based medicine (Sativex) in the treatment of pain caused by rheumatoid arthritis. *Rheumatology.* 2006;45:50–52.
9. Fitzcharles MA, McDougall J, Ste-Marie PA, Padjen I. Clinical implications for cannabinoid use in the rheumatic diseases. Potential for help or harm? *Arthritis Rheum.* 2012;64(8):2417–2425.
10. Katz-Talmor D, Katz I, Porat-Katz B, Shoenfeld Y. Cannabinoids for the treatment of rheumatic diseases: where do we stand? *Nat Rev Rheumatol.* 2018;14:488–498.
11. Fitzcharles MA, Ste-Marie PA, Häuser W. Efficacy, tolerability, and safety of cannabinoid treatments in the rheumatic diseases: a systematic review of randomized controlled trials. *Arthritis Care Res.* 2016;68(5):681–688.
12. Parker J, Atez F, Rossetti RG, Skulas A, Patel R, Zurier RB. Suppression of human macrophage interleukin-6 by a nonpsychoactive cannabinoid acid. *Rheumatol Int.* 2008;28:631–635.
13. Aalborg University Hospital Denmark. CBD treatment in hand osteoarthritis and psoriatic arthritis. https://clinicaltrials.gov/ct2/show/NCT03693833 Accessed March 9, 2020.
14. Croxford JL, Yamamura T. Cannabinoids and the immune system: potential for the treatment of inflammatory diseases? *J Neuroimmunol.* 2005;166(1–2):3–18.

17 Asthma, Chronic Obstructive Pulmonary Disease

ASTHMA, CHRONIC OBSTRUCTIVE PULMONARY DISEASE AND CANNABIS

The effect of cannabis on lung function has long been approached with negativity, as it has primarily been smoked until newer delivery methods have become available. Cannabis has historically served as an asthma treatment in the 1800s, indicating benefits as well as risks for this population of patients.[1] Although smoking is not a good idea for anyone with asthma, smoking cannabis has not been found to be as harmful as anticipated (see "Pulmonary Risks" in Chapter 6). A 2006 case-controlled study of 1,200 participants demonstrated that even heavy smoking of cannabis is not associated with lung cancer and other types of upper aerodigestive tract cancers.[2] A review of cannabis smoking and cancer concluded that, "Results from our pooled analyses provide little evidence for an increased risk of lung cancer among habitual or long-term cannabis smokers."[3] A review of the literature found that short-term cannabis smoking is associated with bronchodilation, while long-term cannabis smoking is associated with increased respiratory symptoms suggestive of obstructive lung disease. This was later shown to be unsubstantiated.[4] The acute bronchodilatory effect of cannabis by inhalation does occur and is transient, lasting approximately 60 minutes. As expected, a review of cannabis smoking reiterated that it is contraindicated in patients with asthma or respiratory disease.

> Several papers have shown the relationship between marijuana use and increase in asthma and other allergic diseases symptoms, as well as the increased frequency of medical visits. This narrative review emphasizes the importance to consider cannabis as a precipitating factor for acute asthma and allergic attacks in clinical practice.[5]

This applies to smoking only and has not been shown for alternative delivery methods.

Cannabinoids are well-known for their anti-inflammatory effects. While most studies thus far on cannabis and asthma have focused primarily on the bronchodilatory effect, some have also observed a reduction in bronchial inflammation.[6,7] THC has long been known to be a bronchodilator. As long ago as the 1970s, cannabis was shown to cause a reversal of exercise-induced asthma and hyperinflation.[8] Still in the 1970s, THC proved to be an effective bronchodilator in a study of human subjects at low doses, 100–200 μg, delivered by aerosolized inhaler. Maximum improvement was seen at approximately 60 minutes and was sustained for at least 3 hours, with

DOI: 10.1201/9781003098201-28

improvement of forced expiratory volume (FEV) 1 lasting for more than 6 hours after dosing.[9]

> Recent large studies have shown that, instead of reducing forced expiratory volume in 1 s {second} and forced vital capacity (FVC), marijuana smoking is associated with increased FVC. The cause of this is unclear, but acute bronchodilator and anti-inflammatory effects of cannabis may be relevant.[10]

Later research proved that this effect is mediated by cannabinoid agonism, with CB1 inhibition of bronchomotor tone.[11] CB2 receptors are thought to be involved in mechanisms for neurogenic inflammation acting through the sensory nerves, thus having potential therapeutic value for allergic asthma.[12]

Both THC and CBD are anti-inflammatory and muscle relaxant, but, contrary to the many claims for the value of CBD, it is not a bronchodilator. A study of the effect of several cannabinoids on pulmonary function in animals showed significant differences between them. THC and THCV inhibited induced tracheal contractions, CBD did not. THC also performed better in suppressing cough. A combination of CBD and THC did not differ from THC alone, indicating a combination might be useful.[13] Some researchers have suggested that CBD and THC may decrease swelling in the lungs and help to open the airways in people with chronic obstructive pulmonary disease (COPD). Smoking anything, of course, poses a risk for those with respiratory disease. A survey of tobacco and cannabis smokers found that cannabis smokers had no more COPD or respiratory symptoms than non-smokers, but that smoking both tobacco and cannabis synergistically increased the risk of respiratory symptoms and COPD.[14]

Vaporizing is a preferred method of delivery as it provides direct medicinal action to the lungs upon inhalation without smoke. Findings from the few studies that do attempt to isolate the respiratory risk associated with vaporizers all demonstrate some level of benefit.[1] A report in 1975 that nebulized inhaled THC could be irritating to asthmatic subjects resulting in cough involved high (20 mg) doses of THC.[8] Conversely, the acute effects of vaporized cannabis on airway function in adults with advanced COPD showed no harm; again, high doses were used. The effect of 35 mg of inhaled vaporized THC cannabis showed no positive or negative effect on airway function, exertional breathlessness and exercise endurance in adults with advanced COPD.[15] In a review of vaporization on respiratory function, the conclusion is that there needs to be more research.

> The possibility that vaporized cannabis might have a salutary effect on breathlessness and exercise performance in symptomatic patients with COPD has not been excluded. . . . Larger randomized clinical trials are needed with a broader study population that includes symptomatic patients with less advanced COPD.[16]

Cannabis itself can provide increased benefit above and beyond the effects of the cannabinoids, due to the selection of cultivars with appropriate terpene content. For example, α-pinene aids in bronchodilation and β-myrcene aids in muscle relaxation. The use of such whole plant material in a vaporizer may yield the most positive results.

PATIENT REPORTS

To move on to patient results from my practice, asthma was present in some of the pediatric cases as well as through all ages. I did treat some patients with COPD in their 70s. The more common situation was that patients with multiple conditions, including asthma, wanted advice about using cannabis with least harm to their asthma or COPD, rather than using cannabis as a direct treatment for their respiratory condition. Here are a few illustrative case reports.

Patient 1: This is a 67-year-old female seen for pain in her back and knees. Asthma was one of the reasons she didn't want to smoke it. She was using an albuterol inhaler up to 3×/day, using 5 mg Norco 2×/day and was also on Celebrex. She used little cannabis. After a year on a CBD/THC 20:1 tincture 2×/day advised for her pain, the pain was the same, but she was down to 1×/day of her inhaler, off the Norco and Celebrex. By the next year, she had added a THC-rich chocolate to help with sleep and found she did not need to use the inhaler at all.

Pearls: This is not primarily an asthma case, but it is a typical asthma case. Patients find relief with their asthma while they least expect it. The gains this patient made by getting off of Norco and Celebrex might overshadow getting off of albuterol, but these all were welcome outcomes. The anti-inflammatory and relaxation benefit of the CBD-rich tincture may have eased her asthma, as bronchodilation would not be expected to result from CBD-rich cannabis.

Patient 2: This is a 72-year-old female with significant back pain due to scoliosis and adult-onset diabetes, also with severe asthma. She was new to cannabis use. Her medications included Singulair, Spiriva, Arcapta, Pulmocort and Brovana nebulizer for her asthma, as well as diabetes medicines, but no pain medicine. She reported that spinal injections were no help for back pain. She had been using a cane to ambulate for 5 years, due to the curvature of her spine, which caused pain in her shoulder. She started on a CBD/THC 1:1 tincture, 10 mg used every night and sometimes during the day. There was no change in her medications, but her back felt better. She continued on this dose for several years and also added topical for joint pain. Her asthma medications remained the same.

Pearls: This is a patient who was in significant pain, yet wanted to avoid opiates due to their negative effect on her impaired respiratory system. She found relief with cannabis, at no risk to her advanced asthma. Unfortunately, her asthma did not improve, but it was not aggravated by this non-smoked cannabis therapy.

Patient 3: This is a 58-year-old male who came in with a primary complaint of insomnia but no history of asthma. He had a 40-year history of using cannabis, currently 4×/day by pipe. He had smoked tobacco for 35 years, but had stopped 5 years prior. I advised an indica tincture or capsule at night for sleep, and to discontinue the nighttime smoked dose. By the next year, he was sleeping better, and still using a pipe 4×/day. He developed lung infections the following year with asthma and cough as sequelae. Inhalers and antibiotics were little help. He was treated with steroids, more inhalers and generally did not get much better. At our next visit, I urged that he stop smoking cannabis and switch to a THC-rich tincture or low-dose edible. I wanted to avoid even vaporizing during his respiratory illness. For a while, he did not use cannabis at all. He had to be hospitalized for his pulmonary condition, which was finally thought to be a case of fungal overgrowth. After 3 years of following this patient with continued wheezing, while continuing to need 3 inhalers and steroids daily, he never did switch to edibles or vaping, but resumed smoking cannabis 2–3x/day.

Pearls: This is a smoker. Although we didn't document it, cannabis likely facilitated this patient getting off tobacco, although stopping cannabis smoking was challenging. To continue to smoke anything with asthma, not even to switch to a vaporizer was a lost opportunity for improved function. Not all patients listen to your advice.

Patient 4: This is a 74-year-old female who presented with insomnia, hypertension and COPD. She had been using cannabis for the past several years as a medical cannabis patient. She had a history of tobacco use, but had stopped 5 years ago. She was also on multiple inhalers, including Spiriva, Asmanex and nebulizers. I advised her to use cannabis by tincture or edible, about 5 mg 2x/day, which allowed her to discontinue Trazodone and Diovan. She said the blood pressure medicine contributed to "gasping for air" and she felt better off of it.

Pearls: This case is an example of a compliant patient, who can benefit from cannabis even with COPD. In cases with COPD we do not expect to see much positive or negative effect on pulmonary function with cannabis use. The patient here was able to discontinue medicines for hypertension and insomnia, but not for COPD, although relaxation and better sleep were contributing to a better quality of life.

Patient 5: This is a 36-year-old male, already a medical cannabis patient for 1 year, with asthma. He reported that vaporizing full flower, a sativa hybrid strain, twice a day allowed him to discontinue Advair. He was still taking Singulair daily with rare use of an albuterol inhaler. He preferred cannabis to Advair as he was a proponent of natural medicines. He stopped tobacco 1 year prior, so the decreased need for Advair may have been due to improved pulmonary function. At our last visit, I advised seeking a strain rich in α-pinene as the effect of terpenes was now becoming more well-known.

Pearls: One might surmise that cannabis replaced Advair in this patient, although his condition likely improved due to stopping tobacco. It's not clear whether vaporizing cannabis was helpful in making that transition, which in itself is significant. I have not found it prevalent that vaporizing such a small amount of cannabis, twice/day, is as effective as pharmaceuticals in most asthma patients.

CANNABIS THERAPY SUMMARY

Cannabis delivery for respiratory disease must be chosen judiciously. While tinctures and edibles pose no risk, it is possible that certified, purified cannabis free of mold, pesticides and solvents delivered through a full flower vaporizer would be most efficacious for such patients. On the rare occasion that a patient was using cannabis primarily for asthma relief, my advice was to vaporize full flower from an α-pinene-rich strain. I actually asked the patients to smell the flowers at the dispensary and choose a pine scented one. Vaporizer pens should be avoided because the oils usually did not contain the terpenes, and because not all brands were free of petrochemical residue. There are some new inhalers in a metered dose form, containing cannabis and selected terpenes that have recently become available. Those with α-pinene would be excellent for treatment of asthma, as they would be bronchodilating. A cannabis inhaler has been marketed that contains 6.5–7 mg THC and 1–2 mg of terpenes in each dispensation.[17] When aerosolized inhalers become more widely available, these would be my first choice for asthma relief.

Cannabis is not ordinarily utilized to treat COPD, but it is good to know that it not only does not harm patients with COPD, but may actually increase their FVC. In some cases, the muscle-relaxant properties of cannabis, especially cultivars with β-myrcene, can bring relief to chest wall and diaphragmatic spasms. Typically, THC-rich cannabis is indicated for bronchodilation, yet CBD-containing products will also aid in muscle relaxation and decrease inflammation in cases of atopic respiratory disease.

REFERENCES

1. Loflin M, Earleywine M. No smoke, no fire: what the initial literature suggests regarding vapourized cannabis and respiratory risk. *Can J Respir Ther.* 2015;51(1):7–9.
2. Tashkin DP. Effects of marijuana smoking on the lung. *Ann Am Thorac Soc.* 2013;10(3):239–247.
3. Zhang LR, Morgenstern H, Greenland S, et al. Cannabis smoking and lung cancer risk: pooled analysis in the International Lung Cancer Consortium. *Int J Cancer.* 2015;136(4): 894–903.
4. Tetrault JM, Crothers K, Moore BA, et al. Effects of marijuana smoking on pulmonary function and respiratory complications: a systematic review. *Arch Intern Med.* 2007;167:221–228.
5. Chatkin JM, Zani-Silva L, Ferreira I, Zamel N. Cannabis-associated asthma and allergies. *Clin Rev Allergy Immunol.* 2019;56:196–206.
6. Williams SJ, Hartley JP, Graham JD. Bronchodilator effect of delta1-tetrahydrocannabinol administered by aerosol of asthmatic patients. *Thorax.* 1976;31(6):720–723.
7. Turcotte C, Blanchet M, Laviolette M, Flamand N. Impact of cannabis, cannabinoids, and endocannabinoids in the lungs. *Front Pharmacol.* 2016;7:317.
8. Tashkin DP, Shapiro BJ, Lee YE, Harper CE. Effects of smoked marijuana in experimentally induced asthma. *Am Rev Respir Dis.* 1975;112(3):377–386.
9. Hartley JP, Nogrady SG, Seaton A. Bronchodilator effect of delta1-tetrahydrocannabinol. *Br J Clin Pharmacol.* 1978;5(6):523–525.
10. Ribeiro L, Ind PW. Marijuana and the lung: hysteria or cause for concern? *Breathe.* 2018;14:196–205.
11. Grassin-Delyle S, Naline E, Buenestado A, et al. Cannabinoids inhibit cholinergic contraction in human airways through prejunctional CB1 receptors. *Br J Pharmacol.* 2014;171:2767–2777.
12. Bozkurt TE. Endocannabinoid system in the airways. *Molecules.* 2019;24(24):4626.
13. Makwana R, Venkatasamy R, Spina D, Page C. The effect of phytocannabinoids on airway hyper-responsiveness, airway inflammation, and coughs. *Pharmacol Exp Ther.* 2015;353:169–180.
14. Tan WC, Lo C, Jong A, et al. Marijuana and chronic obstructive lung disease: a population-based study. *CMAJ.* 2009;180(8):814–820.

15. Abdallah S, Smith BM, Ware MA, et al. Effect of vaporized cannabis on exertional breathlessness and exercise endurance in advanced chronic obstructive pulmonary disease. A randomized controlled trial. *Ann Am Thorac Soc.* 2018;15(10):1137–1138.
16. Tashkin DP. Vaping cannabis and chronic obstructive pulmonary disease. *Ann Am Thor Soc.* 2018;15(10):1137–1145.
17. Russo EB. Taming THC: potential cannabis synergy and phytocannabinoid-terpenoid entourage effects. *Br J Pharmacol.* 2011;163(7):1344–1364.

18 Attention-Deficit Hyperactivity Disorder

ATTENTION-DEFICIT HYPERACTIVITY DISORDER AND CANNABIS

Attention-deficit hyperactivity disorder (ADHD) predominantly appears in young adults although some older adults continue to be affected by it. Evaluating the use of cannabis for this condition is complicated by consideration of its effects in those under 21. One must consider the risk/benefit ratio of the effects of cannabis on youth, as compared with those of the alternatives, often stimulant medications. Treatment with stimulants may lead to insomnia, anorexia or increased stress. As expected, the efficacy of cannabis to help ADHD has mixed reviews. As with all mood disorders, the use of cannabis has historically been considered to be detrimental and classified as a substance of abuse. Some poorly designed studies have tried to associate cannabis use with the development of ADHD. In testing adults who were diagnosed with ADHD and who self-reported use of cannabis, causality between cannabis and ADHD was not found. It was concluded that individuals who began using cannabis regularly before age 16 might have poorer executive functioning (i.e., decision-making, working memory and response inhibition) than users who began later. That's equivalent to saying it seems to be OK for adult use, we don't know about its safety in developing brains, at least under age 16.[1] One study questioned whether continued cannabis use during treatment of comorbid cocaine dependence and ADHD leads to poorer treatment outcome. What they found, however, was significantly better treatment retention among intermittent-moderate cannabis users compared to abstainers and heavy-consistent users (based on % of positive urine samples). They concluded that "The findings suggest that future medication development efforts should consider medication acting at the cannabinoid receptors levels, possibly as partial agonist."[2]

Endocannabinoid activity or dysregulation is implicated in ADHD.[3] Cannabinoid receptor agonists such as THC have been demonstrated to induce dopamine (DA) release in the human striatum.[4] This action is similar to stimulants that directly increase DA levels. Another hypothesis for cannabinoid action is by increasing DA levels indirectly by blocking the action of GABA.[5] Alternatively, cannabinoids may directly activate TRPV1 receptors, which have been found in some dopaminergic pathways, allowing a direct regulation of DA function.[6] However, the enhancement of DA following cannabis use is not a consistent finding. The mechanism by which cannabis may affect ADHD is as yet unclear, and may have less to do with cannabinoids than with terpenes or the combination, because cultivar specificity is an overriding factor in choosing the best medicine for an individual patient.

There are several anecdotal reports of cannabis use in ADHD, often THC-rich strains are utilized.[7,8] One US survey suggested that cannabis was more likely to be

DOI: 10.1201/9781003098201-29

used for the hyperactivity type (type I).[9] In a six-country survey of (illegal) cannabis cultivators, ADHD was the fifth most commonly reported medical reason to grow and use cannabis, 15% of the responders, although use for ADHD was hypothesized to be greater in Northern Scandinavian countries.[10] In a study of 30 ADHD patients using smoked cannabis, 8 patients continued to take stimulants and combined them with cannabis, and 22 patients used it solely. All patients experienced an improvement of a variety of symptoms by cannabis, including improved concentration and sleep and reduced impulsivity. In five cases dronabinol was used, which was also effective.[11] A rare clinical study of a 6-week trial of nabiximols (Sativex), a cannabis extract containing a CBD/THC in approximately a 1:1 ratio, was done in 30 adults with ADHD. The mean number of sprays/day was 4.7, close to 25 mg of cannabinoids, dosed approximately every 3–4 hours. They found no significant memory or cognitive impairment by adding cannabis, but improvement was not statistically significant. But the cannabis extract group reported reduced hyperactivity/impulsivity symptoms as well as improved emotional lability.[12] It could be that low doses of a stimulating THC-rich cultivar would have provided more positive results, and this should be studied.

PATIENT REPORTS

To move on to patient results from my practice, most of these were younger, from 6 years old through the 20s, 30s and 40s. Mostly the cannabis used for this condition is traditionally THC-rich, sativa during the day and indica at night for sleep if needed. I did not note CBD to be particularly useful, nor did the patients stay on it if advised. Smoking or vaporizing were the preferred routes of administration for most of these patients, as is common for their age group. Here are a few illustrative case reports.

Patient 1: This is a 27-year-old male with multiple mood diagnoses, including ADHD, depression, bipolar disorder and anxiety. ADHD was diagnosed at age 6, the remaining diagnoses in his 20s. He had used Adderall in high school, then stopped and resumed 2 years ago, presenting at a dose of 60 mg/day. He was also on Valium for social phobia 10 mg 2x/day, Ambien to sleep and hydrocodone for knee pain. He used a significant amount of cannabis daily, up to 3 ounces/month but didn't have good access. He said, "It makes me feel like a new person when I can get it." I advised him to smoke varying strains during the day in response to his mood, that is, sativa for depression, a relaxing strain for anxiety and an indica edible at night. By the next year, he was down to 40 mg/day of Adderall, was on no Ambien and no Valium, His psychiatrist was supportive of the weaning of his medications. He was off the hydrocodone as well. At his next annual visit, he was off the Adderall and was doing relatively well. He reported that the weaning was challenging, that he got tired and irritated, but cannabis helped. He was smoking quite a bit, 2 ounces/month, 5–6x/day. At this point, he was ready to try some CBD, and his ongoing regimen moved into smoking less, 1 ounce per month, including a CBD-rich strain to relax in the evenings.

Pearls: Patients with ADHD in childhood often have multiple diagnoses and psych meds in adulthood. This patient was heavily medicated, yet ultimately seemed to do better off of everything. With professional guidance, he learned to use less of all of his meds, including cannabis. I believe that using appropriate cultivars was essential to this success.

Patient 2: This is a 40-year-old male with ADHD and bipolar disorder. He had a history of drug use with alcohol and methamphetamine, no longer current. He was a long-time daily cannabis user, smoking a bong several times a day. He was also taking Adderall 40 mg/day, having been on it for 15 years, as well as Lamictal and Prozac. We discussed appropriate strains to reduce his medications. He had access as he was a grower. We decided on a sativa strain to replace Adderall and a CBD/THC hybrid to help him relax. On this regimen he felt well, but still smoked 5×/day. He was off Lamictal and Prozac and had reduced Adderall to 25 mg/day. Over the next 2 years, he got off the Adderall but resumed Prozac 20 mg/day. He continued to smoke about 1 gram/day with a one-month tolerance break annually.

Pearls: As in the previous case, this is a habitual cannabis smoker. Does that mean he's not using it as medicine? When we started working together, he was using it all, 3 medications and cannabis. Now off 2 of the pharmaceuticals, he's comfortable with his herbal lifestyle. In a chronic cannabis user, a tolerance break facilitates ongoing efficacy of the medicine.

Patient 3: This is a 17-year-old female with ADHD, PTSD and exercise-induced asthma. Being a minor, she came in with her mother, who was required to sign the caregiver certificate. She's been on ADHD medications since age 14, now Adderall 15–20 mg/day, also Trazodone 200 mg to help with sleep, Prozac 30 mg and Singulair. We came up with a plan to use an indica edible for sleep, and to use Adderall only in the a.m. at half-dose. During the day, she was to experiment with a THC-rich stimulating strain or hybrid or CBD-rich stimulating strain. These are hard to come by, but a CBD-rich strain with α-pinene and D-limonene might be good for her. At our next visit, she was sleeping well on a 15-mg cannabis chocolate, was off Trazodone, Adderall was at 10 mg/day and Prozac had gone up to 40 mg. By the next year, she was off all her medications, still using the indica chocolate to sleep, eating better and smoking with a water pipe for some nausea. Her regimen has remained the same for years, except that now she dabs 2×/day pre-meals instead of using a bong. I advised her to be wary of excessive use of a concentrate and suggested she try vaping instead.

Pearls: Cannabis helped this young woman during a crucial time in development, from age 17 to 20. She did not abuse it and was able to use different products, one to focus during the day, and another to sleep at night. Note that "dabbing" is a delivery choice that many teens experiment with, and it rapidly can become excessive. It's almost always useful to dissuade young people from this choice.

Patient 4: This is a 10-year-old female with ADHD, also diagnosed with high-functioning autism. Her cognitive skills showed she was learning appropriate for her grade level, but behaviorally she was aggressive, impulsive and poor at taking direction. She was on no medications. At our meeting, she had rapid speech and was unable to sit still for long, yet understood what she was there for. Clearly, this was a case where calming was in order, so we focused on a CBD-rich regimen. We titrated her up to a dose of 35 mg of a CBD/THC 25:1 tincture, taken in the morning and early afternoon. Her weight was low at 70 lb, so this was a high daily dose, 1 mg/lb. It was calming and her behavior improved. She was able to go to a class for the first time in years. Mom wanted to try increasing the dose, and went up to 75 mg 2×/day also with good results. I became concerned about tolerance and suggested a maintenance dose of 50 mg 2×/day, with the possibility of skipping 1–2 doses/week. This worked well for the next year, where two afternoon doses/week were eliminated. She continued with home schooling and benefitted from behavioral therapy, which was now helpful for the first time.

Pearls: The profile for hyperactivity and the type of attention deficit is crucial in understanding whether calming or stimulating effects are best. Whereas THC-rich cannabis may help the majority of ADHD patients focus, for this patient with ongoing impulsivity and aggression, CBD-rich cannabis is a better choice.

CANNABIS THERAPY SUMMARY

There are many factors that are involved in causing an individual's attention deficit symptoms beyond whether hyperactivity is or is not part of the picture. For example, if hyperactivity is present, then a calming effect may be helpful with CBD, which is not ordinarily used to replace a stimulant. One of my patients who had a problem with focus, complained of "burnout" and was on Adderall benefitted from a restorative CBD/THC mix daily. Especially with type A individuals who can tolerate a lot of stress, introducing cannabis as a relaxant is wise. Yet for the inattentive or mixed type of ADHD, a stimulant effect with more THC may be more appropriate. Further, there is often the complication of a patient currently taking pharmaceutical medication, or having to adjust cannabis dosing while stopping his/her medication. In addition, there are many variable effects of cannabis, depending on the strain used and preparation method. The inclusion of α-pinene in choice of cultivar aids focus and is quite helpful with or without hyperactivity. Some of my patients have found success with newly released formulations containing THCV, which can provide focus without psychoactivity. There is always caution in recommending cannabis to youth (see Chapter 10). This is a personal decision, but it may be fair to say that cannabis would be recommended more to treat adult ADHD than for a childhood diagnosis. Perhaps THCV may have a role here. Nevertheless, when faced with the effects of a stimulant versus the effects of cannabis, some parents and youth choose the herbal compound.

REFERENCES

1. Tamm L, Epstein JN, Lisdahl KM, et al. Impact of ADHD and cannabis use on executive functioning in young adults. *Drug Alcohol Depend.* 2013;133(2):607–614.
2. Aharonovich E, Garawi F, Bisaga A, et al. Concurrent cannabis use during treatment for comorbid ADHD and cocaine dependence: effects on outcome. *Am J Drug Alcohol Abuse.* 2006;32(4):629–635.
3. Millichap JG. Altered anandamide degradation in attention deficit hyperactivity disorder. *Pediatr Neurol Briefs.* 2009;23(6):46.
4. Bossong MG, van Berckel BN, Boellaard R, et al. Delta 9-tetrahydrocannabinol induces dopamine release in the human striatum. *Neuropsychopharmacology.* 2009;34(3):759–766.
5. Giuffrida A, Piomelli D. The endocannabinoid system: a physiological perspective on its role in psychomotor control. *Chem Phys Lipids.* 2000;108:151–158.

6. Fernández-Ruiz J, Hernández M, Ramos JA. Cannabinoid-dopamine interaction in the pathophysiology and treatment of CNS disorders. *CNS Neurosci Ther.* 2010;16:e72–91.
7. Strohbeck-Kuehner P, Skopp G, Mattern R. 2008. Cannabis improves symptoms of ADHD. *Cannabinoids.* 2008;3(1):1–3.
8. Hupli AMM. Medical cannabis for adult attention deficit hyperactivity disorder: sociological patient case report of cannabinoid therapeutics in Finland. *Med Cannabis Cannabinoids.* 2018;1:112–118.
9. Loflin M, Earleywine M, De Leo J, Hobkirk A. Subtypes of attention deficit-hyperactivity disorder (ADHD) and cannabis use. *Subst Use Misuse.* 2014;49(4):427–434.
10. Pedersen W. From badness to illness: medical cannabis and self-diagnosed attention deficit hyperactivity disorder. *Addict Res Theory.* 2015;23(3):177–186.
11. Milz E, Grotenhermen F. Successful therapy of treatment resistant adult ADHD with cannabis: experience from a medical practice with 30 patients. www.drmilz.de/wp-content/uploads/Poster-CC-2015.pdf Accessed January 10, 2020.
12. Cooper RE, Williams E, Seegobin S, et al. Cannabinoids in attention-deficit/hyperactivity disorder: a randomised-controlled trial. *Eur Neuropsychopharmacol.* 2017; 27(8):795–808.

19 Autism Spectrum Disorder

AUTISM SPECTRUM DISORDER AND CANNABIS

There are few treatments for autism spectrum disorder (ASD), also generally referred to as autism. Those that are tried, such as antipsychotic medications, have little success with many unwanted side effects. Clearly, a new therapy that might show promise would be welcome. This may come in the form of CBD-rich cannabis.[1] The etiology of ASD is poorly understood, yet endocannabinoid involvement is being explored as a regulatory mechanism. It is thought that the endocannabinoid system is involved in autism, evidenced by decreased anandamide (AEA) levels. Anandamide was measured to be significantly lower in plasma of ASD children compared with levels in control children. The likelihood of manifesting ASD was found to be correlated with decreasing levels of AEA.[2] A possible regulatory mechanism may be increased expression of cannabinoid receptors (CBrs). In support of this hypothesis, high expression of CB2 was documented peripheral blood mononuclear cells of children diagnosed with ASD.[3] Studies on socially impaired mice showed that FAAH blockade reversed social impairment by a CB1 agonism mechanism. In contrast to socially impaired mice, normal mice did not alter their social approach with increasing AEA. The authors conclude that anandamide-mediated endocannabinoid signaling might help to alleviate social impairment in ASD.[4] In practice, we see treatment focused on utilizing CBD or CBD-rich cannabis. We recall that CBD does not bind directly to CBrs, but is expected to increase AEA levels, and exerts anxiolytic effects at serotonin receptors, among other actions.

A review of cannabis use for autism concluded, "Only five small studies were identified that have specifically examined cannabis use in ASD. Studies revealed mixed and inconclusive findings."[5] Nevertheless, there has been a growing body of anecdotal evidence from doctors and parents on the efficacy of cannabis for autism.[6] In a self-reported study of parents administering CBD to their children with ASD for 2 months, there was significant symptomatic improvement. Self-injury, rage, aggression, hyperactivity, sleep and anxiety were improved in almost half or more of the participants. The actual dosage was not reported, but recommended to be at a maximum of 600 mg/day of CBD and 40 mg/day of THC, provided in a CBD/THC 20:1 cannabis oil extract.[7] Small clinical studies have just recently been reported. In a study conducted in Israel, 60 children who were resistant to standard therapy were treated using cannabis oil with a CBD/THC 20:1 ratio for at least 7 months. The dose was up-titrated to effect (maximal CBD dose – 10 mg/kg/day). The researchers found that cannabis treatment improved the functioning of 80% of the children, 50% improved in communication and 40% showed decreased anxiety. According to the primary investigator for the study,

DOI: 10.1201/9781003098201-30

"There are theories for why medical cannabis can alleviate symptoms of autism, but we don't know exactly how."[8] In fact, we do know that CBD is helpful for relaxation and decreasing anxiety, is antipsychotic, anti-inflammatory and anti-convulsant, to name but a few properties but perhaps its action at inhibiting FAAH thereby increasing AEA is most relevant.[9] In a larger recent study, also in Israel, 188 ASD patients were treated with a medical cannabis oil containing 30% CBD and 1.5% THC. Symptoms inventory, patient global assessment and side effects were assessed. After 6 months of treatment, 30% reported a significant improvement, 54% moderate, 6% slight and 9% no change.[10] In another pilot study of only 15 patients, standardized CBD-enriched cannabis extract (with a CBD/THC ratio of 75:1) was given providing an average initial dose of CBD of 2.90 mg/kg/day titrated up to 4.55 mg/kg/day. After 6–9 months the strongest improvements were reported for seizures, attention-deficit hyperactivity disorder, sleep disorders and communication and social interaction deficits. Nine of the ten non-epileptic patients showed improvement equal to or above 30% in at least one of eight categories, six presented improvement of 30% or more in at least two categories and four presented improvement equal to or above 30% in at least four symptom categories. Ten out of the 15 patients were using other medicines, and nine of these were able to keep the improvements even after reducing or withdrawing other medications.[11]

More studies are in the works. The Center for Medicinal Cannabis Research (CMCR) at the UC San Diego School of Medicine is investigating this question. The goals of the trial include determining whether CBD is safe, tolerable and effective in children with autism; whether and how CBD alters neurotransmitters, if it improves brain connectivity, and whether brain inflammation is altered by CBD. Yet another clinical trial testing the effect of cannabidivarin (CBDV) is planned to see whether it is effective to improve behaviors of children with autism by dosing of 10 mg/kg/day of CBDV for 12 weeks.[12] And we must be clear, that the preliminary results of the Israeli studies were obtained using a cannabis extract, not pure CBD. The effects and dosages of pure cannabinoids would not be identical to extracted full-spectrum cannabis oil. There is interest in conducting a clinical trial with Epidiolex, the only FDA-approved form of CBD extracted from cannabis (approved for certain seizure disorders), for outcomes in ASD patients. The lead investigator is an author of a commentary regarding the utility of CBD for ASD. He states, "Ultimately, a physician's decision to utilize CBD in the management of children with ASD will be guided by the limited research findings, her or his clinical expertise and preference, as well as the parent's values and wishes."[13]

PATIENT REPORTS

To move on to patient results from my practice, I saw the greatest benefit with a low percentage THC, CBD-rich product as expected. The patients ranged in age from 5 to 53 years. Most used tinctures due to ease of measuring and supplying the medicine, by the drop. Many were minors or lived in care facilities and had their medicine dispensed to them. Often, I was required to write explicit instructions on dosage and delivery to meet the requirements of the facility. Here are a few illustrative case reports.

Patient 1: This is an adult with autism. He is a 28-year-old male who was very high functioning. He lived in a supportive living environment with caregiver supervision. He was able to talk, but preferred to communicate by writing on a tablet. He also had episodic problems with seizures, rarely onset in the past 2 years, one-two times/ year, for which he was on anti-seizure medications. In this case as the seizures were mostly well-controlled, we focused on cannabis for the autism. His mother brought him in for cannabis to increase seizure control, reduce stress and to help focus. His cognition was good. He was able to write full sentences on his tablet and understand what I told him. When he spoke it was loud, and with a high-pitched whine. He was new to cannabis use. His medications included Xanax and Depakene. This is some of what he wrote to his care team after our visit:

> Hello everyone, I am writing to inform you that I have decided to try a small dose of ACDC which has 1.05% of THC and 18.9% of CBD. My goal is to eventually get off of Depokene in the future. . . . Please see the enclosed business card for more information. You can also see "Weed I" and "Weed II" on UTUBE with Dr. Sanja Gubda.

As you can see, he was quite high functioning, so he was able to give me direct feedback about the effects of the CBD-rich tincture he took. He came in 6 months later reporting increased fatigue and anger on 10 mg 3x/day of the 20:1 CBD mix. He said he thinks it's helping a lot with stress, which was high due to the death of a close family member during this time. He had one seizure during this time, which he was told could be brought on by stress or lack of sleep. We began to titrate his CBD tincture dose upward to 20 mg a.m. and afternoon, and 10 mg at night. We also added a CBD spray in the event of a seizure for immediate relief. With continued anger in the afternoons, we increased his afternoon dose to 45 mg. At our next visit, Zoloft had been added to his medications, and he had a new EEG, which confirmed the diagnosis of generalized epilepsy syndrome. At our next visit, a year later, he reported his seizure medicine had been changed to Lamictal, his CBD dose remained the same. His only complaint was that his sleep was poor due to 3–5x/night nocturia. He reported that he discontinued his nighttime CBD dose on the recommendation of his urologist who thought it might be waking him up, which was likely the case. And a year later, he was stable but wanted to reduce his Zoloft, now 100 mg 2x/day. He thought CBD could help. I did speak with him about strategies for reducing the Zoloft by using 5-HTP, but his CBD dose remained the same.

Pearls: This high-functioning autistic young man knew what he wanted: to get off his medications. The 20:1 tincture helped calm him, and destress him, and possibly even aided his socialization. He was getting regular exercise and taking a class at the community college during this time. But he wasn't able to reduce any of his medications. And as far as nocturia is concerned, it's possible that the CBD-rich cannabis may have exacerbated this known potential side effect of sertraline at high doses. There is evidence that CBD interacts with serotonin receptors.

Patient 2: This is a 16-year-old male with autism and recent signs of aggression, with violent outbursts. He lived in a group home during the weekdays and was at home on weekends. His mother was concerned about the aggression. His medications included Ativan, guanfacine, Lexapro and a lot of Seroquel, 250 mg/day. He was new to cannabis use. During our visit, he was sedated on Ativan and sat in the chair. His communication skills were minimal. His cognition had been measured to be at kindergarten level. He was somewhat overweight with facial acne. I suggested he start on a CBD/THC 20:1 tincture. Unfortunately, the dispenser supplied a THC-rich formula instead, which caused increased aggression. This is the bane of a consultant's existence, having no control over what the client gets to take home. Fortunately, his mother called me with questions and I helped her to realize the problem. Then we did get the right medicine, dosed at 7 mg 2–3x/day. His aggression was much improved, for 2 months, then it returned. I advised increasing the dose, and adding an additional herbal medicine, Damiana, which might counteract the adolescent testosterone effect. By the next year, Seroquel had been discontinued and the patient had lost 30 lb. His cannabis dose was 10 mg 3x/day. I advised mom on an Ativan wean and titrating up the tincture at the same time. By the following year, he was off Ativan, still on Lexapro and guanfacine and on an ongoing dose of 13 mg of tincture 2x/day. He was doing well in the group home and in school. By the time the patient was 21, he was stable on this regimen, was much more relaxed, with little aggression.

Pearls: Beware what product the patient gets from a dispensary or supplier. Especially in this case where THC clearly aggravated aggression, it should be avoided in significant doses. CBD-rich cannabis ultimately facilitated the discontinuance of Seroquel and Ativan. His total dose of 26 mg/day is quite modest, yet it was effective.

Patient 3: This is a 6-year-old male diagnosed with autism at age 3. He was also very restless and was diagnosed with ADHD and anxiety bordering on OCD as well. Several medications were tried, but the parents reported that most did not seem to help. He was taking Buspar 10 mg 2x/day. His weight at time of presentation was 60 lb. He was able to write his name and go to a day program. We titrated him up on a CBD/THC tincture 20:1 from 5 mg 2x/day to 15 mg 2x/day. During this time, he may have reached a saturation plateau, which often happens, showing increased agitation, at 7 mg 2x/day. I advised continuing to titrate up in dose. At 15 mg 2x/day, he was showing less aggression and anxiety. He continued on this dose until mom wanted to try and wean the Buspar. At a dose of 25 mg of tincture in the a.m. and 20 mg after school, he was able to complete the Buspar wean. He was happy, less obsessive and was having no meltdowns. Then we tried adding a small amount of sativa THC to his morning dose, approximately 3 mg. This resulted in a CBD/THC 6:1 mix. More THC was added to help with focus.

Pearls: This was a higher dose per weight than we might ordinarily have to use in autistic children, finally ending up at less than 0.4 mg/kg. This may have been necessary to replace a high dose of Buspar in a 60-lb child. The addition of a higher level of sativa THC is another modification that is often used to help with focus. The inclusion of slightly higher percentages of THC should be studied with autism, yet have not been done, perhaps due to concerns about the effect of THC on developing nervous systems.

Patient 4: This is a 19-year-old male with autism and several other debilitating conditions, including seizure disorder, dystonia, tremor and high levels of iron deposits in the brain, diagnosed as progressive parkinsonian neurological disorder. He spoke occasionally, but sat though most of our visit uncommunicatively. He had a third-grade level of cognition. His weight was 140 lb. Seizure activity was tonic–clonic, onset in the past 6 months and progressed from 1x/month to 2x/day. He was taking Vimpat, Lamictal and amantadine. His parents had started him on a CBD/THC 22:1 tincture at a dose of 16 mg in the a.m. and p.m., with no obvious effect. The family lived out of my area, but the tincture they had access to was acceptable, so I advised increasing the dose. He ended up at a dose of 50 mg 2x/day, while his medications remained the same except for a small increase in amantadine. On this dose, his sei-zures decreased to 1x/month, he was less irritable and his focus in school was good. The dystonia remained the same. Over the course of the next year, these improve-ments continued, except on full moon days, where he became self-injurious with poor sleep. I advised adding 1 mg of indica THC to the nighttime dose, which did help with calming and better sleep on those days.

Pearls: This is another case of needing a higher dose in an autistic patient, yet again with compounding diagnoses. Here, we arrived at about 0.3 mg/kg of cannabi-noids. As earlier, the addition of a small amount of THC was useful in combination with CBD, as in this case to help with sleep. Of note, at this high level of cannabis CBD, 100 mg/day, his dystonia did not improve.

Patient 5: This is a 29-year-old female with several chronic medical problems, including autism, seizure disorder, insomnia with nightmares, deafness, pain and tuberous sclerosis. She was non-verbal. It was unclear what the source of her pain was, but it seemed to keep her up at night. She lived in a group home, with her mother serving as her caregiver. She was new to cannabis use. She was on multiple medica-tions, including Seroquel, Vimpat, Depakote, Keppra, Trazodone and Topamax. She became aggressive most days. I advised a CBD-rich tincture, 20:1 for daytime use, with an indica chocolate before sleep. She couldn't tolerate the chocolate, taking up to 50 mg to achieve sleep, but was spitting it up, so we switched to a 30 mg gummy edible before sleep. This helped her get at least 4–5 hours of sleep. The CBD-rich tincture did help with agitation during the day at a low, 5 mg dose 2x/day, with a seemingly improved mood.

Pearls: This patient's family was so grateful for bringing cannabis into her life. Before she used it, she was up all night moaning, and agitated most of the day. All of the medications she was taking did not take care of her distress. As she was non-verbal, she couldn't articulate what her agitation was expressing, but we know it seemed to be less with cannabis, even with a low dose of CBD. Because her dos-ing was not at the high end, as may be found in other autistic patients, this regimen remained effective for years, not necessitating a tolerance break.

CANNABIS THERAPY SUMMARY

The progress made with almost all autistic patients with the aid of cannabis was remarkable. Interaction with another patient, a 15-year-old girl who was non-verbal at our first meeting, will always stand out in my mind. After a year on a CBD-rich extract given at 100 mg/day in divided doses, mom reported, "She tolerates the can-nabis well. Her verbal communication skills, interpersonal skills, and attention have all significantly improved. Mood swings are still frequent (typically when the effects of cannabis are mostly worn off)." At our 1-year follow-up visit, I was so touched and gratified when this young woman said, "Hello, Dr. Malka," very politely. In treating autism, it is never simple. There are almost always compounding diagnoses.

As a cannabis specialist, and not a neurologist, I am always appreciative of families that come to me with neurologists supportive of the inclusion of cannabis in the patient's care. I have found that most "do not mind" the addition of CBD as long as the patient's prescribed medications are not changed. As you can see, almost all of the autistic patients treated were on a CBD-rich tincture, containing full extract cannabis with a CBD/THC ratio of 20:1. I treated one patient for 5 years using such a protocol with no obvious adverse effects with ongoing improved function. I assume that as in all cases of cannabis therapy, the full-spectrum extract is preferable to pure CBD. It is always a challenge, to work in concert with the patient's care team. In most cases, my advice is offered in response to the parents' requests, and I always encourage them to review any treatment plan we enact with the other physicians involved in the case. There is often a need to monitor the effects closely for the first year, necessitating monthly–bimonthly follow-up.

REFERENCES

1. Khalil RB. Would some cannabinoids ameliorate symptoms of autism? *Eur Child Adolesc Psychiatry*. 2012;21:237–238.
2. Karhson DS, Krasinska KM, Dallaire JA, et al. Plasma anandamide concentrations are lower in children with autism spectrum disorder. *Mol Autism*. 2018;9:18.
3. Siniscalco D, Sapone A, Giordano C, et al. Cannabinoid receptor type 2, but not type 1, is up-regulated in peripheral blood mononuclear cells of children affected by autistic disorders. J *Autism Dev Disord*. 2013;43(11):2686–2695.
4. Wei D, Dinh D, Lee D, et al. Enhancement of anandamide-mediated endocannabinoid signaling corrects autism-related social impairment. *Cannabis Cannabinoid Res*. 2016;1(1):81–89.
5. Agarwal R, Burke SL, Maddux M. Current state of evidence of cannabis utilization for treatment of autism spectrum disorders. *BMC Psychiatry*. 2019;19:328.
6. Kurz R, Blaas K. Use of dronabinol (delta-9-THC) in autism: a prospective single-case-study with an early infantile autistic child. *Cannabinoids*. 2010;5(4):4–6.
7. Barchel D, Stolar O, De-Haan T, et al. Cannabidiol use in children with autism spectrum disorder to treat related symptoms and co-morbidities. *Front Pharmacol*. 2018;9:1521.
8. Aran A, Cassuto H, Lubotzky A. Cannabidiol based medical cannabis in children with autism: a retrospective feasibility study. *Neurology*. 2018;90(15 Supple):P3.318.
9. Polega S, Golubchik P, Offena D, Weizman A. Cannabidiol as a suggested candidate for treatment of autism spectrum disorder. *Prog Neuro-Psychoph*. 2019;89:90–96.
10. Bar-Lev Schleider L, Mechoulam R, Saban N, Meiri G, Novack V. Real life experience of medical cannabis treatment in autism: analysis of safety and efficacy. *Sci Rep*. 2019;9:200.
11. Fleury-Teixeira P, Caixeta FV, Ramires da Silva LC, Brasil-Neto JP, Malcher-Lopes R. Effects of CBD-enriched cannabis sativa extract on autism spectrum disorder symptoms: an observational study of 18 participants undergoing compassionate use. *Front Neurol*. 2019;10:1145.
12. Montefiore Medical Center. Cannabidivarin (CBDV) vs. placebo in children with autism spectrum disorder (ASD). https://clinicaltrials.gov/ct2/show/NCT03202303 Accessed March 14, 2020.
13. Salgado CA, Castellanos D. Autism spectrum disorder and cannabidiol: have we seen this movie before? *Glob Pediatr Health*. 2018;5:1–5.

20 Autoimmune Disorders

AUTOIMMUNE DISORDERS AND CANNABIS

Endocannabinoids play an important role in immune regulation.[1] The concept that dysregulation of the endocannabinoid system (ECS) can play a role in autoimmune diseases is now an accepted fact. A review of the ECS and the immune system reminds us that it is an important modulator of the autonomic nervous system, inflammation, the immune system and microcirculation, all important in the pathophysiology of autoimmune disease.

> The effect of cannabinoids on immune functions appears to be transient which would allow the inhibitory effects to be overcome when the immune system needs to be activated during infections. This is supported by the downregulation of cannabinoid receptor expression when the immune cells are activated.[2]

In fact, the biphasic activity of cannabinoids lends itself well to modulatory effects, such as immune stimulation or inhibition when needed, such as in autoimmune disease. One author points out that while exogenous cannabinoids may have inhibitory effects on some immune cells,

> A number of recent studies have demonstrated that the endocannabinoids may have some stimulatory impact on the immune system and may actually be important in homeostasis or control of immune reactions. This apparent contradiction may be due in part to a biphasic response relative to the cannabinoid ligand concentration.[3]

Immune modulation involves a complex interdependent regulatory system, not least of which includes activity of T cells, B cells, macrophages, cytokines, among others. Cannabinoid agonists have effects on all main cellular subsets of the immune system, including, but not limited to, B cells, T cells, NK cells, macrophages, mast cells, generally causing a reduction in pro-inflammatory cytokines and an increase in anti-inflammatory cytokines. Cannabinoids can influence the balance between inflammatory and regulatory T cells, promoting immune regulation.[4] Immune effects modulated by cannabinoids are thought to be dose-dependent. THC can have modulating effects on both cell-mediated and humoral immunity.[5] A review of cannabinoid effects on immunity presents much of the relevant literature.[6] Immunomodulatory effects attributed to THC have been linked primarily to activation of CB2 receptors.[7] In early studies (1989) of experimental autoimmune encephalitis mice, THC-treated animals had mild clinical symptoms with a survival greater than 95%, compared with a 98% death rate in the placebo group. The better survival was accompanied by markedly reduced central nervous system inflammation. Future research in this model in suppressing neuroinflammation seems to indicate best result is achieved with a CBD/THC mix.[8] It is possible that THC alone, as

DOI: 10.1201/9781003098201-31

an immunosuppressant, would have fared better in a non-neurodegenerative immune dysfunction model. In another study, THC attenuated the severity of the autoimmune response in this experimental model of autoimmune diabetes by reducing the expression of tumor necrosis factor and cytokine microRNAs.[9] A study of the effects of cannabis on peripheral blood mononuclear cells of patients with chronic abdominal pain revealed an immunosuppressive effect via deactivation of pro-inflammatory and pro-mitogenic pathways. However, long-term cannabis exposure in two patients resulted in reversal of this effect.[10] This is an important observation, reminding us that the cannabinoid receptor (CBr)-dependent functions of THC or any cannabinoid will downregulate with tolerance development.

A review of the in vitro and in vivo effects of CBD on these immune cells is long, yet not conclusive. Some proposed mechanisms include CBD action directly or indirectly at CBrs, acting through ion channels and TRPV1 receptors, causing suppression of all of the aforementioned cell types as well as lymphocytes and mediators, and CBD-induced alterations in miRNA expression, to name but a few. The authors conclude:

> Overall, the data overwhelmingly support the notion that CBD is immune suppressive and that the mechanisms involve direct suppression of activation of various immune cell types, induction of apoptosis, and promotion of regulatory cells, which, in turn, control other immune cell targets.[11]

In addition, the anti-inflammatory and antioxidative effects of CBD affect inflammatory immune disease. As with all cannabinoids, these effects are considered to be biphasic, with the potential for opposing effects at other doses. Much of the in vitro information and animal studies were conducted at high levels (i.e., 20 mg/kg of pure CBD). Both CBD and THC showed an immunomodulatory effect on lymphocytes isolated from venous blood of human volunteers. At relatively high concentrations, they were found to inhibit proliferation, with CBD showing higher immunosuppressive effects than THC.[12] We don't yet know what to expect with CBD-rich cannabis used at lower doses. In animal models of inflammation, CBD reduced cell-mediated joint destruction in a rheumatoid arthritis model, and reduced plasma levels of pro-inflammatory cytokines in a mouse model of diabetes.[13]

There is a need for long-term outcome studies of the effect of cannabinoids and cannabis on human immune system function. There are rare few autoimmune conditions that have been somewhat researched, such as rheumatoid arthritis and Crohn's disease. These are discussed separately (see Chapters 16 and 34). A review of cannabis studies on autoimmune disease summarizes:

> Several clinical trials in multiple sclerosis, inflammatory bowel disease, and fibromyalgia suggest cannabis' effectiveness as an immune-modulator. . . . Although lacking clinical research, in vitro and in vivo experiments in rheumatoid arthritis, diabetes type 1, and systemic sclerosis demonstrate a correlation between disease activity and cannabinoids.[14]

One report of 200 patients with lupus (SLE) concluded that those who used marijuana showed poorer compliance with their standard therapeutic regimen and an increase in neuropsychiatric SLE.[15] For most other autoimmune diseases, we have to infer cannabis therapeutic action while we await human studies.

PATIENT REPORTS

To move on to patient results from my practice, there was a wide range of products used for this condition. Most of the patients with autoimmune disease were in their 30s–60s at the time of presentation. Some patients chose to use mostly THC, some mostly CBD, some topical and all combinations thereof. It was always necessary to educate patients about the therapeutic aspects of cannabis in regulating the disease, and not just the pain. Those that took cannabis regularly, daily, not just when there was pain had better outcomes. Here are a few illustrative case reports.

Patient 1: This is a 51-year-old female in chronic pain since age 35 due to ankylosing spondylitis. She had back stiffness with decreased range of motion, degenerative disc disease with spurring and increasing sacroiliac pain. She was HLA-B27 positive. She had been on Enbrel for 5 years with no apparent help. Currently, she was on Humira, rare Tramadol as needed and Lexapro. She had been using cannabis for the past 3 years. She was using a homemade THC-rich tincture of unknown concentration 4–6×/day. Her cannabis use and condition remained stable over the next 2 years. When she started going to a dispensary, she was better able to specify dosage and tincture contents, and ended up on a CBD/THC 2:1 or 1:1 tincture during the day and indica at night. Over the next 2 years, her condition worsened somewhat due to a torn labrum in her hip. This led to worsening sacroiliac pain for which she received nerve block injections. Her medications and cannabis remained the same. Sometimes she added smoking by pipe.

Pearls: This patient was moderately stable over the 5 years she was a patient. It's unclear if her condition would have been worse off the cannabis. As with any medical therapy, in patients with chronic degenerative conditions, often remaining stable is a sign of therapeutic efficacy. Of note is the absence of opiate pain medication in this patient with significant pain.

Patient 2: This is a 38-year-old female with multiple autoimmune conditions, including rheumatoid arthritis, lupus and mixed connective tissue disorder. She was on methotrexate, Celebrex, morphine sulfate 15 mg at bedtime and oxycodone prn. She was new to cannabis use. I suggested a CBD/THC tincture for the day and an indica for the night. She followed my advice immediately and soon was sleeping better. She took about 5 mg of the CBD/THC 20:1 tincture 2×/day and 15 mg of indica by tincture at night. She was able to get off the morphine, and was taking one Norco/day for pain. She was newly started on 5 mg of prednisone. After several years, she was managing her inflammatory conditions with a CBD/THC 20:1 edible, about 10 mg 4×/day.

Pearls: I wish I could have put her on a higher dose of cannabis, to try and avoid the prednisone and achieve better endocannabinoid regulation, and daytime pain relief. The custom of using cannabis as a rescue medicine, and not as a balancing-daily-used at the right dose medicine is frustrating. She was disabled and low-income. It is likely that she could not afford to use more cannabis.

Patient 3: This is a 64-year-old female with multiple immune dysfunction diagnoses, including lupus, fibromyalgia, interstitial cystitis, irritable bowel syndrome, rosacea and also had poor sleep. She had been on Plaquenil for 21 years, and also took gabapentin for peripheral neuropathy. She was new to cannabis use. She began to use an indica edible to help with sleep and found it effective at 10 mg. She didn't enjoy the psychoactivity, so I advised adding some CBD. This was my advice for the next 2 years, but because she was sleeping well, she didn't want to alter her regimen. She sometimes was able to use 5 mg of THC to sleep, which reduced the psychoactivity.

Pearls: This is typical of patients who come in with a specific goal in mind. In this case, to sleep better. She was satisfied. She saw no obvious reason to invest in more cannabis as an immune modulator. Perhaps as more human trials are completed, a stronger case for cannabis therapeutic use will emerge.

Patient 4: This is a 69-year-old female with a 2-year history of polymyalgia rheumatica. She had been experimenting with cannabis for the past year, without professional advice. She was vaping once/day. She reported that edibles made her groggy. She was currently taking prednisone 7 mg/day, down from 20 mg/day at the beginning of her condition, and amitriptyline at night. She was prescribed methotrexate, but hadn't started it. I advised a CBD/THC 1:1 tincture, 10 mg 3×/day. She found that tolerable, with no disorienting or sedating side effects. After 1 year while on the tincture, she was able to wean the prednisone and was off. She still had some pain, so we continued the tincture 2×/day for the next year.

Pearls: It seems like 2 years to get off prednisone is typical with this diagnosis. Did cannabis help her condition? We don't know, although the outcome was as desired, less pain and less medication. In this case, becoming educated about a form of cannabis that she could tolerate was key to compliance, especially in the elderly. Pain management often requires THC. Finding the right amount of CBD to combine it with to reduce side effects is always an individualized process.

Patient 5: This is a 42-year-old female with lupus who had been using cannabis for 2 years during which time she was able to discontinue Plaquenil. She was also taking 600 mg/day of naproxen and a low dose of Prozac. She was only using an edible of unknown dose, in the evenings ¼ of a cookie. She reported that she tried a CBD-rich candy, but it didn't help her joint pain. She said her liver function tests returned to normal on cannabis, and off the Plaquenil. Over the next year, she switched to smoking less than a joint/day with an improvement in her condition, having only one flare-up. This continued for several more years. At our last visit, her usage by smoking had increased to 2 joints/day, mostly due to stress at home, while the lupus remained in remission.

Pearls: This is typical of a younger adult patient, even one new to cannabis, that they try and prefer smoking to other delivery methods, and usage can increase with stress. It is unclear how long her remission would have lasted off cannabis, perhaps the results would have been the same. But stress is a known trigger for autoimmune disorders, and regulating it with cannabis was likely helpful. That's the benefit of using a THC-rich cannabis, as opposed to a drug that primarily targets immune function such as Plaquenil, that it has multiple useful effects for such patients.

CANNABIS THERAPY SUMMARY

All autoimmune diseases have endocannabinoid regulation, we might even say dys-regulation. As seen in more detail with immune-related arthritis (i.e., RA), gastro-intestinal disease (i.e., Crohn's disease) or nervous system disorders (i.e., multiple sclerosis), we are faced with symptom management that can happen at relatively low doses of cannabis and/or the possibility of disease modification, which most likely would need higher doses of cannabis, not routinely achieved. Most of these patients had a component of pain and/or insomnia likely due to pain, for which some THC-rich cannabis was used. Most patients ended up on a regimen that included cannabis with some CBD during the day and more THC at night. Several patients with auto-immune conditions added THCA to their regimens with benefit due to its immu-nomodulatory effect. This is a therapeutic avenue that deserves more investigation. The challenge with autoimmune patients is to educate them about using cannabis regularly, and not just when there is an autoimmune flare-up and not to stop when the pain is reduced. Managing endocannabinoid dysregulation is an ongoing process requiring ongoing treatment.

REFERENCES

1. Katchan V, David P, Shoenfeld Y. Cannabinoids and autoimmune diseases: a systematic review. *Autoimmun Rev.* 2016;15(6):513–528.
2. Pandey R, Mousawy K, Nagarkatti M, Nagarkatti P. Endocannabinoids and immune regulation. *Pharmacol Res.* 2009;60(2):85–92.
3. Croxford JL, Yamamura T. Cannabinoids and the immune system: potential for the treatment of inflammatory diseases? *J Neuroimmunol.* 2005;166:3–18.
4. Almogi-Hazan O, Or R. Cannabis, the endocannabinoid system and immunity-the journey from the bedside to the bench and back. *Int J Mol Sci.* 2020;21(12):4448.
5. Klein TW, Cabral GA. Cannabinoid-induced immune suppression and modulation of antigen-presenting cells. *J Neuroimmune Pharmacol.* 2006;1:50–64.
6. Oláh A, Szekanecz Z, Bíró T. Targeting cannabinoid signaling in the immune system: "high"ly exciting questions, possibilities, and challenges. *Front Immunol.* 2017;8:1487.
7. Cabral GA, Rogers TJ, Lichtman AH. Turning over a new leaf: cannabinoid and endo-cannabinoid modulation of immune function. *J Neuroimmune Pharmacol.* 2015;10(2): 193–203.
8. Al-Ghezi ZZ, Miranda K, Nagarkatti M, Nagarkatti PS. Combination of cannabinoids, 19-tetrahydrocannabinol and cannabidiol, ameliorates experimental multiple sclerosis by suppressing neuroinflammation through regulation of miRNA-mediated signaling pathways. *Front Immunol.* 2019;10:1921.
9. Li X, Kaminski NE, Fischer LJ. Examination of the immunosuppressive effect of delta 9-tetrahydrocannabinol in streptozotocin-induced autoimmune diabetes. *Int Immunopharmacol.* 2001;1(4):699–712.
10. Utomo WK, de Vries M, Braat H, et al. Modulation of human peripheral blood mono-nuclear cell signaling by medicinal cannabinoids. *Front Mol Neurosci.* 2017;10:14.
11. Nichols JM, Kaplan BLF. Immune responses regulated by cannabidiol. *Cannabis Cannabinoid Res.* 2020;5(1):12–31.
12. Zgair A, Lee JB, Wong JCM, et al. Oral administration of cannabis with lipids leads to high levels of cannabinoids in the intestinal lymphatic system and prominent immuno-modulation. *Sci Rep.* 2017;7:14542.

13. Tanasescu R, Constantinescu CS. Cannabinoids and the immune system: an overview. *Immunobiology.* 2010;215:588–597.
14. Katz D, Katz I, Porat-Katz BS, Shoenfeld Y. Medical cannabis: another piece in the mosaic of autoimmunity? *Clin Pharmacol Ther.* 2017;101(2):230–238.
15. Jalil B, Sibbitt Jr. W, Cabacangun R, et al. Medical marijuana related outcomes in patients with systemic lupus erythematosus. ACR/ARHP Annual Meeting. 2014. https://acrabstracts.org/abstract/medical-marijuana-related-outcomes-in-patients-with-systemic-lupus-erythematosis/ Accessed June 15, 2020.

21 Back Pain, Neck Pain

BACK PAIN, NECK PAIN AND CANNABIS

Pain is the most common diagnosis for which patients seek to use medical cannabis. This has been confirmed in several countries and states. In California, a survey was done as far back as 2007.[1] It found the most prevalent pain complaint in the patient population was back pain, with low back pain being the most common, but thoracic and cervical pain were significant as well. A survey of medical cannabis patients in three US states revealed that 64% had been diagnosed with chronic pain. Among this group, the vast majority, 91%, reported back or neck pain. Medical cannabis was reported as being effective in treating their symptoms in 75% of these patients.[2] In a survey of the therapeutic role of cannabis for back pain due to degenerated discs, it was found that 65% of the patients stated their symptoms "much improved," with an additional 29% reporting slight improvement. Seventy-six percent were "very satisfied" with their therapeutic use of cannabis.[3] Cannabis is especially helpful for neuropathic pain, such as that caused by the pressure of a disc upon a nerve, as well as neuroinflammation. It can provide relief from the pain itself, reduce inflammation, often reduce the amount of opiate medication used and it can help with the side effects of other medications, such as nausea, dizziness or gastrointestinal upset.[4]

As is evident, this is the category of patient that comprises the majority of medical cannabis patients, who are often able to reduce their use of opiates and other medications. This type of pain can often become chronic, leading to opioid dependence. A recent survey in Australia of patients with chronic non-cancer pain who also were taking opiates showed 77% had back or neck pain.[5] Here, recreational cannabis was not found to reduce pain in participants taking the oral morphine equivalent of 75 mg/day of opiates. This study underscores the importance of proper use of cannabis with medical supervision, especially when high doses of opiates are already on board, that is, a few puffs on a "joint" will likely not be strong enough to impact the effects of high-dose opiates. The very complex manner by which cannabis and cannabinoids affect pain in general is discussed in other pain sections (see Chapters 25, 39 and 40).

Studies of cannabis treatment of back pain show a range of efficacy. In a study done in Israel, patients with refractory low back pain without symptom relief from analgesics and at least two narcotics were followed for 12 months. Cannabis was smoked at a recommended rate of 4 doses per day up to 20 grams per month. There were no differences in MCT (medical cannabis therapy) response between post-surgical patients, disc patients and spinal stenosis patients in this study. Pain scores decreased from 8.4 to 2.0, range of motion improved and over half of the patients stopped opiate therapy. The authors concluded that MCT appears to be highly effective in this population of patients:

> The improvement in life quality is mostly in the physical compound score. The high patient compliance and high rates of return to work, as well as the opiate sparing effect,

might indicate that MCT therapy should be considered also in chronic back pain patients, who have not failed opiate therapy for such a prolonged period.[6]

A study of patients with severe low back pain due to failed back surgery syndrome achieve effective analgesia in less than 50% of the cases. An experiment using a spinal cord stimulator in combination with a cannabinoid preparation containing a suspension of THC (19%) and CBD (<1%), 50–100 mg/day or more, was taken for 12 months. The mean pain perception decreased from 8.1 at the first visit to 4.7 at the end. There were improvements in sleep and mood as well.[7]

THC-rich cannabis has dominated the public arena for treatment of pain because it is an effective analgesic and it has been the most well-known. Currently, CBD is gaining popularity in pain management, which may or may not be warranted. The overly attributed efficacy of CBD for pain management has not clearly been confirmed when in pure form, and is more effective for neurogenic or inflammatory pain as a cannabis extract. A review of the actions of CBD versus THC for pain management is discussed in other pain sections. In a report of cannabis medicinal extracts (CME) to treat neurogenic symptoms including pain, they concluded that "Intoxication seemed to be primarily associated with THC CME, but even here was usually of tolerable intensity. CBD CME appeared to have analgesic and antispasticity properties in its own right."[8] CBD also shows promise as a therapy for disc disease. This was studied in an animal model. Intradiscal injection of CBD immediately after injury significantly attenuated the effects, with the higher dose (120 nmol) being the most effective.[9] Multiple studies seem to indicate that cannabis extracts with THC and CBD combined seem to do best at managing pain with the least adverse effects.[10] Neuropathic pain patients receiving Sativex (approximately a CBD/THC 1:1 mix) experienced a 14% reduction in pain, and in another study 36% of patients in the THC/CBD spray treatment group achieved at least a 30% improvement in pain scores, compared to 20% in the placebo group.[11,12] There are several clinical trials in progress to study cannabinoid dosing and composition effects specifically for back pain. The analgesic effects of vaporized THC cannabis, placebo cannabis, oxycodone and placebo oxycodone on patients with chronic back and neck pain are being investigated.[13] Vaporized cannabis 5.6% CBD/3.7% THC is being compared with the action of dronabinol in subjects with neuropathic back pain.[14]

Let's not forget other potential aspects of back or neck pain, especially after an injury, such as muscle spasms and inflammation, for which cannabis is highly effective. This is covered in detail in another section (see Chapter 37). Cannabis use for back pain illustrates the application of multiple delivery systems, including widespread use of topical products, which are non-psychoactive. Many of such patients have been prescribed a muscle relaxant, an opiate pain medicine and an anti-inflammatory. Cannabis can and does replace all of these as a single herbal medicine.

PATIENT REPORTS

To move on to patient results from my practice, the most prevalent cases were of mild back or neck pain, with adult patients of all ages. These are simple to treat. I have included some reports of more significant pain later as well. The entire range of products was used in my patient population for pain relief. Of course, as expected, the therapy varied with the level of pain. These patients simply smoked or vaporized as needed and/or used topical cannabis. The more complicated cases used greater amounts of cannabis including edibles. Here are a few illustrative case reports.

Patient 1: This is a 56-year-old female who had a 10+ year history of cannabis use. She smoked it 2×/day for hip and sciatic pain, which she had for over 20 years, and for sleep. She was on no pain medicine, but did use up to 1,200 mg of ibuprofen on some days. I advised trying vaporizing, but she chose to continue to smoke it and added topical for her back and hip. She said "It provides better relief and is not as hard on my body as ibuprofen." Her ibuprofen use decreased. For sleep, she occasionally added an indica chocolate.

Pearls: This represents the mild end of the pain spectrum, for someone who is an experienced cannabis user and not fearful of the psychoactive effects of cannabis, but really preferred them. She did learn about other uses besides smoking, such as topicals and edibles. Her ibuprofen use remained rare, while her cannabis use increased.

Patient 2: This is a 53-year-old male with a history of head and neck pain and poor sleep due to several issues. He had a prior injury to his skull, neck and jaw. This was treated with two cervical disc replacements, jaw alignment and acupuncture. His main pain medicine was cannabis, for which he had a 30-year history. He was also on gabapentin and Celebrex. His preferred usage was by pipe 2×/day. I advised an indica edible to help sleep, which he did. This reduced his smoking to 1×/day. He reported feeling better with longer sleep and more relaxation in his neck.

Pearls: Insomnia due to pain actually results in more pain, more muscle spasm and is an important symptom to manage, especially in back or neck pain. Often muscle tension from sleeping unmedicated overnight contributes to poor sleep and waking up in pain. Even without insomnia, overnight cannabis medication is useful for this type of pain.

Patient 3: This is a 50-year-old returning patient, already using cannabis for low back pain, sleep and mood. This is a classical presentation, of a typical adult patient, with the three most prevalent conditions. It is not unusual to see this triad. This patient was unusual in that she had multiple other issues, including alcohol dependence, just recently stopped 3 months prior, and tobacco dependence, although she was trying to cut down. She did not have cannabis dependence, even though she had been using it for 40 years, she was using only one joint/day. She did not like pharmaceuticals and was taking no medications. She was seeing a chiropractor regularly for diagnosed lumbar spondylosis. Over the 5 years we worked together, she continued to smoke one joint/day, she reduced tobacco somewhat, stayed off alcohol and added topical cannabis to her regimen. Her mood and back pain stabilized off alcohol using a small amount of cannabis.

Pearls: As back pain is the most common pain condition reported for medical cannabis, it is likely that a majority of patients may present with multiple other issues as well, which all need advisement. To arrive at a regimen that amounts to one joint/ day plus added topical is a satisfactory outcome for this patient, although after 40 years, one may be tempted to conclude that this practice was somewhat of a "crutch," utilized to treat all challenging health issues. This may be the case, but perhaps the benefits outweigh the risks, notwithstanding the continued smoking method.

Patient 4: This is a 39-year-old male with low back pain, hip and knee pain, depression and insomnia. Obesity was a concern. At 360 lb he was advised to lose weight. His back MRI showed spondylolysis and spondylolisthesis. His medications included hydrocodone, 10 mg 3×/day, SOMA 2×/day, Prozac 60 mg/day and Voltaren 75 mg 2×/day. He had a cannabis history of smoking 2×/day for 20 years. I advised the addition of a CBD/THC tincture 2–3×/day for increased pain management to hopefully allow opiate reduction. Over the next 2 years, he focused on weight loss and was able to wean off Prozac with a loss of 135 lb. He continued to smoke, use tinctures and vaporize mostly CBD-rich products, as well as use topical on his knees, and then proceeded to get off opiates. His pain reduced while he lowered his opiate and antidepressant medicines.

Pearls: This is a somewhat younger patient who is used to smoking cannabis. It's rewarding to be successful in introducing other forms of delivery and CBD-rich benefits to this age group. It was successful in reducing two pharmaceutical medications and in reducing pain. Contrary to expectations of cannabis use resulting in appetite stimulation, in this case the patient was able to achieve much weight loss. Expanding the cannabis formulary for previous recreational cannabis users is a common experience as a cannabis consultant.

Patient 5: This is an 80-year-old female with chronic back pain due to osteoarthritis, osteoporosis and injury. She had fallen a few years earlier and fractured three vertebrae. Her medications included Norco 5 mg 5×/day, a fentanyl patch 50 μg, Requip and Cymbalta. She was new to cannabis use. I advised an opiate wean with a CBD/THC 1:1 tincture, but she preferred to use topical generously, on her back, knees and hands. She felt her symptoms were much better, with less pain. Her opiate dose did not change. By the following year, she was on a fentanyl patch 100 μg, and off Norco. She was still using topical. I continued to suggest an internal tincture, but to no avail for several years.

Pearls: Elderly patients may have more fear of cannabis, even CBD-rich cannabis, than opiates. They are often even leery of topicals. Opiates are common in chronic back pain cases, but they are not all successfully substituted (see Chapter 40).

CANNABIS THERAPY SUMMARY

We see the whole spectrum of products at varying doses applied for cannabis therapeutic use in this category of patient. This is likely due to the severity of symptoms, the age, familiarity with cannabis and the provision of professional guidance. Cannabis is helpful for muscle spasm of the back or neck muscles, pain and inflammation. It can be used internally and/or topically, applied directly to the affected area, to provide relief without psychoactive effects. Another back pain patient achieved ongoing relief with a CBD-rich transdermal patch that lasted for several days. For those using full flower, it is useful to look for strains containing β-myrcene, which provides added muscle relaxation, commonly found in indicas. Products containing THCA add anti-inflammatory benefits. Often the issue of insomnia due to pain needs to be addressed as well for further pain management and relaxation.

REFERENCES

1. Nunberg H, Kilmer B, Pacula RL, Burgdorf JR. An analysis of applicants presenting to a medical marijuana specialty practice in California. *J Drug Policy Anal*. 2011;4(1): Article 1.
2. Piper BJ, Beals ML, Abess AT, et al. Chronic pain patients' perspectives of medical cannabis. *Pain*. 2017;158(7):1373–1379.
3. Bhattacharyya M. Back pain due to degenerated disc: any therapeutic role of cannabis. *Orthop Proc*. 90(B):supp II. February 21, 2018. https://online.boneandjoint.org.uk/doi/abs/10.1302/0301-620X.90BSUPP_II.0900224d Accessed March 15, 2020.
4. Hill KP, Palastro MD, Johnson B, Ditre JW. Cannabis and pain: a clinical review. *Cannabis Cannabinoid Res*. 2017;2(1):96–104.
5. Campbell G, Hall WD, Peacock A, et al. Effect of cannabis use in people with chronic non-cancer pain prescribed opioids: findings from a 4-year prospective cohort study. *Lancet Public Health*. 2018;3(7):e341–e350.
6. Yassin M, Garti A, Robinson D. Effect of medicinal cannabis therapy (MCT) on severity of chronic low back pain, sciatica and lumbar range of motion. *Int J Anesth Pain Med*. 2016;2(1.5):1–6.
7. Mondello E, Quattrone D, Cardia L, et al. Cannabinoids and spinal cord stimulation for the treatment of failed back surgery syndrome refractory pain. *J Pain Res*. 2018;11:1761–1767.
8. Wade DT, Robson P, House H, Makela P, Aram J. A preliminary controlled study to determine whether whole-plant cannabis extracts can improve intractable neurogenic symptoms. *Clin Rehabil*. 2003;17:18–26.
9. Silveira JW. Protective effects of cannabidiol on lesion-induced intervertebral disc degeneration. *PLoS One*. 2014;9(12):e113161.
10. Johnson JR, Burnell-Nugent M, Lossignol D, et al. Multicenter, double-blind, randomized, placebo-controlled, parallel-group study of the efficacy, safety, and tolerability of THC:CBD extract and THC extract in patients with intractable cancer-related pain. *J Pain Symptom Manage*. 2010;39(2):167–179.
11. Nurmikko TJ, Serpell MG, Hoggart B, et al. Sativex successfully treats neuropathic pain characterized by allodynia: a randomised, double-blind, placebo-controlled clinical trial. *Pain*. 2007;133:210–220.
12. Serpell M, Ratcliffe S, Hovorka J, et al. A double-blind, randomized, placebo-controlled, parallel group study of THC/CBD spray in peripheral neuropathic pain treatment. *Eur J Pain*. 2014;18:999–1012.
13. University of Colorado, Denver. A double-blind, placebo-controlled crossover study comparing the analgesic efficacy of cannabis versus oxycodone. https://clinicaltrials.gov/ct2/show/NCT02892591 Accessed March 10, 2020.
14. University of California San Diego. A randomized, cross-over controlled trial of dronabinol and vaporized cannabis in neuropathic low back pain. https://clinicaltrials.ucsd.edu/trial/NCT02460692 Accessed March 10, 2020.

22 Brain Trauma

BRAIN TRAUMA AND CANNABIS

Brain trauma results in neurological damage and in the case of stroke, ischemia followed by secondary changes with ongoing neuronal deficits. Following a traumatic brain injury (TBI), the brain attempts to compensate and recover in multiple ways, including activating the endocannabinoid system. The search for pre- and post-injury therapeutics has yielded few, if any, products for clinical use. The potential for cannabinoids to be therapeutic agents as neuroprotectants is widely known and is not new. A US government patent applied for in 1999 and issued in 2003 – titled Cannabinoids as Antioxidants and Neuroprotectants – states, "The cannabinoids are found to have particular application as neuroprotectants, for example in limiting neurological damage following ischemic insults, such as stroke and trauma."[1] In a review of cannabinoids effect on brain trauma, the authors suggest, "Given that cannabinoids are able to attenuate excitotoxicity, inflammation, and oxidative stress, they have been proposed as promising candidates to become effective neuroprotective therapies, including the brain damage in neonatal ischemia."[2]

Over the past few years, the endocannabinoid system has been examined for its neuroprotective role. Cannabinoid receptors (CBrs) are influenced by endocannabinoids and THC. Although anandamide (AEA) is present in very low levels in the brain, its concentration increases upon injury. Activation of CB1 receptors reduces excitatory neurotransmitter release, blocks the expression of pro-inflammatory genes and reduces reactive-oxygen species (ROS). Activated CB2 receptors influences macrophages, decreases pro-inflammatory cell formation, promotes anti-inflammatory cell development, all of which results in reducing inflammation and limiting brain cell death.[3] The mechanisms are still being elaborated. Most studies have shown an upregulated expression of both CB1 and CB2 receptors in stroke, with neurons (for CB1) and microglial/macrophages, astrocytes and neutrophils (for CB2) being the most common cells for these responses. Upregulation of CB2 receptors has been found in TBI in newborn animals.[4]

The dose of THC to prevent against neuronal damage can be very low. Prior administration of THC provided impairment protection in two mouse models of central nervous system injury. A very low dose of THC (0.002 mg/kg) reduced injury-induced cognitive deficits in mice.[5] THC (1 mg/kg i.p.) or AEA (1–10 mg/kg i.p.) was found to reduce the infarct volume through a CB1-dependent mechanism.

Our findings demonstrate the potential of a single treatment with a very low dose of THC to induce pharmacological pre- and postconditioning and protect the brain from the development of cognitive deficits due to epileptic seizures and CO [carbon monoxide] intoxication and probably from other insults that involve excitotoxicity.[6]

DOI: 10.1201/9781003098201-33

The time window for protective intervention with THC was found to be short, 4 hours in rodents. The authors conclude that preconditioning with low dose THC can be done for 1–7 days before the insult and postconditioning treatment can be applied for at least 3 following days.

CBD and THC affect brain injury by additional mechanisms as well. In early animal studies, the effects of THC and CBD both reduced glutamate toxicity in a CBr-independent manner.[7] CBD has also been shown to be protective against global and focal ischemic injury through various mechanisms. It is a potent antioxidant and anti-inflammatory agent.[8] The antioxidant power of CBD was found to be even greater than that of THC. In animal studies, CBD (3 mg/kg) had a long-lasting neuroprotective effect when administered both pre- and post-ischemia, whereas only pre-ischemic treatment with THC (10 mg/kg) reduced the infarction size. CBD showed the neuroprotective effect until 6 hours after cerebral ischemia in mice. In a more recent study, repeated treatment with CBD from 1 to 3 days post-injury, after cerebral ischemia improved the functional deficits, but not after 5 days. The authors conclude: "Mice with activated CB receptors showed a marked increase in neurogenesis at the sight of damage in vitro suggesting that endocannabinoid tone plays an active role in the regeneration of damaged neurons following a stroke."[9] How this translates to humans regarding the timing and dose of cannabinoids needed for brain trauma repair and/or prevention has yet not been determined. Several synthetic cannabinoid agonists have been tested in TBI patients. In one report, dexanabinol (also known as HU-211), which has been shown to have potent neuroprotective activity, was tested in a phase III clinical trial. A 150-mg dose of dexanabinol was given within 6 hours of injury. It was proven to be safe, but had no effect on parameters at 6-month follow-up.[10] Another cannabinoid agonist – KN38–7271 – at a higher dose was administered within 4.5 hours of injury. Patients received 1,000 μg, 500 μg or placebo. Survival rates within 1 month of injury were significantly better in the treatment groups, but these effects were not seen at 6 months.[11] This protocol may not be the best way to approach treatment after a TBI. It is unlikely that a one-time dose could have anti-inflammatory, antioxidant and neuroprotective effects of sufficient duration to address the ongoing damage after a head injury. A longer dose of cannabinoids would be needed. In fact, that is indicated in a study of patients with ongoing cannabis use. In a 3-year retrospective study of patients, who had sustained a traumatic brain injury, decreased mortality was reported in individuals with a positive THC screen. Mortality in the THC (+) group (2.4%) was significantly decreased compared with the THC (–) group (11.5%).[12]

Another category of cannabinoids likely useful for neuroprotection are cannabinoid acids, but research has yet to be done on humans. One such cannabinoid, THCA, has been noted clinically to reduce seizures, which may translate to efficacy for TBI (see Chapter 46). Both THCA and CBDA may show promise for anti-inflammatory and neuroprotection without psychoactivity and may provide additive effects to other cannabinoids.[13,14] Cannabis, as opposed to pure cannabinoids, holds even greater neuroprotective promise with the inclusion of terpenes, such as β-caryophyllene for its anti-inflammatory properties, or terpinolene for its antioxidant properties. Not only does cannabis have neuroprotective properties, but its effects are also useful for minimizing other common side effects of brain injury, including nausea, pain and anxiety. The use of medical cannabis may provide many patients with an increased quality of life.

PATIENT REPORTS

To move on to patient results from my practice, few patients with a history of brain trauma consulted me. Those I saw ranged in age from a teen to an older adult with a case of long-term post-concussion sequelae. The benefits of cannabis for this condition are not well-known among patients. More often, the desire to avoid the potential for disorienting effects dissuades people with this condition from considering its use. Most present with post-injury symptoms, such as headache or insomnia. Here are a few illustrative case reports.

Patient 1: This is a 28-year-old male with a head injury 2 years prior due to a motorcycle accident. His ongoing symptoms since the accident include chronic headache, depression, weight loss, left-sided numbness pain and paresthesias and a left foot injury from landing on his left side. He ambulated with a cane due to R-sided weakness. An MRI of the brain was taken 3 years post-injury. It showed abnormality of the right frontal lobe and left parietal lobe. He complained of memory problems saying that he felt like there were "crumbled walls in my head." He was already a medical cannabis patient at our first meeting, and had been using THC oil, CBD oil and raw cannabis in the form of unheated hashish. These he began within 6 months of his injury. He was on no medications. I advised him that he could use an unheated cannabis tincture to get the same effects as the cold extracted hash for cannabinoid acid intake. At our next visit, he was making his own cold extracted tincture of unknown concentration taking a few sprays several times per day. He was also vaporizing a sativa hybrid for appetite and mood. He continued to have appetite and vomiting issues. I advised him to increase his unheated tincture dose to one dropperful 3×/day. He continued on this regimen for the next few years, using tincture and raw cannabis, frozen juiced ice cubes and vaporizing 5×/day. By the third year of this regimen, he stated he was feeling better, had less pain, better mood and was walking without a cane.

Pearls: The use of cannabinoid acids as anti-inflammatory agents is well-documented, but not widely used clinically. It is due to patients like this that we are reminded to consider their use for brain trauma among other neuroprotective uses. This patient was a grower and was able to produce his own medicine. Cannabinoid acids are not yet widely available in dispensaries.

Patient 2: This is a 15-year-old female who had a fall from a horse 2 years prior with resultant concussion and brain trauma. She had chronic headaches and ongoing anxiety after her injury. I have no information about head MRI results, and to the best of my knowledge, no EEG was done. She was seeing a counselor. She came in with her mother, both interested in how cannabis could help. She had not used it previously. She had just weaned of off several medications, including gabapentin, sertraline, Lyrica and quetiapine. She still had problems with sleep several nights a week. I advised a low dose of an indica edible as needed for sleep, and urged follow-up with a neurologist and counseling for possible PTSD. By our next visit, she was sleeping well on 15 mg of an indica chocolate before bed, using no other medications, and still having some anxiety daily. She said she was feeling better. This year we focused on anxiety and added a CBD/THC 4:1 tincture used in the a.m. and after school. This did help her anxiety. On follow-up several years later, the headaches were gone, sleep was improved while some anxiety remained.

Pearls: By the time I get to see patients, they are well past their original brain injury; so the goal is usually to treat ongoing symptoms, in this case insomnia, headache and anxiety, all of which improved. If patients are referred to cannabis use as soon as possible after injury, it's possible that these symptoms can be mitigated early on.

Patient 3: This is a 57-year-old female who had a concussion 20 years prior due to a fall from a seizure, with resultant brain trauma and now a severe daily headache. She was new to cannabis use. She was on multiple medications, including Lamictal, carbamazepine and lorazepam, which controlled the seizures, leaving her only with absence seizures 1–3x/week resulting in loss of speech for minutes to hours. She also took Serax to sleep and opiates for joint pain 2x/day. She had been told by her health professional to try CBD-rich cannabis at the start of her headache, which did not help. We started her on a THC-rich edible, 30 mg in the morning, added to 20 mg of a CBD-rich tincture in the a.m. She continued to complain of poor sleep, so we added an indica edible before bed. Her headaches improved significantly and sleep improved as well. She was able to reduce to a CBD/THC 1:1 tincture, not daily, but prn migraine, and added the use of a vape pen most days as needed for pain. Her medications did not change.

Pearls: This is not a case of current brain trauma, but of ongoing headaches post-concussion. It is notable that her headaches decreased from daily to weekly. This patient found that she did not need to use as high a daily dose of cannabis as at the start of therapy as her symptoms improved. She was on approximately 50 mg of mixed CBD/THC products for less than 2 years before improvement led to a much-reduced dose. This is certainly indicative of post-concussion headache improvement, but may give insight into dosing needed to calm brain inflammation.

Patient 4: This is a 53-year-old male with a history of brain trauma and concussion in the past from football. He also had osteoarthritis and chronic pain of the neck and spine with some scoliosis. His ongoing post-concussion symptoms included extreme fatigue, confusion, dizziness, headaches, nausea and loss of appetite. He was using THC-rich cannabis by smoking 3x/day. He was on no medications but did see a chiropractor. He stated, "All medications have had a negative effect, making things worse. Cannabis has been the only thing that helps, but only slightly." Over the 3 years we worked together, I advised adding some CBD by tincture, to increase his dosage without increasing confusion or dizziness, and some added topical for neck pain. He did got relief from the topical but was not interested in CBD.

Pearls: This is a case of THC-rich cannabis being used for its immediately felt effects, in alleviating mood and fatigue and reducing pain. It was hard to impress upon this patient with a long history of cannabis use and cognitive dysfunction after brain trauma the value of the "less dramatic" effects that cannabis may offer. It was unfortunate that cannabis helped "only slightly" yet we were not able to safely titrate his dose upward without causing more disorientation, as he was habituated to THC-rich cannabis and did not want to change.

CANNABIS THERAPY SUMMARY

The intriguing question of how to use cannabis as a neuroprotectant immediately post-TBI in humans has yet to be answered, as well as the very real challenge of its legality and availability in likely a hospital setting. Unfortunately, cannabis still being a Schedule I drug makes its dispensation at this crucial time of need unlikely. A more promising avenue may be the dispensation of a CBD-predominant hemp extract or the CBD cannabinoid itself now that hemp has been decriminalized federally. According to animal studies with pure CBD, therapeutic results were achieved with 3 mg/kg of CBD given 1–3 days post-injury. This would be a good starting place in human therapeutics, but there are no signs that such therapy is likely to be available anytime soon, at least not until it becomes FDA approved for such purpose. As far as symptomatic treatment of headache, sleep and/or nausea is concerned, we see success with typical doses for these conditions, ranging from 10 to 30 mg of cannabinoids from cannabis per dose, with the caveat that it is only THC-rich cannabis that helps sleep. And let's not forget the benefit of cannabinoid acids, barely tested for neuroinflammation, yet expected to be beneficial, without added psychoactivity.

REFERENCES

1. Hampson AJ, Axelrod J, Grimaldi M. Cannabinoids as antioxidants and neuroprotectants. 2003. National Center for Biotechnology Information. PubChem Database. Patent-US6630507. https://pubchem.ncbi.nlm.nih.gov/patent/US6630507 Accessed on March 3, 2020.
2. Fernández-Ruiz J, Moro MA, Martínez-Orgado J. Cannabinoids in neurodegenerative disorders and stroke/brain trauma: from preclinical models to clinical applications. *Neurotherapeutics*. 2015;12:793–806.
3. Mechoulam R, Panikashvili D, Shohami E. Cannabinoids and brain injury: therapeutic implications. *Trends Mol Med*. 2002;8(2):58–61.
4. Fernández-Ruiz J, Moro MA, Martínez-Orgado J. Cannabinoids in neurodegenerative disorders and stroke/brain trauma: from preclinical models to clinical applications. *Neurotherapeutics*. 2015;(4):793–806.
5. Schurman LD, Lichtman AH. Endocannabinoids: a promising impact for traumatic brain injury. *Front Pharmacol*. 2017;8:69.
6. Same Y, Asaf F, Fishbein M, Gafni M, Keren O. The dual neuroprotective: neurotoxic profile of cannabinoid drugs. *Br J Pharmacology*. 2011;163:1391–1401.
7. Hampson AJ, Grimaldi M, Axelrod J, Wink D. Cannabidiol and D9-tetrahydrocannabinol are neuroprotective antioxidants. *Proc Nat Acad Sci*. 1998;95:8268–8273.
8. Hayakawa K, Mishima K, Fujiwara M. Therapeutic potential of non-psychotropic cannabidiol in ischemic stroke. *Pharmaceuticals*. 2010;3:2197–2212.
9. Luvone T, Esposito G, De Filippis D, Scuderi C, Steardo L. Cannabidiol: a promising drug for neurodegenerative disorders? *CNS Neurosci Ther*. 2009;15(1):65–75.
10. Maas AI, Murray G, Henney 3rd H, et al. Efficacy and safety of dexanabinol in severe traumatic brain injury: results of a phase III randomised, placebo-controlled, clinical trial. *Lancet Neurol*. 2006;5:38–45.
11. Firsching R, Piek J, Skalej M, et al. Early survival of comatose patients after severe traumatic brain injury with the dual cannabinoid CB1/CB2 receptor agonist KN38–7271:

a randomized, double-blind, placebo-controlled phase II trial. *JNLS A Cent Eur Neurosurg*. 2012;73(4):204–216.

12. Nguyen BM, Kim D, Bricker S, et al. Effect of marijuana use on outcomes in traumatic brain injury. *Am Surg*. 2014;80(10):979–983.

13. Russo EB. Cannabis therapeutics and the future of neurology. *Front Integr Neurosci*. 2018;12:51.

14. Russo EB, Marcu J. Cannabis pharmacology: the usual suspects and a few promising leads. *Adv Pharmacol*. 2017;80:67–134.

23 Cancer

CANCER AND CANNABIS

The benefit of cannabis for cancer patients has traditionally been centered upon palliative relief of nausea, vomiting and loss of appetite that may be a consequence of chemotherapy or radiation therapy (see Chapters 14 and 38). In fact, cannabis has often proven more effective than any other medication for these symptoms, and has long been prescribed in the form of dronabinol, an FDA-approved form of THC since 1975. Other potential palliative effects of cannabinoids include treatment of cancer-induced pain and peripheral neuropathy that may result from chemotherapy.[1] In addition, cannabis is used to treat the depression and fatigue that may accompany cancer. For a cancer patient, cannabis has a number of potential benefits, especially in the management of symptoms. In a review of cannabis use in cancer care, the author summarizes:

> Cannabis is useful in combatting anorexia, chemotherapy-induced nausea and vomiting, pain, insomnia, and depression. Cannabis might be less potent than other available antiemetics, but for some patients, it is the only agent that works, and it is the only antiemetic that also increases appetite . . . and it could prove useful in chemotherapy-induced neuropathy.[2]

An observational study of 2,970 cancer patients reported the benefits of cannabis after a 6-month study. While 25% died and almost 20% stopped the treatment, of the remaining 60% who responded, 96% reported an improvement in their condition. The authors conclude: "In addition to pain relief, similar to findings in other prospective studies, the most improved symptoms reported by patients in our cohort were nausea and vomiting, sleep disorders, restlessness, anxiety and depression, pruritus and headaches."[3] Some of the improvement in symptoms may be due to some patients having completed chemotherapy during this period. "Cannabis as a palliative treatment for cancer patients seems to be well tolerated, effective and safe option to help patients cope with the malignancy related symptoms."[3]

Yet in addition to all of the aforementioned, some patients request advice on how to use cannabis to treat the cancer itself. There are many anecdotal reports of success with high-potency oils, some by patients using an oil referred to as "Rick Simpson oil," yet long-term follow-up is generally unavailable, even anecdotally. There have been no large-scale clinical trials to verify these positive reports. The course of treatment with cannabis for its antiproliferative effects is experimental, complex, expensive and requires continual reinforcement. I have worked with several patients in this regard, mostly in the event that they are determined to follow this course anyway and I cannot deter them. I prefer to recommend cannabis as an adjunctive therapy to potentially augment other therapies they may be doing under the supervision of their oncologist. On rare occasion, some patients prefer to use cannabis as a stand-alone

DOI: 10.1201/9781003098201-34

therapy, or unfortunately, as a last-ditch effort when all else has failed. The research that has guided me is providing advice presented in the following.

Cannabis and cannabinoids are generally thought to have antitumoral properties. Cannabinoid receptors are upregulated in tumor tissue. the endocannabinoid system (ECS) can be overactivated in cancer and may be pro-tumorigenic. Conversely, the activation of cannabinoid receptors reduces tumor growth. The upregulation of endo-cannabinoid degrading enzymes has been observed in aggressive human tumors and cancer cell lines.[1] Yet, in some cases, low doses of cannabinoids actually stimulate cancer cell growth in vitro.

> There is mixed evidence on the effects of cannabinoids on cancer: in vitro and in vivo studies and clinical data showed both antineoplastic and protumoral activity. However, studies performed to investigate marijuana smoking effects on carcinogenesis and tumour growth produced contradictory results.[4]

Depending on concentration, cannabinoids may either inhibit or stimulate cancer cell growth in vitro and potentially in vivo. "It has been demonstrated in vitro that cannabinoids can exhibit a stimulatory activity in nanomolar concentration and an inhibitory activity in micromolar concentration (biphasic response), which significantly exceeds concentrations usually detected in blood of marijuana smokers."[5] This underscores the need for judicious consideration of cannabis as a cancer therapy, with specific regard to appropriate dosing.

> A number of plant-derived, synthetic and endogenous cannabinoids are now known to exert antiproliferative actions on a wide spectrum of tumor cells in culture. More importantly, cannabinoid administration to mice curbs the growth of various types of tumor xenografts, including lung carcinoma, glioma, thyroid epithelioma, skin, and pancreatic carcinoma, lymphoma and melanoma.[6]

It is important to remember that the function of the ECS in animals is far different from in vitro or xenograft studies.

The antiproliferative effects of cannabinoids differ depending on the type of cancer and within cell lines of the same type of cancer. As far as the properties of specific cannabinoids are concerned, a study of several of these showed surprising results with xenografts produced by breast carcinoma cells injected into mice. Cannabidiol was the most effective overall, followed by CBC and CBG. THCA was effective as well, with potency similar to THC. The least effective was CBDA.[7] One review article summarizes the results for in vivo studies for the aforementioned types of cancers. For gliomas, both CBD and THC were studied and shown to be effective. For prostate xenografts, a synthetic cannabinoid agonist was studied and shown to be effective. Breast carcinoma, as earlier, showed multiple cannabinoids being effective. Lung carcinoma treated by THC in mice was found to be effective, also in limiting metastasis. In skin carcinoma, a study with a CB2 agonist was found to be effective with limitation of metastasis as well. Lymphoma studies of mouse cell lines showed THC to be effective.[8] Pancreatic cancer in vitro studies demonstrated tumor growth-inhibiting effects with CBD, THC and synthetic derivatives.[9] A recent report found that THC did not show anticancer activity in colorectal cancer cell lines, but that CBD was somewhat successful, and synthetic cannabinoids more so.[10]

A rare clinical trial with human subjects was done with intratumoral injection of THC into nine patients with glioma, with daily injection into a brain cavity at the site of debulking. Total doses ranged from 0.80 to 3.29 mg for 10–64 days. The result was decreased tumor cell proliferation and increased apoptosis.[11] The study proposes that cannabinoid inductions of glioma cell death may occur by two mechanisms:

[A] process of programmed cell death called apoptosis and an impairment of tumor vascularization and therefore blood (i.e., nutrient and oxygen) supply. Remarkably, this antiproliferative effect seems to be selective for tumor cells, supporting the notion that cannabinoid receptors regulate cell survival and cell death pathways differently in tumor and non-tumor cells.[6]

The fact that cannabinoids only seem to induce apoptosis in cancer cells, while not harmful to normal cells does imply the possibility of a cannabinoid cancer-targeted therapy. Intratumoral injection, however, is not the same as taking oral concentrated cannabis oil, which goes into the general circulation.

In recent years, the focus has shifted from using THC-enriched oils to treat cancer to CBD-rich oils or combinations with THC. There are several proposed mechanisms of action for CBD that have been proposed. There include stimulation of reactive oxygen species (ROS) production, inhibition of degradation of anandamide (AEA) and downregulation of gene expression of Id-1, a key regulator of the metastatic potential of breast cancer.[5] In a study of immune-competent mice, treatment with CBD significantly reduced breast tumor mass as well as the size and number of lung metastasis. The tumor acquired resistance to the inhibitory properties of CBD (1 or 5 mg/kg) by approximately day 25, and by the end of the study (day 30), this effect was not statistically significant.[12] This brings up the real and complicating issue of resistance to treatment developing over time. A review of the effects of CBD concludes: "Collectively, these preliminary data demonstrate that, besides its well known pro-apoptotic anti-proliferative and anti-invasive actions, CBD may also exert anti-angiogenic effects, thus further strengthening its potential application in cancer therapy."[13]

As far as mixed cannabinoid effects are concerned, these are most promising. "The anti-tumor activity of THC on glioma cells is enhanced by cannabidiol Interestingly, the anti-cancer effects of cannabidiol (CBD) may occur completely independently of cannabinoid receptor activation."[14] In a clinical study of a combination of THC and CBD in 21 patients with glioblastoma, 83% had 1 year survival rate compared with 53% in the placebo group.[15]

Thus, THC/CBD-balanced preparations, obviously if well produced and standardized, could be considered a therapeutically safer option than dronabinol or nabilone, whose therapeutic windows are usually very narrow. Other constituents of cannabis, especially terpenes have been proposed to exert synergic therapeutic actions with phytocannabinoids.[16]

Regarding cannabis in combination with antineoplastic drugs, two studies are of interest. THC and temozolomide provided strong antitumoral action in glioma xenografts, and gemcitabine and several cannabinoid agonists synergistically acted upon pancreatic cancer cells. It has also been indicated that anandamide and HU-210 may enhance the efficacy of paclitaxel and 5-fluorouracil.[1]

I concur with a recent review which summarizes: "Cannabinoids can palliate some cancer symptoms but it is unclear how effective they are compared to or combined with conventional therapies, or even whether cannabis, purified cannabinoids, or synthetic cannabinoids are more effective."[14]

PATIENT REPORTS

To move on to patient results from my practice, most of the patients seen with cancer were middle-aged or older, about 40–90 years old. I have seen two types of patients here: those who want to treat the symptoms of cancer and those who want a therapeutic regimen to reduce the cancer itself. All too often, these patients come in too late in their process, that is, at stage IV, or when other therapies have stopped working. Here are a few illustrative case reports.

Patient 1: This is a 59-year-old female with glioblastoma, recently diagnosed, who just had surgical removal of the tumor 1 month earlier. She was about to start radiation and chemotherapy. At first, she just wanted to use cannabis for palliative reasons, that is, nausea from chemotherapy, help with sleep, etc. I advised a CBD/THC 1:1 mix, 10 mg 2×/day for mood and nausea, and up to 40 mg THC indica at night as needed for sleep. She then got in touch with someone who sold high-dose oil to treat cancer and followed a protocol resulting in CBD/THC 1:4 ratio, 1,000 mg at night for 2 months, then reduced to 125 mg at night for maintenance. She continued to use a 1:1 edible, approximately 10 mg 2×/day. Chemotherapy was due to end shortly. Her MRI was clear and she was feeling well. By the end of her second year, her maintenance regimen, 125 mg at night continued, the MRI was normal, but she was feeling tired. I was concerned that her maintenance dose wasn't quite high enough, especially now that chemotherapy ended, so I suggested she raise it to 200 mg at night. By the end of the third year, her MRI was still normal, but her nighttime dose was only 150 mg. The fatigue continued. I again advised going up to 200 mg at night, which she did. During the fourth year, recurrence in the lungs manifested on the 150 mg nightly dose of CBD/THC 1:1. The patient is considering increasing cannabis again while pursuing other anticancer options. At last follow-up, she had had a recurrence on the 150 mg maintenance dose, but now 5 years post-diagnosis is still managing her cancer.

Pearls: Glioblastoma is one of the rare cancer types that have had human trials, with promising results. I do encourage glioblastoma patients who want to use cannabis as a cancer therapy to add it as an adjunct to their traditional treatment. The problem is in getting patients to understand that maintenance on cannabis is required, as we don't have enough information to ensure that the tumor won't come back after the cannabis is withdrawn. Indeed, it is with patients such as these that we can learn if cannabis can improve longevity. This patient has well exceeded the median 15–16-month survival rate for her cancer.

Patient 2: This is a 61-year-old female also with glioblastoma, similar to the previous case, having completed surgery and radiation and was undergoing chemotherapy. This patient was referred by a dispensary who gave her a CBD/THC 1:3 tincture. She was taking 12 mg 2×/day. She wanted to use cannabis therapeutically to treat her cancer. We immediately began an upward titration protocol of a CBD/THC 1:3 oil to reach 200 mg 2×/day plus 300 mg at night, which she did for 3 months. She reported that the chemotherapy was stopped due to high liver enzymes. Her MRI showed the tumor had shrunk to half its previous size during this time. I then advised a maintenance protocol for 6 months of 300 mg/day of the same oil, which she did. The MRI showed no tumor. We then went to a maintenance protocol of 200 mg/day ongoing, with MRI checks every 2 months. As with the previous patient, there has been a recurrence on the maintenance dose.

Pearls: As the previous case, cannabis therapy is shown to be a potentially useful adjunct to standard treatment of glioblastoma. Time will tell what the appropriate maintenance dose is and how long it must continue. These first two patients tell us that the maintenance dose must be increased, or that the extension of survival with the aid of cannabis may be less than or equal to about 5 years.

Patient 3: This is an 88-year-old female with rectal cancer diagnosed 3 months earlier. She did not want surgery, as recommended, which would necessitate a colostomy. She did do 1 month of radiation treatment. She was new to cannabis use. Her daughter came in with her to help with facilitating a plan. We began a protocol titrating up to 250 mg by suppository every night of a CBD/THC 1:4 mix. Fortunately, we had a source of custom-made suppositories made from concentrated cannabis oil. It took 1 month to titrate up to full dose, which she stayed on for 3 months. She tolerated the cannabis effects well, sleeping through its nightly time of action. There was no evidence of a tumor at this time. We then began a maintenance protocol of a 125-mg suppository at night with a CBD/THC 2:3 ratio. She followed-up 1 year later, reporting that she stopped using the suppositories because they were inconvenient, and wanted to use oral cannabis instead. There was still no tumor. I advised her to continue suppositories, as she would be altered from oral therapy and would probably not like it, but she chose to discontinue cannabis therapy. She passed on 1 year later with metastatic cancer.

Pearls: This case illustrates the efficacy of suppository delivery, especially relevant to pelvic/rectal conditions. Due to avoidance of second-pass metabolism, we can avoid some of the disorienting effects from the 11-OH-THC metabolite and provide THC directly to the rectal area. In addition, there is some evidence that rectal absorption is more efficient than oral absorption, so we can use a lower dose. In retrospect, a mix with a higher concentration of CBD might have been more appropriate in this case as CBD has been shown to be effective in colon cancer cell lines. As far as efficacy for rectal cancer is concerned, all we can conclude is that this patient had 1 year of no tumor growth while on this protocol. Due to the patient's advanced age, it is remarkable that she was compliant with over 1 year of cannabis therapy, especially by daily suppository use.

Patient 4: This is a 70-year-old male with prostate cancer, already treated with radiation and Lupron. He said it was localized to the prostate, but was an aggressive type. He had been using cannabis for the past 2 years to help manage hypertension originally, but recently started on high-dose oil to treat the cancer. He was taking 500 mg cannabinoids/day of a CBD/THC 4:1 mix for the past month. He wanted advice on how to proceed. I advised continuing on the high-dose therapy for 2 more months, for a 3-month period total, then moving to a maintenance dose. He did 2 more months of a CBD/THC 1:1 oil with a total of 600 mg cannabinoids/day, then reduced it to 240 mg/day for 8 more months. He was putting the oil into capsules and distributing it by dosing 4×/day. At the same time, the Lupron treatment continued for 2 years. Meanwhile, his PSA levels were being monitored. They were low, and his cancer was stated to be in remission or gone. I advised continuing on 50 mg/day of the 1:1 oil, divided into twice daily dosing for maintenance for an indefinite time. The patient stopped cannabis at this time, as it was causing alteration in perception during the day, and he thought he was fine. When his PSA began to rise, off Lupron, off cannabis, he contacted me again for advice. He then took 100 mg/day of the 1:1 oil for 3 months and went back to 50 mg/day. His PSA plateaued on 100 mg, and slightly raised again on 50 mg. We came up with a suppository plan for 50 mg/day for maintenance to reduce psychoactivity, which was easily tolerated. He has reported that his PSA is stable on this regimen.

Pearls: Did this patient need to use cannabis at all? I don't know. But he was determined to do so. He already started on the high-dose oil before he consulted me. He made his own decisions throughout, to do maintenance, to stop maintenance, to resume maintenance, because it is possibly preventive for recurrence. I am not a cancer specialist, nor do I claim to be. At all times, I advised cannabis as an adjunct therapy, and the patient was being regularly followed by a urologist. When his PSA rose off the cannabis, I suggested it may be an "off the anti-inflammatory (cannabis)" bounce. This might happen after high- or even moderate-dose cannabis is withdrawn. We don't know. There is much to be learned about parameters of, and its reestablishment as cannabis therapy is reduced.

Patient 5: This is a 59-year-old female patient who I'd been seeing for ongoing neuroendocrine tumors. Her original diagnosis was over 9 years ago, treated by surgery. She complained of chronic problems with nausea, appetite and sleep. She took alprazolam or zolpidem as needed for sleep. Her ongoing therapy included Sandostatin injections 1×/month for carcinoid tumor symptoms such as excessive sweating. She reported previously following a high-dose "Rick Simpson oil" (THC-rich) protocol to treat the cancer. Her tumor growth seemed now to be arrested. She followed an erratic cannabis protocol over the next year, using low doses of CBD-rich oil most of the time to control nausea, but did report a 3-month period of high-dose use. I recommended that she stay on at least 50 mg/day of a CBD/THC 2:1 mix as a maintenance dose. She preferred to continue to treat symptoms, most often vaping an indica strain for appetite, relaxation and sleep. At our last visit, there was indication of growth of liver tumors, after which she did pass on.

Pearls: The concept of a moderate dose of cannabinoids for preventive maintenance following cancer is difficult to sell patients on, because there are no controlled trials of their effectiveness, no established protocol of either dose or composition and during periods of "remission" the need for prevention is not evident. Yet, especially when patients have used high-dose cannabis as part of their anticancer therapy, it is risky to not have a maintenance period of at least several years. Unfortunately, this patient did not remain on a maintenance protocol, yet used cannabis for symptom control. Hopefully, there will be clinical trials to support this policy at some time in the not-too-distant future.

Patient 6: This is a 63-year-old female with a 2-year history of metastatic small cell lung cancer and squamous cell carcinoma of the head and neck. She had previously done chemotherapy and a course of high-dose cannabis oil, "Rick Simpson oil," that a family member made for her. She used 400–500 mg of THC-rich cannabinoids/day, which she had just finished after 6 months. Now she was using about 1 ounce/month by smoking or vaporizing. Other medications included oxycodone 10 mg/day, Ativan and blood pressure medicines. I advised her to discontinue smoking and stay on a maintenance cannabis therapy with a CBD/THC mix of at least 100 mg/day. She ended up using 50–75 mg of a CBD/THC 3:1 oil at bedtime. Over the next year, the cancer was stable, with no new metastases, nor new tumor growth. She did have neck lymph nodes surgically removed. She still complained of daily fatigue, some nausea and peripheral neuropathy. Oxycodone and Ativan were discontinued. At our next annual visit, she reported using 40 mg of the oil each night and was still smoking 2–4 joints/day. She had a 40-pack year history of tobacco smoking, which stopped when her cancer was diagnosed. She passed on 2 years after our last visit.

Pearls: The efficacy of high-dose cannabis oil for metastatic lung cancer has been supported by some anecdotal reports. Again, what is missing is the importance of a maintenance dose, which we still don't know will be successful in the long term. Much more research needs to be done on this issue.

CANNABIS THERAPY SUMMARY

I have reported here on several cases among many that I have had experience with using cannabis as a therapy for the cancer itself. Two other patients with pancreatic cancer that I have seen also utilized cannabis as an adjunct with limited success. At this time, one has passed on after 4 years and one is still effectively combatting the cancer. It is undisputable that cannabis therapy for nausea, mood, pain, appetite and pain is a useful adjunctive therapy, but for the treatment of cancer we have much to learn. In general, an oral dose of 800 mg/day of cannabinoids for at least 3 months is indicated as antiproliferative therapy, or 500 mg/day by rectal administration. There are also patients who have applied concentrated topical cannabis to areas affected by cancer, such as to the breasts or the skin, although the absorption of cannabis oil through the skin is likely inefficient. How are we to evaluate whether cannabis as an anticancer therapy is even useful? The projection of success and/or extension of life and quality of life depends upon the type of cancer, the composition of the cannabis, that is, whether THC-dominant, CBD-dominant or a mix, the stage of the cancer and whether the patient is following the standard treatment protocol and is using cannabis as an adjunct or as an alternative. I have counseled that as an adjunct it might be considered, but not to replace other therapies. There is just so much that we don't know about effects of high-dose cannabis in patients with cancer, that this course is difficult to recommend even to patients who plead with the clinician for a chance to try. And it seems that most don't appreciate the need for a sufficient ongoing maintenance therapy, advised even when the cancer is in remission. As far as symptom mediation is concerned, the doses and cannabis advised are the same as in non-cancer patients, in the 10 mg dose range, or by vaporization as needed.

REFERENCES

1. Velasco G, Sánchez C, Guzmán M. Towards the use of cannabinoids as antitumour agents. *Nat Rev Cancer.* 2012;12(6):436–444.
2. Abrams DI. Integrating cannabis into clinical cancer care. *Curr Oncol.* 2016;23(S2):S8-S14.
3. Bar Lev Schleider L, Mechoulam R, Lederman V, et al. Prospective analysis of safety and efficacy of medical cannabis in large unselected population of patients with cancer. *Eur J Intern Med.* 2018;49:37–43.
4. Bifulco M, Laezza C, Pisanti S, Gazzerro P. Cannabinoids and cancer: pros and cons of an antitumour strategy. *Br J Pharmacol.* 2006;148(2):123–135.
5. Śledziński P, Zeyland J, Słomski R, Nowak A. The current state and future perspectives of cannabinoids in cancer biology. *Cancer Med.* 2018;7(3):765–775.
6. Guzman M. Cannabinoids: potential antitumoral agents? *Cannabinoids.* 2006;1(2):15–17.
7. Ligresti A, Moriello AS, Starowicz K, et al. Antitumor activity of plant cannabinoids with emphasis on the effect of cannabidiol on human breast carcinoma. *J Pharmacol Exp Ther.* 2006;318:1375–1387.
8. Sarfaraz S, Adhami VM, Syed DN, Afaq F, Mukhtar H. Cannabinoids for cancer treatment: progress and promise. *Cancer Res.* 2008;68:(2).
9. Sharafi G, He H, Nikfarjam M. Potential use of cannabinoids for the treatment of pancreatic cancer. *J Pancreat Cancer.* 2019;5(1):1–7.
10. Raup-Konsavage WM, Johnson M, Legare CA, et. al. Synthetic cannabinoid activity against colorectal cancer cells. *Cannabis Cannabinoid Res.* 2018;3(1):272–281.
11. Guzmán M, Duarte MJ, Blázquez C, et al. A pilot clinical study of Δ9-tetrahydrocannabinol in patients with recurrent glioblastoma multiforme. *Br J Cancer.* 2006;95:197–203.
12. McAllister SD, Murase R, Christian RT, et al. Pathways mediating the effects of cannabidiol on the reduction of breast cancer cell proliferation, invasion, and metastasis. *Breast Cancer Res Treat.* 2011;129(1):37–47.
13. Massi P, Solinas M, Cinquina V, Parolaro D. Cannabidiol as potential anticancer drug. *Br J Clin Pharmacol.* 2013;75(2):303–312.
14. Bowles DW, O'Bryant CL, Camidge DR, Jimeno A. The intersection between cannabis and cancer in the United States. *Crit Rev Oncol Hematol.* 2012;83(1):1–10.
15. GW pharmaceuticals achieves positive results in phase 2 proof of concept study in glioma www.globenewswire.com/news-release/2017/02/07/914583/0/en/GW-Pharmaceuticals-Achieves-Positive-Results-in-Phase-2-Proof-of-Concept-Study-in-Glioma.html Accessed January 10, 2020.
16. Guzmán M. Cannabis for the management of cancer symptoms: THC version 2.0? *Cannabis Cannabinoid Res.* 2018;3(1):117–119.

24 Cardiovascular Disease, Hypertension

CARDIOVASCULAR DISEASE, HYPERTENSION AND CANNABIS

Cannabis and cannabinoids have extensive, complex effects on the cardiovascular system. As with all tightly regulated homeostatic systems, endocannabinoid involvement is widespread and acts by both stimulatory and inhibitory functions. A review of the cardiovascular effects of cannabinoids summarizes: "Cannabinoids, through central and local mechanisms, affect key cardiovascular parameters in health and disease, such as heart rate, blood pressure, vascular and cardiac contractility and inflammation."[1] Cannabinoids have a whole host of actions in the cardiovascular system, including vasoactivity, cardiac performance, ischemia-reperfusion, endothelial and smooth muscle cell migration, angiogenesis, vascular wall, inflammation and atherogenesis. The complex effects of cannabinoids on cardiovascular actions are mediated through multiple cannabinoid receptors (CBrs) – vascular and myocardial. Non-CBrs are also targeted, including intracellular ion channels and transporters, as well as targets on cardiac myocytes, vascular smooth muscle and endothelial cells. Endocannabinoids often perform opposing functions to maintain cardiac homeostasis. A review points out that cannabinoid agonists such as AEA and THC evoke effects such as hypotension, bradycardia and depressed cardiac contractility, but these are less pronounced/absent in normotensive animals and augmented in hypertensive ones.[2] Endocannabinoid regulation of atherosclerosis in animal models indicate CB2 receptor activity is involved. Cannabinoids also attenuate inflammatory responses and the interaction between activated endothelium and inflammatory cells. A review of the topic points to a mouse model of atherosclerosis, in which THC resulted in significant inhibition of plaque development in a CB2-dependent manner.[3] It further points out that selective CB2R agonists have been shown to be cardioprotective not only in limiting atherosclerosis but also in animal models of myocardial infarction, stroke and stenosis.

Cannabinoid effects on blood pressure are contradictory. Regarding endocannabinoid regulation, a review states: "The ECS may become over-activated and may contribute to hypotension/cardiodepression through cardiovascular CB1 receptors. . . . Intriguingly, the ECS may also be activated as a compensatory mechanism in various forms of hypertension."[2] As far as vasodilation and blood pressure effects are concerned, are cannabinoids vasodilators or vasoconstrictors? The confusing answer is both. The vasodilatory effect of endocannabinoids may involve CB1 and TRPV1 receptors. "Cannabinoids elicit hypotension and bradycardia via peripherally located CB1 receptors. Those receptors mediate presynaptic inhibition of norepinephrine release from peripheral sympathetic nerve terminals with major impact on blood pressure regulation. However, vascular cannabinoid receptors may also directly

DOI: 10.1201/9781003098201-35

mediate vasodilation."[4] Conversely, "THC can produce vasoconstriction in a CB1 and endothelial dependent manner. The acute effects of THC including intoxication and tachycardia are quite subject to tachyphylaxis, and will often diminish with chronic administration."[5] Decreased cardiac contractility with cannabinoids has also been suggested to explain decreased blood pressure in rodent studies.[6] In a study of heavy cannabis users before and after cessation, they found:

> Systolic blood pressure increased from a mean of 129.6 mmHg during cannabis use to a mean of 139.8 mmHg during abstinence. Diastolic blood pressure increased from a mean of 74.8 mmHg during cannabis use to a mean of 81.8 mmHg during abstinence.[7]

One might infer that we are looking at a 10-point or less reduction in blood pressure in chronic cannabis users. Clinically, this is within the range that I have seen most often in my patient population.

As far as the response of heart rate to THC or THC-rich cannabis is concerned, it may stay the same, or increase, or decrease. "A review of almost 200 articles describing almost 400 different tests demonstrated that an increase in HR [heart rate] was the most consistent result, and almost all studies with the measurement of this parameter proved statistically significant."[8] This review found that increases in HR associated with smoking one cannabis cigarette ranged from 20% to 100%, with the peak occurring 10–30 min after the onset of smoking. It is unclear where the 100% statistic comes from, that is, doubling the heart rate, as this is not seen clinically. The same review goes on to say that chronic use results in a decrease in heart rate. Furthermore, "Because tolerance develops to the acute cardiovascular effects of cannabis with repeated use, it is plausible that a rebound increase in heart rate and blood pressure would be observed following abrupt cessation of heavy use."[8] Indeed, small HR variability can be seen during a withdrawal phase. It's not possible to anticipate a single response by an individual to a homeostatic modulator such as THC. The challenge of interpreting studies on the cardiovascular effects of cannabis has been limited by study bias, individual variability, dosage inconsistency and tolerance of subjects.

It is not only cannabinoid agonists such as THC that are cardioprotective, but CBD is also active in this arena. CBD acts largely in a non-CBr manner. It is known to affect the cardiovascular system, in part by binding to adenosine receptors. Adenosine receptors affect the regulation of coronary blood flow and oxygen consumption by cardiac muscle. CBD was beneficial in animal models of myocardial infarction, stroke, cardiomyopathies and autoimmune myocarditis.[9]

> In vivo administration of CBD before cardiac ischemia and reperfusion also reduces ventricular arrhythmias and infarct size. CBD also causes both acute and time-dependent vasorelaxation in isolated arteries in rats and humans. There is also evidence from animal studies that CBD modulates the cardiovascular response to stress.[10]

In a study of the effect of 600 mg of pure CBD (likely translatable to lower doses of CBD-rich cannabis) on cardiovascular function, they found a small blood pressure decrease of 6 mmHg and increased HR by 10 beats per minute.[8]

A study of the acute and chronic effects of CBD on human cardiovascular function in healthy males was carried out using 600 mg of CBD for 7 days. They found that developed in response to chronic CBD administration, but CBD's ability to lower blood pressure persisted during stress.[12] The authors also point out that not only CBD but also THCV and THC may have some protective effects against ischemia/reperfusion injury by anti-inflammatory effects via the CB2 receptor.

There have been several poorly designed studies that seem to have a bias toward cannabis as having negative cardiac outcomes, such as increased risk for myocardial infarction, but this has largely been refuted (see "Cardiovascular Risks" in Chapter 6).[11] A review of the effect of cannabis on cardiovascular function concluded:

> The cardiovascular effects of marijuana largely depend on several factors, including composition of the plant . . . and the route of administration (inhalation route can lead to rapid increases in plasma levels with more rapid decline, whereas oromucosal administration of marijuana extracts, such as nabiximols, or pure THC can result in lower, but more stable levels).[9]

PATIENT REPORTS

To move on to patient results from my practice, they ranged in age from 40s with simple hypertension to the 80s with more severe heart disease. The question was often whether cannabis was contraindicated, rather than how it might be therapeutic. While it is true that naive users should be made aware that inhalation methods might cause transient heart palpitations or tachycardia, this is by no means prohibitive in that slowly increasing dosage, other delivery methods and products with CBD can circumvent this problem. Here are a few illustrative case reports.

Patient 1: This is an 81-year-old female, on hospice, with multiple medical problems of such significance that her anxiety complaints had been overlooked. She had congestive heart failure (CHF) and severe dyspnea, and was on supplemental oxygen. She also had glaucoma, insomnia and anxiety. She was on several heart medications and eyedrops. She was new to cannabis use. With CHF and her breathing issues, inhalation of cannabis was contraindicated, but we were able to start her on a CBD-rich tincture. She ended up using a low dose, about 1–2 mg 2×/day, which she said helped her to relax. I also advised an indica tincture before bed. Her dispensary recommended a 10-mg indica mint that she took before bed to give her 7 hours of sleep, and a 5-mg sativa mint that she took every morning to improve appetite. She had gained 5 lb over the year. And she was supplementing with a CBD-rich mouth spray as needed for anxiety or agitation. I advised her to increase her daily tincture dose to 3 mg 2×/day. On follow-up with this patient's family, I learned that 3 years subsequent to our last visit she passed away. This is what her daughter had to say.

> My mother passed away peacefully on cannabis. She was helped so much by your wisdom and she was able to get off Hospice as well as morphine. She dealt as best she could with her Congestive Heart Failure and lack of sleep from it by staying calm and sleeping with cannabis. . . . [S]he had to go back on Hospice, again, the nurses could only offer morphine and lorazepam and she could never tolerate the morphine and was

sick and totally crazy on it hallucinating and screaming in her hospital bed at home. I finally went back to her cannabis and she was comfortable on tinctures and passed in peace at home.

Pearls: Several things of interest are apparent in this case. First, she exceeded her hospice projection and was able to see me for 2 years in a row. Second, she was able to take THC-rich sublingual mints for sleep and appetite, which were fine with her CHF, because they were a low-enough dose and have a moderate time of onset. CHF is a condition that needs careful supervision. In the case of this elderly patient, dispensary suggestions could have been dangerous for her health. It turned out OK, but could just as easily not have. In some states with a more cautious medical cannabis protocol, this would have been avoided as the physician must specify what specific cannabis medicine the patient is approved for. She came seeking help for anxiety, and found better sleep and appetite as well. As per the addendum, we see here where cannabis acts effectively for palliative care, perhaps better than anything else that she could have taken.

Patient 2: This is a 69-year-old male who was using cannabis to aid in blood pressure control. He had been using it for 50 years, just a few puffs a day, mostly by pipe. He was on two blood pressure medications, Benicar and isradipine, which he said "makes him sick." His blood pressure range was 125–165/60–95 on the medication and cannabis. He said the cannabis helps to lower it 15–20 points. I would describe him as a type A personality, high strung, and indeed in this patient, relaxation did seem to lower his blood pressure. He did not tolerate several additional hypertension medications that he'd been prescribed. He also had clonazepam for anxiety, which he rarely used. Over the next few years, his blood pressure started to spike, and labetalol was added. He continued to have spikes in the afternoons, after which cannabis use brought it down, which he reported was by 30 points. He did not deviate from smoking it 2× daily.

Pearls: Do we know how much help cannabis was to this patient's hypertension? Probably not, as he smoked 2×/day with or without blood pressure spikes. Yet, over 5 years, he reported that he believed it was helping to reduce it. Presumably, his ability to destress was linked to cannabis use, even though he also did yoga and exercise. This is a case of a specific type of patient who has stress-induced blood pressure increases. We would not expect to see a 30-point decrease in other forms of hypertension.

Patient 3: This is a 60-year-old male with complaints of heart palpitations and stress. He had been using cannabis for 45 years, an average of 2 puffs/day. The heart palpitations came on in the evenings, and he'd had them since his 20s. He said they felt like an irregular heartbeat. His EKG was normal, and on exam his heart was normal in rate and rhythm. He reported that 1 puff made them go away. He was on no medications. I advised him to have no more than 1 puff per episode, as he was a very light user, and 2 puffs could potentially exacerbate the palpitations. Over the 4 years we worked together, he actually continued at 1 puff 1–2×/evening.

Pearls: One of the undesirable side effects of THC is the possibility of increasing heart palpitations, especially in users with no tolerance. This is an example of almost microdosing, where the amount of cannabis used is not enough to cause a negative effect. It is commonly found that the dose of cannabis is of great importance in endocannabinoid-related homeostasis.

Patient 4: This is a 78-year-old male who came in wanting to use cannabis to decrease inflammation, especially in his cardiovascular system. He was concerned about lipids but didn't want to take statins. He also wanted to treat his blood pressure that averaged in the 150s/70s. He had been using a small amount of cannabis tincture for several months. I counseled him on several health maintenance actions, including decreasing caffeine and salt, increasing water, getting more exercise and using a CBD-rich tincture daily. Over the next few years, his lipid levels improved, but blood pressure did not, as expected for CBD-rich cannabis. Ultimately, he began 10 mg of lisinopril, which brought his blood pressure down to 130/70. Cannabis use changed to about 5 mg of indica at bedtime as he also reported some insomnia. Sleep improved with cannabis, so he continued THC as a daily anti-inflammatory. He was quite pleased that his only prescribed medication was a low dose of lisinopril.

Pearls: Little attention has been paid to the anti-inflammatory potential of cannabis, not only in reducing cardiac inflammation, but in serving a lipid-lowering function. Low doses of cannabinoids are not proven to have such function. But for many cardiovascular conditions, improved sleep, less stress, and taking "preventive" measures proactively, such as a small amount of daily cannabis, may contribute to improved health.

CANNABIS THERAPY SUMMARY

Although the endocannabinoid system and THC are known to affect a multitude of cardiovascular regulatory mechanisms, it is not often that cannabis is used as a therapeutic regimen for cardiovascular conditions. The most common condition we see it used for is hypertension, with a lowering of blood pressure from 10 to 30 points. This is often achieved with modest doses of THC such as a few puffs of THC-rich cannabis, most effectively in cases of stress-induced blood pressure fluctuations. We also know that cannabis is cardioprotective for inflammation, ischemia and cardiomyopathy, yet dosing for these outcomes has rarely been documented and has yet to be determined. In using cannabis to treat cardiovascular conditions, it is important to avoid selected risk, such as the acute effect of THC in naive users, which may precipitate increased heart rate or palpitations. Clinically we advise avoidance of high doses of THC in patients susceptible to these negative effects. One of the caveats we give to patients at risk for MI, angina or low cardiac output is to avoid inhalation methods and use low doses of oral methods with slower onset. Of course, this caveat does not apply to CBD-rich cannabis, which can be safely applied for most dosing protocols.

REFERENCES

1. Bondarenko AI. Cannabinoids and cardiovascular system. *Adv Exp Med Biol.* 2019;1162:63–87.
2. Pacher P, Steffens S. The emerging role of the endocannabinoid system in cardiovascular disease. *Semin Immunopathol.* 2009;31(1):63–77.

3. Mach F, Montecucco F, Steffens S. Cannabinoid receptors in acute and chronic complications of atherosclerosis. *Br J Pharmacol.* 2008;153(2):290–298.
4. Bonz A, Laser M, Kullmer S, et al. Cannabinoids acting on CB1 receptors decrease contractile performance in human atrial muscle. *J Cardiovascular Pharmacol.* 2003;41(4):657–664.
5. Russo E. Synthetic and natural cannabinoids: the cardiovascular risk. *Br J Cardiol.* 2015;22:7–9.
6. Cunha P, Romão AM, Mascarenhas-Melo F, Teixeira HM, Reis F. Endocannabinoid system in cardiovascular disorders: new pharmacotherapeutic opportunities. *J Pharm Bioallied Sci.* 2011;3(3):350–360.
7. Vandrey R, Umbricht A, Strain EC. Increased blood pressure following abrupt cessation of daily cannabis use. *J Addict Med.* 2011;5(1):16–20.
8. Malinowska B, Baranowska-Kuczko M, Schlicker E. Triphasic blood pressure responses to cannabinoids: do we understand the mechanism? *Br J Pharmacol.* 2012;165(7):2073–2088.
9. Pacher P, Steffens S, Haskó G, Schindler TH, Kunos G. Cardiovascular effects of marijuana and synthetic cannabinoids: the good, the bad, and the ugly. *Nat Rev Cardiol.* 2018;15(3):151–166.
10. Jadoon KA, Tan GD, O'Sullivan SE. A single dose of cannabidiol reduces blood pressure in healthy volunteers in a randomized crossover study. *JCI Insight.* 2017;2(12):e93760.
11. Mittleman MA, Lewis RA, Maclure M, Sherwood JB, Muller JE. Triggering myocardial infarction by marijuana. *Circulation.* 2001;103(23):2805–2809.
12. Sultan SR, O'Sullivan SE, England TJ. The effects of acute and sustained cannabidiol dosing for seven days on the haemodynamics in healthy men: a randomised controlled trial. *Br J Clin Pharmacol.* 2020;86(6):1125–1138.

25 Chronic Pain

CHRONIC PAIN AND CANNABIS

Chronic pain is a condition where patients are often focused on primarily managing their pain, significant pain, above and beyond the underlying causative condition(s). In this case, they seek help for the condition of "pain management," which is multifactorial. Cannabis holds a special role in this arena due to its myriad of potential effects, including, but not limited to, analgesia, anti-inflammatory, antinociception, mood management, muscle relaxation and synergy with opiates (see Chapter 40). The effect of cannabis and cannabinoids on pain have been well-documented in multiple reviews.[1-6] Chronic pain is the most common reason patients approved for medical cannabis report that they use it. Currently, 60–90% of patients in state-level medical cannabis registries list pain as their qualifying condition for the medical program.[7-9] In a survey of chronic non-cancer pain patients published in 2003, only 15% reported having used cannabis for pain relief.[10] This lower number is likely more representative of a non-medically approved population. Trends have shown an increase in cannabis use for pain in the past 20 years. In a recent study of medical cannabis, patients with chronic pain almost half smoked cannabis, one-quarter vaporized, with edibles and sublinguals making up the remainder. This illustrates how much smoking is still preferred, but also how little direction these patients received in utilizing chronic long-acting dosing, that is, tinctures of edibles 2–3x/day. "Respondents described in great depth how medical cannabis improved their treatment of chronic-pain and enhanced their quality of life."[9]

Chronic pain is often complex and can result from nociceptive, inflammatory, peripheral and/or centralized pain mechanisms. Pain isn't pain until it reaches the brain. Prior to that, it is nociception. Cannabinoid mechanisms of action involve not only cannabinergic pathways, but action on multiple other receptors and a multitude of non-neuronal cells (see Chapter 39 for mechanism).[3] Cannabis manages chronic pain in part, by preventing peripheral nociception from reaching the brain. In addition to changes in pain perception, there is also the possibility of change in attitude. Often patients report that their condition may remain unchanged, but "it doesn't bother them as much," or their perspective is altered, so they're not as focused on the pain.

The effectiveness of CBD versus THC versus a mix for pain really depends upon the type of pain, the patient's mood, whether synergy with opiates is a factor and whether central or peripheral mechanisms are involved among other things. Also vital is the patient's tolerance to cannabis, whether they are naive or experienced, and what level of adverse effects they have with THC. The much hoped for efficacy of THC for pain management has been limited by proven efficacy for chronic but not acute pain, although there are still conflicting reports, some indicating that dosage is critical, especially for new-onset pain. Dose escalation of inhaled cannabis showed no efficacy at a low dose, reduced pain at a moderate dose and increased pain at a high dose.[11] The

DOI: 10.1201/9781003098201-36

efficacy of cannabis-based products is expected to be more effective at a lower dose than for pure THC or CBD, especially for significant pain. To investigate this, a study of dosage efficacy in a standardized cannabis plant extract (Cannador) for acute pain after surgery provides some insight. Cannador capsules containing THC was given as a one-time dose providing 5, 10 or 15 mg. There was a linear dose–response curve, with only 25% of patients requesting more analgesia at the highest, 15 mg dose. The 5-mg dose had no clinical effects on pain.[12] It might be inferred from this and other studies, that a 10–20 mg dose of a THC-rich preparation would provide significant analgesia. Of course, these results would not apply in chronic cannabis users who have developed a tolerance. Even with chronic pain, most studies show a pain reduction of about 30% with THC, or THC-rich cannabis, generally not close to being adequate. In a recent study of patients use of cannabis for pain, an average reduction of 3 points on a 10-point scale was recorded, with THC-rich cannabis being the most effective.[13] But of course, the type of chronic pain is relevant to the success one has with cannabis, neuropathic and inflammatory pain giving a higher success rate.

On the other hand, the overly attributed efficacy of CBD for pain management has not clearly been confirmed when in pure form, and has been found to be more effective for neurogenic or inflammatory pain as a cannabis extract. An analysis of patients with severe chronic pain treated with a CBD/THC oromucosal spray (nabiximols) showed best results for neuropathic pain as compared with nociceptive or mixed pain.[14] In the aforementioned study, regarding patients use of cannabis for pain, CBD content was only associated with gastrointestinal pain relief.[13] In a report of cannabis medicinal extracts (CME) to treat neurogenic symptoms including pain, they concluded that, "Intoxication seemed to be primarily associated with THC CME, but even here was usually of tolerable intensity. CBD CME appeared to have analgesic and anti-spasticity properties in its own right."[15] In contrast, using purified CBD, it was reported that CBD showed no analgesic action of its own in a clinical study using a daily dose of 450 mg CBD.[2]

With severe or chronic pain requiring higher chronic cannabis dosages, it may be that the presence of CBD brings an advantage to pain management, either in detracting from tolerance to THC, amplifying THC effects, managing comorbid symptoms and likely all of the above. In a trial of the efficacy, safety and tolerability of a CBD/THC approximately 1:1 ratio compared with a THC extract, in patients with intractable cancer-related pain, the THC group showed a non-significant change, whereas the CBD/THC group showed a reduction of more than 30% from baseline pain. The actual amount of cannabinoids taken by sprays of the extract had a wide range and reached high but similar doses, from 3 to 16 sprays/day, which is equivalent to 16–83 mg/day, divided into 4 doses/day. Extracts with THC and CBD combined seem to do best at managing pain with the least adverse effects.[16]

In a review of cannabis use for chronic pain, the authors found that patients preferred to use cannabis plant products versus purified oral cannabinoids to treat their chronic pain, stating:

> This evidence indicates that the tolerability and efficacy profiles of oral cannabinoids are inferior when compared to those of the cannabis plant. This has been noted by chronic pain patients who prefer use of the whole plant rather than oral cannabinoids.[17]

The effectiveness of full extract cannabis is, of course, a product of synergy minimally between the cannabinoids and the terpenes and is known to be more effective at lower doses than pure cannabinoids. This is known as the "entourage effect."[18] Much of this synergy is due to the intrinsic effects of the terpenes in cannabis. For example, β-myrcene has opioid-type analgesic effects, β-caryophyllene, β-myrcene, α-humulene and α-pinene are anti-inflammatory, while D-linalool has anesthetic properties.[3,18]

PATIENT REPORTS

To move on to patient results from my practice, patients with chronic pain constitute a large portion of those who seek cannabis use. While in general these patients were older adults, in their 50s–80s, there are exceptions for the rare youth that have chronic pain. There are so many cases of cannabis treating a wide range of pain, acute and chronic, that it's impossible to relate all of the interesting cases. I've chosen the ones related here to illustrate the applicability to all ages and its unique ability to simultaneously treat emotional and physiological pain. A psychological shift is almost required to break a chronic pain pattern. Chronic pain patients with opiate dependence issues who want to use cannabis to decrease their opiate dose are presented in a separate section (see Chapter 40). Here are a few illustrative case reports.

Patient 1: This is a 56-year-old female with severe chronic low back pain for the past 4 years. She was referred by her pain management specialist for additional help, having had spinal injections, neurostimulator implantation, opiates and lumbar laminectomy and fusion. She was diagnosed with arachnoiditis and pseudo-meningocele and was experiencing daily pain on a 75 µg fentanyl patch. Her pain management specialist did not want to keep increasing her opiate dose. In his notes he stated, "I'm not sure what I can offer her, as she has had a variety of treatments already. We discussed alternative therapies with referral to Dr. Malka to discuss options." Her other medications included Restoril, Neurontin, Wellbutrin, Klonapin, Zoloft, Pristiq, tizanidine, Celebrex and Norco prn. She was not new to cannabis use, saying "It takes away her symptoms almost immediately." She was using edibles and smoking cannabis. After consultation with me she was able to wean off the fentanyl patch using 25 mg of THC-rich edibles day and night, yet continued all her other medications. She was still seeking further physiological therapy after several years on cannabis. A "nerve cutting" procedure was planned shortly after our last visit, yet she continued to report that cannabis "has been the best pain reliever I've had ever."

Pearls: Cannabis was a "comfort" to this patient. Her chronic pain condition, using multiple medications, continually seeking new solutions, was ongoing. But her ability to accept her condition and better manage it was helped by cannabis which she felt so positively about. Sometimes the best we can do is help the patient manage their pain, if not reduce it. With appropriate dosing of cannabis, she was able to get off the fentanyl patch, and continue Norco prn.

Patient 2: This is a 70-year-old male with a spinal cord injury below C6–7, 30 years prior. He was quadriplegic but had some use of his hands. He experienced pain in his arms, shoulders and upper back and muscle spasms in his legs. He had been using cannabis for 10 years as his main pain management tool. He also took baclofen 10 mg 2×/day, among other medications, but none for pain. His typical regimen was vaping 6×/day, with sativa during the day and indica before bed. His sleep was good, and his mood was remarkably good. He remained active in community affairs via computer. He did become bedridden during the time we worked together, due to non-healing decubitus ulcers, yet remained in good spirits until his passage 4 years after we met.

Pearls: This is a good example of medicating emotional as well as physical pain. I suspect that this patient's positive outlook on life was facilitated by cannabis in a way that opiates would have detracted from. Cannabis allowed him to be interactive and not as withdrawn as opiates might have done.

Patient 3: This is an 81-year-old female with severe back pain, due to spondylosis throughout, multiple osteoporotic compression fractures, scoliosis and degenerative disc disease. She was referred by her pain management physician. Her medications included Percocet 3×/day and Celebrex 200 mg 2×/day. She was new to cannabis use. She described her chief complaint as "Pain, Pain, Pain." As is the case often with naive elderly patients, she was slow to reach a therapeutic level of cannabis. She began using a daily 3 mg dose of a CBD tincture and 1 mg of indica at night. Over the next year, she was able to increase to 5 mg of tincture 1–2×/day. Her back compression fractures were an ongoing problem, with the added complication of bilateral hip replacements over the past year. Her pain continued. Finally, 2 years after we met, at our fourth visit, she progressed to the dose I originally advised, 10 mg of a CBD-rich tincture daily and continued 1 mg of indica at night. She continued on Percocet 3×/day if needed.

Pearls: Reaching a therapeutic level of cannabis with the elderly takes much repetition, repeated follow-ups and a support system, in this case her primary care physician, who referred her to me. I believe cannabis was helpful for this patient's pain, as her opiate prescription did not increase with time, while her condition deteriorated. That is an appropriate goal.

Patient 4: This is a 67-year-old male who was referred by his osteopath for advice on how to use cannabis for pain. He had multiple kinds of pain – a brachial tumor causing pain, abdominal pain due to diverticulitis, emotional pain due to PTSD also contributing to insomnia and degenerative disc disease throughout his back. He was taking oxycodone 10 mg 3×/day and diazepam 5–10 mg at night. He agreed to follow my instructions on an opiate and benzodiazepam wean. He started using a CBD/THC 1:1 tincture 10 mg 3×/day, and added a 30 mg indica capsule at bedtime. At a 2-month follow-up, he was down to oxycodone 5 mg 2×/day, right on schedule. He said his pain was better than on the higher dose of oxycodone. But he still wasn't sleeping well. He continued to take diazepam 5 mg, down from 10 mg at night. We tried adding vaporized cannabis to his nightly regimen, and continuing the diazepam at 5 mg. By the next year, he was sleeping well on 10 mg indica plus vaping as needed, while continuing the 1:1 tincture 10 mg 2–3×/day. He was using oxycodone 5–10 mg in a 24-hour period. His back pain and brachial pain were still a problem. Sleep was better, but his pain management was equivalent to what it had been when he came in 1 year ago. He was planning ongoing osteopathic visits as well as a surgical consult.

Pearls: I'd be so pleased if all patients would be this compliant! This is a rare case of a patient truly being committed to his stated desire, of wanting to not progress with opiate use. He did exactly as instructed, came in every 2–3 months for follow-up, and we achieved our goal. His pain did not improve, but he was sleeping better and feeling hopeful. Pain management will continue to be an issue for this patient, cannabis will not do it all.

Patient 5: This is a 57-year-old male with chronic pain throughout his neck and back for the past 13 years. He had a cervical fusion from C4 to C7. He also had an injury to his thoracic spine and pain in both shoulders. He'd been on opiates for the past 13 years, currently on Nucynta 125 mg 2×/day and tizanidine 4 mg 2×/day. He was new to cannabis use. After 1 year on a low dose of cannabis, 5 mg of a CBD/THC 4:1 tincture, his muscle spasms improved and he was able to stop the muscle relaxant. By the next year, he had been diagnosed as HLA-B27 positive and was thought to have ankylosing spondylitis. Lyrica was an added medicine. He was becoming adjusted to a lifelong chronic pain diagnosis. He was making an attempt to wean the Nucynta, and was down to 75 mg 2×/day. His cannabis use remained the same, not really enough to manage his pain. I advised an increase in THC dose, that is, a 1:1 tincture, for the third year in the row. He was then lost to follow-up. I'm not sure if it was because he hadn't followed my instruction or another reason.

Pearls: It is challenging when patients do not follow advice on required dosing protocols needed for success. Especially with chronic pain patients, if the pain is not improving, they are likely not to continue cannabis therapy. Unfortunately, it was likely that the patient's not reaching therapeutic levels of cannabis to manage his pain deterred him from continuing it even for its other benefits, that is, muscle relaxation and opiate reduction.

CANNABIS THERAPY SUMMARY

There are so many benefits of using cannabis to treat chronic pain that it's no surprise that it is the most prevalent condition for which medical cannabis patients seek counsel. It's important to remember that CBD alone is not expected to be antinociceptive, but due to its anti-inflammatory and neuroprotective effects, it may stand alone for inflammatory and neuropathic pain by reducing the cause of the pain. As far as analgesia is concerned, some THC is required. The research seems to indicate that a CBD/THC mix of approximately 1:1 may prove superior to THC alone for overall quality of life and success of treatment. The chronic pain cases presented here are all in adults, but in the rare case that a child has chronic pain, mixed cannabinoid dosing with small amounts of THC can prove useful. A 10-year-old child with chronic pain used a 5-mg dose of CBD/THC in a 1:1 ratio before bed with pain relief at least overnight. There are several factors that contribute to this including the benefits just mentioned, but also CBD does increase the availability of anandamide, contributes to mood management and relaxation and mitigates the psychoactive effects of THC. THC, on the other hand, is directly analgesic, is synergistic with opiates, helps sleep, can provide stimulation and some cultivars have antidepressant effects, and in this case, altered perception may be a bonus. The dose will vary depending on the severity of pain and the patient's tolerance. Often a 10–20 mg dose of a mixed extract or edible used 3×/day can provide 24-hour relief. Strains that contain β-caryophyllene would be beneficial, especially for inflammatory pain due to its intrinsic anti-inflammatory properties. Topicals can safely add to pain relief and are safe for all ages.

REFERENCES

1. Hill KP, Palastro MD, Johnson B, Ditre JW. Cannabis and pain: a clinical review. *Cannabis Cannabinoid Res.* 2017;2(1):96–104.
2. Karst M, Wippermann S. Cannabinoids against pain. Efficacy and strategies to reduce psychoactivity: a clinical perspective. *Expert Opin Investig Drugs.* 2009;18(2):125–133.
3. Russo EB, Hohmann AG. Role of cannabinoids in pain management. In: Deer R, et al. eds. *Comprehensive Treatment of Chronic Pain by Medical, Interventional, and Integrative Approaches.* New York, NY: Springer New York; 2013:181–197.
4. Elikotti J, Gupta P, Gupta K. The analgesic potential of cannabinoids. *J Opioid Manag.* 2009;5(6):341–357.
5. Lynch ME, Campbell F. Cannabinoids for treatment of chronic non-cancer pain: a systematic review of randomized trials. *Br J Clin Pharmacol.* 2011;72(5):735–744.
6. Aggarwal S. Cannabinergic pain medicine: a concise clinical primer and survey of randomized-controlled trial results. *Clin J Pain.* 2013;29(2):162–171.
7. Reinarman C, Nunberg H, Lanthier F, Heddleston T. Who are medical marijuana patients? Population characteristics from nine California assessment clinics. *J Psychoactive Drugs.* 2011;43(2):128–135.
8. Sexton M, Cuttler C, Finnell JS, Mischley LK. A cross-sectional survey of medical cannabis users: patterns of use and perceived efficacy. *Cannabis Cannabinoid Res.* 2016;1.1.
9. Piper BJ, Beals ML, Abess AT, et al. Chronic pain patients' perspectives of medical cannabis. *Pain.* 2017;158(7):1373–1379.
10. Ware MA, Doyle CR, Woods R, Lynch ME, Clark AJ. Cannabis use for chronic non-cancer pain: results of a prospective survey. *Pain.* 2003;102(1–2):211–216.
11. Wallace M, Schulteis G, Atkinson JH, et al. Dose-dependent effects of smoked cannabis on capsaicin-induced pain and hyperalgesia in healthy volunteers. *Anesthesiology.* 2007;107:785–796.
12. Holdcroft A, Maze M, Dore C, Tebbs S, Thompson S. A multicenter dose-escalation study of the analgesic and adverse effects of an oral cannabis extract (Cannador) for postoperative pain management. *Anesthesiology.* 2006;104(5):1040–1046.
13. Li X, Vigil JM, Stith SS, et al. The effectiveness of self-directed medical cannabis treatment for pain. *Complement Ther Med.* 2019;46:123–130.
14. Überall MA. A review of scientific evidence for THC:CBD oromucosal spray (nabiximols) in the management of chronic pain. *J Pain Res.* 2020;13:399–410.
15. Wade DT, Robson P, House H, Makela P, Aram J. A preliminary controlled study to determine whether whole-plant cannabis extracts can improve intractable neurogenic symptoms. *Clin Rehabil.* 2003;17:18–26.
16. Johnson JR, Burnell-Nugent M, Lossignol D, et al. Multicenter, double-blind, randomized, placebo-controlled, parallel-group study of the efficacy, safety, and tolerability of THC:CBD extract and THC extract in patients with intractable cancer-related pain. *J Pain Symptom Manage.* 2010;39(2):167–179.
17. Romero-Sandoval EA, Fincham JE, Kolano AL, Sharpe BN, Alvarado-Vazquez PA. Cannabis for chronic pain: challenges and considerations. *Pharmacotherapy.* 2018;38(6):651–662.
18. Russo EB. Taming THC: potential cannabis synergy and phytocannabinoid-terpenoid entourage effects. *Br J Pharmacol.* 2011;163(7):1344–1364.

26 Depression, Bipolar Disorder

DEPRESSION AND CANNABIS

The debate about whether cannabis helps depression or might cause it has been going on for as long as cannabis has been considered a drug of abuse. Many ill-conceived studies have tried to show that cannabis can harm your mood, especially in youth. This has not been borne out with adjustment for other risks. In the National Longitudinal Survey of Youth of 1979, 8,759 adults (age range 29–37 years) were interviewed in 1994 for marijuana use and current depression. After adjusting for differences in baseline risk factors, past year marijuana use while young did not significantly predict later development of depression.[1] A large study done in Sweden observing over 45,000 individuals stated:

> [T]here was no increased risk of future depression among cannabis users at age 18 to 20. With the large number of cases, and control for important background factors, we believe our study adds to previous findings supporting the hypothesis that cannabis use does not increase the risk of depression."[2]

In a longitudinal cohort study of 8,598 Swedish men and women, cannabis users had no increased risk of depression and anxiety at follow-up. "Adjusted for all confounders (alcohol and illicit drug use, education, family tension, place of upbringing), the associations were no longer statistically significant."[3] A 2005 Australian study of thousands of cannabis users found normal rates of depression once other factors such as alcohol use, gender, illness, etc. were accounted for.[4] Over 4,400 adults completed the Center for Epidemiologic Studies Depression scale and cannabis use. Daily users reported less depressed mood and more positive effect than non-users. They found that medical users reported more depressed mood and more somatic complaints than recreational users.[5] Still the debate continues, highlighting the need to disseminate the flaws in studies uncorrected for bias.

Clinical depression is hypothesized to be linked to endocannabinoid (EC) dysregulation. A deficiency in the EC tone leads to a depressive-like phenotype in experimental animal models of depression. Depressed patients as well have been found to have reduced levels of endogenous cannabinoids.[6] Postmortem studies of patients with major depression have revealed a decrease in CB1 receptors in the glial cells of the brain gray matter. Changes in EC tone may differ from minor to major depression with downregulation of the system involved in major depression, while an upregulation is elicited in minor depression.[7]

Cannabinoids have been found to have antidepressant properties depending on the type of cannabis used and its dosage, as expected. To review the effects of THC on

DOI: 10.1201/9781003098201-37

the endocannabinoid system, we recall that it is a cannabinoid (CB) agonist, and its stimulation of CB receptors shows a bidirectional dose–response curve, so its effect on depression is likely to be dose-dependent. Interaction with TRPV1 channels, serotonin 5-HT1A receptors and enhancement of adenosine signaling could explain the positive effects not only by CBD, but may be influenced by THC as well.[6] In an animal study using CB agonists, low doses of the agonist elicited antidepressant-like behavior and enhanced 5-HT neurotransmission, while high doses opposed those effects and attenuated 5-HT neurotransmission. They concluded "It is becoming apparent that the correct dosage is important in mood control."[8] These results were confirmed with later tests using THC.[9] In investigating the effects of other cannabinoids, also in animals, it was found:

High doses 1.25, 2.5, and 5 mg/kg, both Δ9-THC and Δ8-THC showed a U-shaped dose response with only Δ9-THC showing significant antidepressant-like effects at 2.5 mg/kg. Other cannabinoids studied include CBG and CBN, which did not produce antidepressant-like actions, while CBC and CBD exhibited significant effect only at 20 and 200 mg/kg, respectively.[7]

These are very high doses and not likely to be reached clinically in people. In mice, high doses of CBD (50 mg/kg) were found to exert fast and maintained antidepressant-like effects. CBD significantly enhanced serotonin and glutamate levels, which were prevented by 5-HT1A receptor blockade.[10] A proposal that these cannabinoids may exert their effects at much lower doses as antidepressants by slowing tryptophan degradation was confirmed in studies of peripheral blood cells in vitro, concluding, "Effects of THC and CBD to increase tryptophan concentrations in unstimulated PBMC (peripheral blood mononuclear cells) in the nanomolar concentration range, may give some explanation for the observed well-being after smoking marijuana."[11]

Human studies are few, but indicate that lower doses of THC may be clinically therapeutic. One report reviewed a 2002 study, in which healthy volunteers smoking cannabis showed a positive correlation with the ratings on a scale of depression indicating an antidepressant effect. This report also recounted that of the 75 patients treated with 2.5–7.5 mg of dronabinol per day, almost 80% showed improvement of depressed mood.[12]

In a survey of medical cannabis users, a 50% reduction in depression was noted following cannabis use. Two puffs were sufficient to reduce ratings of depression. Contrary to expectation, they found CBD/THC combination strains CBD (>9.5%)/ low THC (<5.5%) were associated with the largest changes in depression ratings.[13] But strain identification was not delineated. It is now thought that the terpene profile that determines many strain characteristics is also most important in mood effects. Cultivar selection is important, because strains that are too sedating may contribute to the lethargy of depression, and could accentuate dysfunctional symptoms. In general, sativa dominant strains are more uplifting. However, it's not merely the THC that makes a specific cultivar useful for depression and fatigue. The terpene, α-pinene, can boost energy and is said to improve concentration. Not as alerting as α-pinene, D-limonene is thought to contribute to a calm, clear-headed and mood-elevating experience. Terpene content has rarely been delineated in studies of cannabis and depression, presenting woefully incomplete study designs for the most part. These studies have contributed to reviews such as the following, which concluded that "There is no credible evidence regarding the effectiveness, or harms of marijuana for the treatment of depression."[14] The conflicting results of cannabis effect on depression depends on several variables. The internal endocannabinoid tone of the patient, the dose, chronicity and type of cannabis used, and the type of depression, minor or major, with any other confounding factors.

BIPOLAR DISORDER AND CANNABIS

Bipolar disorder is often treated with mood stabilizers, so it is reasonable to predict that a dysregulated EC system might be involved. One review of the subject hypothesizes that "Cannabinoids, especially when used in combination, have several characteristics in common with drugs known to benefit this disorder, including antidepressants, antipsychotics, anticonvulsants (mood-stabilizers) and anxiolytics."[15] The range of possible benefit versus harm exists as in the case of depression. In comparing bipolar I subjects with and without a history of cannabis use disorder, it was found that those who used cannabis had significantly better neurocognitive performance, particularly on measures of attention, processing speed and working memory. Of note, almost half of those with a cannabis use history were in the "remote" past. They suggest that as "Similar results have also been found in schizophrenia in several studies. These data could be interpreted to suggest that cannabis use may have a beneficial effect on cognitive functioning in patients with severe psychiatric disorders."[16] Another group concludes that patients with bipolar disorder who use cannabis have been shown to have higher illness severity and poorer outcome. Yet they note that patients report improvement with cannabis.[17] The only study that was actually done with bipolar patients while using cannabis found that bipolar patients using cannabis showed significant improvement in total mood disturbance.[18]

The glaring problem with all of these reports is that no concerted use of an appropriate strain of cannabis was part of the treatment. As we know, different strains would be required for the depressive phases and the manic phases. The difference in outcome between medical patients who might have advice on appropriate use of cannabis and the less informed use by recreational patients would be a useful comparison, and not yet done.

PATIENT REPORTS

To move on to patient results from my practice, patients ranged in age from 16 years old to the 80s. Depression is not an uncommon theme for cannabis patients to present with. Often it is accompanied by a co-diagnosis of anxiety, which really would indicate a separate avenue of therapy, but there are some types of products that could be used for both. In many cases the use of antidepressants is reduced with cannabis therapy. Bipolar disorder was a less common diagnosis and showed yet a different type of therapy as beneficial. Here are a few illustrative case reports.

DEPRESSION

Patient 1: This is a 52-year-old male with multiple psychiatric diagnoses, including major depressive disorder versus bipolar II, anxiety and ADHD. He had a history of suicidality, with current despair, but no active plan. He also had a history of treatment failure on electric shock therapy. He had been doing counseling for the past 4 years. His medication history was extensive and changed even during the 2 years we worked together. During this short time, these included Neurontin, Latuda, Adderall, Buspar, lamotrigine, Prozac and Klonapin. Fortunately, I received regular updates from his psychiatrist who was aware of his desire to replace some medications with cannabis. His reaction to pharmaceuticals was an ongoing challenge. He complained of memory loss, so lamotrigine was discontinued. Buspar was ineffective, and his suicidal ideation was exacerbated by Klonapin, also discontinued. He was new to cannabis use. I advised a CBD/THC 1:1 tincture in the a.m. and a 4:1 tincture in the afternoon. He ended up using a CDB/THC 1:1 chocolate at way too high a dose, typically 30 mg 3–4x/day. On follow-up, I again stressed the need for a higher CBD ratio in the afternoons, and explained that he should be using no more than 25 mg 2x/day. This time his symptoms improved somewhat, on a 1:1 chocolate in the a.m., and a 20:1 tincture 2x/day. At our third visit he had weaned off of all medications, had begun walking for exercise, suicidality was decreased, yet depression was still an issue.

Pearls: It's best to work in conjunction with a patient's mental health professional in serious psychiatric cases. He reported to his psychiatrist that he was taking a CBD-rich cannabis, which was not exactly the case. Unfortunately, I did not catch this patient's overuse of cannabis medicine until our 1-year follow-up. I anticipated that a cannabis naive person would not escalate to 120 mg of edible use per day. Of greater consequence was the myriad of psychiatric medicines that he was going on and off of. Perhaps cannabis did help him discontinue these medications. It is unclear how he did the following year as our visits ended.

Patient 2: This is a 66-year-old female with a history of depression, anxiety, insomnia, and pain from an elbow injury. She had been using cannabis for the past several years by a tincture of unspecified composition. Her medications included Abilify 5 mg, venlafaxine 150 mg/day, propranolol 60 mg/day and bupropion 150 mg/day, some of which she had been on for 10 years. I advised the addition of a few puffs of a sativa strain during the day for depression and pain. She did this over the next year, using a bong or vaporizing, and ended an abusive relationship. The next year was more of the same, complicated by two abdominal surgeries for prior colon issues. Finally, she settled on a CBD-rich strain, 2 puffs 3–4x/day and discontinued all antidepressants, continuing on propranolol. She reported feeling very emotional, but was looking forward to a more stable year as she recently further decreased stress by retiring.

Pearls: It could be that anxiety was the more pressing diagnosis, in that a CBD-rich strain was most effective for this patient. It is often an overlapping diagnosis that needs treatment, and cannabis effectiveness is a trial-and-error process unique to the individual. Confirming her current mental health status by medications prescribed, that is, 3 antidepressants, was potentially misleading. It could be that anxiety was really what was undertreated. Encouraging the patient to find an effective strain could be risky in mental health, as THC often helpful for depression, can exacerbate anxiety, but increasing the CBD content is usually a safer course.

Patient 3: This is a 50-year-old female patient with multiple mental health diagnoses, including depression, anxiety, ADHD as well as insomnia and menopausal mood dysphoria. She had been using cannabis for the past 7 years by smoking. She experimented with several strains to "reduce stress." She was on no medications. I advised she try counseling and continue using a relaxing strain. By the next visit she had done so, and was also on newly prescribed Zoloft 50 mg/day. She was not doing counseling any longer. She had started using a water pipe, found sativa too stimulating for her anxiety and was also using a CBD-rich strain during the day. The Zoloft seemed to be helping with depression. She continued to experiment with products, now using a CBD/THC 1:1 edible or smoking for daytime use and an indica before bed. We discussed using 5-HTP to replace the Zoloft as she wanted to get off of medication. By our fifth year of consultation, she was off Zoloft, sleeping well and using a CBD-rich tincture daily and an indica vape pen at night.

Pearls: As the previous case and as is often the case, multiple diagnoses make it difficult to know whether a relaxant or a stimulant is needed. In fact, this is a good example of a patient with serotonin dysfunction, often found in menopausal cases, associated with both depression, anxiety and sleep disturbance. The combination of 5-HTP and cannabis strains/products that changed to accommodate shifting mood issues was helpful for her. In this case, her shifting therapeutic protocol was likely useful to accommodate the fluctuating hormones of the menopausal transition.

Patient 4: This is a 16-year-old male who came in with his mother with multiple mood issues, including depression, anxiety, ADHD and anger. He had been on ADHD medications in childhood, and more recently taking Effexor 225 mg/day and Seroquel 200 mg in the a.m. and 300 mg in the p.m. He reported that they made him feel suicidal and stopped them. He then was hospitalized for suicidal ideation, and now was primarily feeling anger. His father had died 4 years earlier and the anger was prevalent after that. He started to use cannabis on his own instead of the medications, and his mother wanted advice on how to use it responsibly. I advised a CBD/ THC 2:1 tincture for daytime use and a relaxing strain in the evenings after school. The patient did not follow my advice, and settled upon smoking sativa 2×/day and an indica before bed. He said neither the tincture nor vaporizing gave him as good an effect. He said he continues to be depressed until he smokes. He started counseling but stopped. He was performing well in a home school independent study format. Mom was supportive of what he was doing. I was not. I advised him to resume counseling and to consider cannabis as a medicine, not as an escape. I suggested a low-dose edible sativa mint for daytime use to reduce the smoking habit. I doubt he complied. That was our last visit. He was soon to turn 18 and likely able to continue to use cannabis without his mother's supervision.

Pearls: This is a not uncommon example of an attempt to teach a young person to use cannabis with respect as a medicine. It also illustrates the need to become an ally of the overwhelmed parent caregiver. Whenever a minor is recommended cannabis, it is up to the caregiver to monitor its use. I told mom that we could cancel his recommendation if he did not follow her restrictions, but she wanted him to be legal, as she knew he would continue to use it anyway. Was I complicit in allowing poor use of the medicine? Probably. Would he have been better off without my input? I doubt it. At least his suicidal ideation was apparently gone. I hope it helped him control his anger and alleviate depression, as that was our intention. But he had a long way to go before he was using it to his best advantage. CBD would really have been calming and useful for him. If we had been in a state where his access was defined by a prescribed dose, there would have been more control over what he legally could take.

BIPOLAR DISORDER

Patient 1: This is a 37-year-old female with a history of bipolar disorder and anxiety. She had been on multiple medications that she wished to discontinue by using cannabis more effectively. She just weaned herself off Lithobid, Klonapin, Trazodone, Zoloft and Seroquel. She had been using cannabis for 17 years, currently smoking it daily, but was unsure about which strains would be best. Her mood was unstable with depression currently dominant. We agreed she would add a CBD-rich strain, Harlequin, for anxiety and mood stabilization, and discussed diet and exercise for depression. At our next visit, she was back on Abilify and lithium, and smoking cannabis in the evenings. She was under the care of a psychiatrist. Over the next year, she weaned off Abilify, tried a CBD tincture, but preferred CBD by vape pen. Her mood was stabilizing as she continued with a diet and exercise plan. At our last visit, the bipolar tendencies were less of a problem with ongoing bouts of anxiety. She continued to use a CBD-rich product, switching to tincture, CBD/THC 20:1 at a dose of 25 mg 2×/day.

Pearls: I learned from this patient that CBD is effective in mood stabilization. Often anxiety and depression are concurrent, and apparently in this case, treating anxiety with CBD also helped to stabilize her mood.

Patient 2: This is a 16-year-old male with primarily anger issues, yet had been treated for bipolar disorder and ADHD. He also slept poorly, waking throughout the night. His diagnoses also included substance abuse disorder, primarily for his use of "marijuana" to help with sleep. His medication history over the past few years included Lexapro, Wellbutrin, Intuniv, Vyvanse, Seroquel and Depakote. He was recently prescribed Abilify, which he was not taking. He had been hospitalized in the past year for suicidal ideation. He was currently seeing a psychotherapist. He came in with his mom who knew he was using cannabis and wanted help with boundaries. During our visit, he was hostile, restless and so angry that he punched the walls. I advised a CBD-rich tincture for daytime use and an indica tincture before bed. I advised him to avoid using smoking as a delivery method. Mom reported that a CBD/THC 20:1 tincture was helpful in controlling rage, and that an indica edible before bed did help with sleep but felt too strong. He switched to vaporizing indica before bed. Progress was slow. His explosive episodes decreased from 1×/week to 1×/month, but he was still verbally abusive. At our next visit, he was doing better in school, sleeping through the night by vaporizing before bed and continued to use a CBD-rich tincture 2×/day, in the a.m. and after school. By this time, he was 17 and mom had questions about smoking cannabis. He wanted to do it on weekends with his friends. The fact that he was discussing it with is parents was positive.

Pearls: Again, we find that a CBD-rich product was helpful for mood stabilization. In this case, bipolar disorder was one of a multitude of mental health diagnoses, yet recently there was an issue with suicidal ideation, which seemed to have resolved as his sleep and mood improved. Treating insomnia was integral to mood improvement. The patient himself said he could focus better at school after a good night of sleep.

Patient 3: This is a 61-year-old female with a long history of treatment-resistant bipolar disorder. Her therapeutic history included multiple medications, electric shock therapy, several suicide attempts and hospitalizations, counseling and naturopathic and spiritual therapies. At our first visit, she was already a medical cannabis patient, smoking a few times/day to help stabilize her mood. She was off all pharmaceutical medications. She reported still dealing with depression and anxiety, but was able to manage it. I advised a CBD/THC strain that might be more balancing than the THC-rich strain she was using. She continued to smoke or vaporize a few times/day for the next several years, settling on a CBD-rich vape pen during the day and a smoked indica in the evenings. Insomnia remained a complaint, so ultimately, she used an indica in the evenings. At the time of our last visit, she had been using cannabis and off medications for 6 years, which she said worked best, along with continued counseling.

Pearls: Here is a case illustrating a CBD/THC mix in a patient who preferred inhalation. This is more difficult to come by smoked, as raw flower with this ratio is not always available in dispensaries. It is more common to find CBD-rich and CBD/THC 1:1 varieties premixed in a vaporizer pen. These often do not retain the terpenes, necessitating raw flower to provide a true indica to aid with sleep.

CANNABIS THERAPY SUMMARY

It is now evident that the dispute of old, as to whether cannabis can help or exacerbate depression, has been approached with incomplete information about the components of cannabis that is crucial to the answer. Typically, cultivars that are uplifting or stimulating produce the best results, those that have THC and appropriate terpenes, such as α-pinene and D-limonene. If in fact one is using an indica with a lot of β-myrcene, the risk for lethargy and possible "inertia" goes up. Such a cultivar would be useful in the evening for insomnia. Surprisingly, CBD has a role in treating many depressed patients, possibly because they have a co-diagnosis with anxiety, and/or a combination with the right terpenes could blunt some of the psychoactivity from THC while still being uplifting. The dose and delivery method seems to vary according to patient preference, the younger patients preferring smoking or vaporization, while the older ones are satisfied with oral methods. Keep in mind that it is rare to find ingestible products that have retained and have specified terpene content. This is best achieved by full flower or when you can find it, extracts that list the terpene content.

The choice of cannabis for bipolar disorder appears to be different from that of depression, although this is purely anecdotal as no studies have been done to confirm this. CBD-rich cannabis may be useful as a mood stabilizer, with the addition of THC varying as to whether a manic or depressive phase is underway. The terpene content for bipolar patients is somewhat similar to that of depression, as D-limonene is uplifting, while not necessarily stimulating. An important property of cannabis for depression and bipolar disorder is that it can change one's perception, and very often, it is this shift alone that provides relief.

REFERENCES

1. Harder VS, Morral AR, Arkes J. Marijuana use and depression among adults: testing for causal associations. *Addiction.* 2006;101(10):1463–1472.
2. Manrique-Garcia E, Zammit S, Dalman C, Hemmingsson T, Allebeck P. Cannabis use and depression a longitudinal study of a national cohort of Swedish conscripts. *BMC Psychiatry.* 2012;12:112.
3. Danielsson AK, Lundin A, Agardh E, Allebeck P, Forsell Y. Cannabis use, depression and anxiety: a 3-year prospective population-based study. *J Affect Disord.* 2016;193:103–108.
4. Swift W, Gates P, Dillon P. Survey of Australians using cannabis for medical purposes. *Harm Reduc J.* 2005;2:18.
5. Denson TF, Earleywine M. Decreased depression in marijuana users. *Addict Behav.* 2006;31(4): 738–742.
6. Micale V., Tabiova K., Kucerova J., Drago F. Role of the endocannabinoid system in depression: from preclinical to clinical evidence. In: Campolongo P, Fattore L, eds. *Cannabinoid Modulation of Emotion, Memory, and Motivation.* New York, NY: Springer; 2015.
7. El-Alfy AT, Ivey K, Robinson K, et al. Antidepressant-like effect of delta 9-tetrahydrocannabinol and other cannabinoids isolated from Cannabis sativa L. *Pharmacol Biochem Behav.* 2010;95(4):434–442.
8. Bambico FR, Katz N, Debonnel G, Gobbi G. Cannabinoids elicit antidepressant-like behavior and activate serotonergic neurons through the medial prefrontal cortex. *J Neurosci.* 2007;27(43):11700–11711.
9. Bambico FR, Hattan PR, Garant JP, Gobbi G. Effect of delta-9-tetrahydrocannabinol on behavioral despair and on pre-and postsynaptic serotonergic transmission. *Prog Neuropsychopharmacol Biol Psychiatry.* 2012;38(1):88–96.
10. Linge R, Jiménez-Sánchez L, Campa L, et al. Cannabidiol induces rapid-acting antidepressant-like effects and enhances cortical 5-HT/glutamate neurotransmission: role of 5-HT1A receptors. *Neuropharmacology.* 2016;103:16–26.
11. Jenny M, Schröcksnadel S, Überall F, Fuchs D. The potential role of cannabinoids in modulating serotonergic signaling by their influence on tryptophan metabolism. *Pharmaceuticals (Basel).* 2012;(8):2647–2660.
12. Blass K. Treating depression with cannabinoids. *Cannabinoids.* 2008;3(2):8–10.
13. Cuttler C, Spradlin A, McLaughlin RJ. Naturalistic examination of the perceived effects of cannabis on negative affect. *J Affect Disord.* 2018;235:198–205.
14. Campos-Outcalt D, Hamilton P, Thiagarajan W, Celaya M, Rosales C. Arizona Department of Health Services Medical Marijuana Advisory Committee Report. Medical marijuana for the treatment of depression: an evidence review. 2012. www.azdhs.gov/medicalmarijuana/documents/debilitating/Debilitating-Conditions-Depression.pdf Accessed April 5, 2020.
15. Ashton CH, Moore PB, Gallagher P, Young AH. Cannabinoids in bipolar affective disorder: a review and discussion of their therapeutic potential. *J Psychopharmacol.* 2005;19(3):293–300.

16. Braga RJ, Burdick KE, DeRosse P, Malhotra AK. Cognitive and clinical outcomes associated with cannabis use in patients with bipolar I disorder. *Psychiatry Res.* 2012;200(2–3):242–245.
17. Gruber SA, Sagara KA, Dahlgren MK, et al. Marijuana impacts mood in bipolar disorder: a pilot study. *Mental Health Subst Use.* 2012;5:228–239.
18. Sagar KA, Dahlgren MK, Racine MT, et al. Joint effects: a pilot investigation of the impact of bipolar disorder and marijuana use on cognitive function and mood. *PLoS One.* 20186;11(6):e0157060.

Depression, bipolar disorder ...

27 Fibromyalgia, Chronic Fatigue Syndrome

FIBROMYALGIA, CHRONIC FATIGUE SYNDROME AND CANNABIS

Fibromyalgia (FM) is a syndrome consisting not only of pain and muscle tension but also may include insomnia, depression, anxiety, headaches, fatigue and irritable bowel syndrome (IBS). In chronic fatigue syndrome (CFS), fatigue is the prominent symptom. Pathogenesis, while not known for either of these, is hypothesized to be different. They may present with several symptoms in common, such as fatigue, pain, depression and insomnia. Clinically, the diagnosis may overlap both conditions, or fibromyalgia may progress to CFS in some patients. Cannabis is proving to be an efficient single medicine for fibromyalgia, providing relief otherwise requiring multiple pharmaceutical medications. In a 2014 survey of 1,300 fibromyalgia patients done by the National Pain Foundation and National Pain Report, 62% of respondents found cannabis very effective compared to 8–10% for the three FDA-approved pharmaceuticals for this condition.[1]

Cannabis therapeutic research has focused primarily on fibromyalgia. No reports of efficacy for CFS have yet been published. Due to the fact that cannabinoids have demonstrated the ability to block spinal, peripheral and gastrointestinal mechanisms that promote pain in headache, fibromyalgia, IBS and related disorders, a syndrome of "clinical endocannabinoid deficiency" has been suggested as a mechanism.[2,3] This reflects the possibility that the "endocannabinoid tone" is lower in individuals prone to these conditions, including FM, hence exogenous cannabinoids may be helpful in bringing homeostasis. Other hypotheses of cannabinoid therapeutic action include reduced sensitization of nociceptive sensory pathways and alterations in cognitive and autonomic processing, or that they may preferentially target the affective qualities of pain.[4] And the muscle relaxant, anti-inflammatory, sleep inducing and mood-altering qualities of cannabis all contribute to its effectiveness.

Cannabis is thought to be helpful for fibromyalgia by inference from studies using purified THC or nabilone, a synthetic analogue. Electrically induced pain in several fibromyalgia patients was attenuated after doses of 10–15 mg THC. All patients who completed the THC therapy over 3 months had pain relief of greater than 50%.[5] Similar results were found in a study with a larger sample size. Participants received 7.5 mg of THC for 7 months. The result was a reduction of pain from an average of 7.9 to 4.4, slightly less than a 50% change.[6] The dosage was less here, possibly indicating that maximal pain relief was not reached, but chronic pain data indicates only a 30% improvement with cannabis, so these are impressive results. Studies conducted with nabilone were not as significant. In 40 fibromyalgia patients who received nabilone

DOI: 10.1201/9781003098201-38

from 0.5 to 2 mg/day the visual analogue scale (VAS) score for pain was reduced by approximately two points. Improvements in anxiety and the Fibromyalgia Impact Questionnaire were noted.[7] Another study documented help with sleep, but not with pain using 0.5 mg nabilone at bedtime.[8] Apparently a higher dose was required for pain management.

The results of a study looking at associations between cannabis use and opioid use and/or unstable mental illness in FM patients referred to a FM clinic was published in 2012. Cannabinoids were being used by 13% of all patients, of whom 80% used cannabis and 24% used prescription cannabinoids. They misleadingly concluded that "Opioid drug – seeking behavior and current unstable mental illness were also strongly associated with herbal cannabis use in the entire cohort, although this association disappeared when we restricted analysis to the FM patients only."[9] They note that for such results "data not shown." The title of the article heralds the association of negative psychosocial parameters associated with cannabis use in FM patients. What they found, in fact, was that with the inclusion of non-FM pain patients presenting to this clinic, such associations arose, yet in the FM cohort no statistically significant associations were found. As always, it is imperative to read research concerning cannabis use with discernment, as ongoing bias in study design and reporting remains an issue.

Recently, a small study of 20 FM patients using vaporized cannabis was conducted. Here they used a THC-rich strain, a CBD-rich strain, a balanced approximately CBD/THC 1:1 strain and, interestingly, a placebo with terpenes left in, but cannabinoids taken out. The 1:1 strain resulted in a 30% decrease in pain scores compared to placebo. They also found that THC-containing strains caused an increase in pressure pain threshold, while the CBD-dominant strain did not.[10] In a survey of 28 actual cannabis users, levels of use from rare to several times daily were assessed. VAS scores showed a statistically significant reduction of pain and stiffness, enhancement of relaxation, an increase in somnolence and feeling of well-being. Patients noted reduced pharmaceutical use as well when they started using cannabis.[11] In another recent survey, 84% of the participants with fibromyalgia reported consuming cannabis with a mean dose of 15–50 gram per month, mostly by smoking and/or vaporizing. Ninety-four percent reported pain improvement and 93% reported better quality of sleep.[12]

An interesting discussion of CFS is found in the literature, with potential applications for cannabis. The author discusses the diagnosis myalgic encephalomyelitis/chronic fatigue syndrome (ME/CFS) and hypothesizes:

> Cannabis's ability to keep producing effective results when other medications have failed may lie in three factors: the many different strains of the plant, the many routes of application available, and the many systems it affects suggests . . . that when used skillfully, Cannabis may be able to, in effect, nudge the body out of illness states that it's become mired in.[13]

In my experience, with CFS patients, this often entails a high sensitivity to even the smallest doses of cannabis.

PATIENT REPORTS

To move on to patient results from my practice, this is a diagnosis most often found in middle-aged to older adults, with my patients aged in their 40s, 50s and 60s. I rarely encountered fibromyalgia as a single presenting diagnosis. Often symptoms included several aspects of the syndrome, such as insomnia, mood disorders, migraine headache and, of course, pain. Here are a few illustrative case reports.

Patient 1: This is a 42-year-old female patient with multiple medical diagnoses, including bipolar disorder versus PTSD, fibromyalgia, insomnia and shoulder bursitis. She had been using cannabis for 11 years, focused mainly on chronic shoulder pain from an old injury. Her only current medication was Benadryl used occasionally for sleep, although she had previously used Voltaren, Vicodin and Ativan, now replaced with cannabis. She was vaporizing or smoking 3×/day and using topical. Over the next few years, she used mostly indica by vaporizing in the evenings, and topical as needed. During this time, she also started to have intestinal cramping and was diagnosed with IBS. A death in the family caused resurgence of depression and she was started on Lexapro, at which time her cannabis use also increased fourfold. I advised her to begin a CBD/THC tincture and reduce her smoking.

Pearls: Be aware of covert fibromyalgia syndrome challenges. It wasn't until our fourth year of working together that the patient told me she had been diagnosed with fibromyalgia 10 years earlier. Shoulder pain was the motivating issue for her cannabis use. Indeed, over the ensuing years, we did have to address many of the syndrome's symptoms, such as insomnia, joint pain, IBS, depression and anxiety. It would have been better to advise a CBD/THC 1:1 mixture for ongoing stabilization and prevention of exacerbation at the outset.

Patient 2: This is a 64-year-old male with multiple diagnoses, including fibromyalgia, sleep apnea with insomnia, PTSD, depression and neck pain. He also had recovered from a previous myocardial infarction. He was currently on medical leave from work for multiple medical conditions, including repetitive use injury of hands, inability to concentrate and fatigue, among others. His medications included Topamax, lisinopril, Zetia, Provigil and nightly Remeron and Xanax. He also used a CPAP machine for sleep. He was new to cannabis use. I advised nightly indica use for sleep. By the next year, he had used little cannabis as he did not like THC, and was now growing his own CBD-rich strain. He ended up preparing a CBD topical for various body aches and continued the same medications with the addition of Cymbalta.

Pearls: This is an example of a patient who remains uncomfortable with his use of cannabis, allowing CBD only, and then, only as a topical. We were only able to help him topically, but it was of enough value that he was a returning patient. Topicals are not expected to correct an endocannabinoid deficiency as they have no central effects. Typically, with only topical use for FM, we find very little improvement, adjustment in pharmaceuticals or mood, as is the case here.

Patient 3: This is a 45-year-old female patient diagnosed with fibromyalgia with a history of Lyme disease. She also complained of insomnia, depression, anxiety and myalgias. She was on multiple medications, including Norco 10 mg, 8/day, SOMA

4/day, Valium 10 mg at night, Zoloft and Trazodone. She had been using cannabis for 2 years, consisting of daily edibles and tinctures. CBD had just become available, so I advised including it in her tincture 3×/day. Over the next year, she vaporized a CBD/THC 2:1 strain and used a CBD-rich tincture. She was able to wean off Norco and SOMA, yet continued the Valium at night. She continued to complain of chronic pain "all over," yet preferred the CBD-rich cannabis to THC, and in error had switched to a higher content CBD strain. I again advised a CBD/THC 2:1 or 1:1 mix for better pain management.

Pearls: While I was pleased with the Norco and SOMA wean, we do not want the patient to have unnecessary ongoing pain. CBD is often promoted as a better alternative to THC for pain, which is not the case. Patients need to be educated about the safety and efficacy of combination mixtures and find the dose that offers the best pain management with the least psychoactivity.

Patient 4: This is a 65-year-old female patient with fibromyalgia, chronic fatigue and dizziness. She did not like the effects of THC and had tried a CBD/THC 2:1 tincture, but said it made her feel "too stoned." She was not receiving much benefit from topicals over the past year. She had been experimenting with cannabis for 4 years. Her medications included Celebrex, valacyclovir, Cymbalta and Requip. We tried the only thing left to try which was a CBD/THC 20:1 mix either by vaporizing or tincture. She found that using tincture by spray 5×/day did bring some relief. At the time of our last visit, she was still experiencing burning pain over her whole body, and had been diagnosed with low back disc disease.

Pearls: Sensitive people, such as those with chronic fatigue, or environmental sensitivity can be extremely intolerant to THC above minimal doses. Unfortunately, we don't get the same level of pain relief with low THC cannabis, but we do get muscle relaxation, some pain management and reduced anxiety.

Patient 5: This is a 54-year-old female with multiple conditions, including ME/CFS, POTS (postural orthostatic tachycardia syndrome), daily migraine, fibromyalgia, joint pain, neck pain, insomnia, dizziness, nausea and chronic Lyme disease. Her medications included low doses of clonazepam, Ativan and Topamax. She unfortunately took 5–10 mg of Maxalt daily. She was also on thyroid medication and Cortef in the a.m. She was new to cannabis use, but desperate because her chronic conditions continued to worsen. Because I predicted she would be sensitive to THC, I advised one puff of a CBD/THC 1:1 vape pen at the start of a headache and a regimen of raw juiced cannabis and a CBDA/THCA tincture, approximately 10 mg 3×/day. She tried the raw juice, but said it gave her constipation. She tried smoking indica before bed, with no help for sleep. When she tried vaporizing a CBD/THC 1:1 oil, even one puff caused her heart to race and increased dizziness. This occurred with all combinations until she tried a CBD/THC 18:1 mix, which she used several times a day with some improvement. The migraines decreased to 2–3×/month, thus allowing her to decrease Maxalt, pain and nausea improved and she was hopeful for continued improvement.

Pearls: Again, we see that extremely sensitive individuals cannot tolerate even minimal amounts of THC. One puff of an 18:1 mix may provide 0.2 mg of THC. Did she need THC at all? Presumably yes for the most effective treatment of migraines. At the time of this case, pure CBD was not widely available, yet this is a rare case in which I would recommend it if it were (keeping in mind that without the terpenes, a higher dose might be required). Whether that microdose of THC was helping her migraines more effectively than pure CBD would have done is an interesting question.

CANNABIS THERAPY SUMMARY

The type of cannabis used for FM covers the whole scope of what's available, depending on whether you're treating pain, daytime fatigue, headache, IBS and/or nighttime insomnia. It is interesting that most of the patients I saw preferred CBD-rich products as they were uncomfortable with much THC. Although the limited research on FM indicates that THC would be helpful, we find that CBD is helpful as well. Because FM has components of inflammation, this is not surprising. Although CBD would not be expected to correct for an EC deficiency, perhaps that is not an underlying mechanism of great significance or microdoses of THC may actually help correct such a deficiency. The dosing ranged from minimal amounts up to the common doses of approximately 10 mg of tincture 3x/day. As usual, the THC-rich indicas do serve best as a sleep aid, here, by inhalation, but a longer acting dose by edible may be more efficacious. And for CFS patients who usually show extreme sensitivity to medications, we do see that microdoses of a CBD-rich product brought benefit, although more may be preferable. In such sensitive patients, adding a dose of THCA might prove useful as it is anti-inflammatory, immune modulating and non-psychoactive. Anecdotally, if supplied in raw juiced form, it may counteract the fatigue of chronic disease.

REFERENCES

1. National Pain Report. Marijuana rated most effective for treating fibromyalgia. 2014. http://nationalpainreport.com/marijuana-rated-most-effective-for-treating-fibromyalgia-8823638.html Accessed April 20, 2020.
2. Russo EB. Clinical endocannabinoid deficiency (CECD): can this concept explain therapeutic benefits of cannabis in migraine, fibromyalgia, irritable bowel syndrome and other treatment-resistant conditions? *Neuroendocrinol Lett.* 2004;25:31–39.
3. Russo EB. Clinical endocannabinoid deficiency reconsidered: current research supports the theory in migraine, fibromyalgia, irritable bowel, and other treatment-resistant syndromes. *Cannabis Cannabinoid Res.* 2016;1(1):154–165.
4. Walitt B, Klose P, Fitzcharles MA, Phillips T, Häuser W. Cannabinoids for fibromyalgia. *Cochrane Database Syst Rev.* 2016;7:CD011694.
5. Schley M, Legler A, Skopp G, et al. Delta-9-THC based monotherapy in fibromyalgia patients on experimentally induces pain, axon reflex flare, and pain relief. *Curr Med Res Opin.* 2006;22:1269–1276.
6. Weber J, Schley M, Casutt M, et al. Tetrahydrocannabinol (delta 9-THC) treatment in chronic central neuropathic pain and fibromyalgia patients: results of a multicenter survey. *Anesthesiol Res Pract.* 2009;2009:1–9.
7. Skrabek RQ, Galimova L, Ethans K, Perry D. Nabilone for the treatment of pain in fibromyalgia. *J Pain.* 2008;9(2):164–173.
8. Ware M, Fitzcharles M, Joseph L, Shir Y. The effects of a nabilone on sleep in fibromyalgia: results of a randomized controlled trial. *Anesth Analg.* 2010;110:604–610.

9. Ste-Marie PA, Fitzcharles MA, Gamsa A, Ware MA, Shir Y. Association of herbal cannabis use with negative psychosocial parameters in patients with fibromyalgia. Arthritis Care Res (Hoboken). 2012;64(8):1202–1208.

10. van de Donk T, Niesters M, Kowal MA, et al. An experimental randomized study on the analgesic effects of pharmaceutical-grade cannabis in chronic pain patients with fibromyalgia. *Pain.* 2019;160(4):860–869.

11. Fiz J, Durán M, Capellà D, Carbonell J, Farré M. Cannabis use in patients with fibromyalgia: effect on symptoms relief and health-related quality of life. *PLoS One.* 2011;6(4):e18440.

12. Habib G, Avisar I. The consumption of cannabis by fibromyalgia patients in Israel. *Pain Res Treat.* 2018;Article ID 7829427.

13. Johnson C. Marijuana as medicine for ME/CFS and FM IV: the doctor speaks – treatment #I. Health Rising website. August 21, 2019. www.healthrising.org/blog/2019/08/21/marijuana-as-medicine-for-me-cfs-and-fm-iv-the-doctor-speaks-treatment-pt-i/ Accessed April 20, 2020.

28 Gastrointestinal Disorders (Upper)

GASTROINTESTINAL DISORDERS (UPPER) AND CANNABIS

Cannabis can be useful for several upper gastrointestinal (GI) disorders, including ulcers, slow transit time, dysphagia or reflux. In researching the effects of cannabis on the upper GI tract, there have been many animal studies done using very high levels of THC or cannabis extracts, not necessarily relevant to common cannabis dosing. High levels of endocannabinoids are found throughout the digestive system. Both the CB1 receptor and the CB2 receptors can be found in the gut.[1] The endocannabinoid system (ECS) seems to play many roles in the GI tract. These include regulation of stomach acid, motility, visceral sensation, inflammation, pain and satiety. Cannabinoids have been shown to regulate relaxation of the lower esophageal sphincter, gastric acid secretion, gastric emptying, gastrointestinal motility and fluid secretion. Cannabinoids can protect the gastric mucosa by virtue of their antisecretory, antioxidant, anti-inflammatory and vasodilatory effects.[2,3]

As far back as 1978, it was shown that acute and long-term cannabis treatment reduced the rate of gastric ulceration in rats subjected to restraint-induced stress. In a human study, smoking cannabis for more than 2 days a week was associated with low gastric acid output.[4] Cannabis also protects against non-steroidal anti-inflammatory drug-induced gastric damage. In animal studies, THC protected against diclofenac-induced gastric hemorrhagic streaks through both oral and ip routes at 0.64 and 0.06 mg/kg, respectively.[5] In another study, it was found that oral cannabis (but not systemic) administration decreased gastric damage caused by naproxen. Complete protection occurred with a 10 mg/kg of cannabis extract, while at 3 mg/kg there was 80% inhibition of the lesions.[6] What's interesting here is that the authors did not describe heating their ethanolic cannabis extract. Possibly they were actually testing a THCA-rich extract, and not THC. In fact, cannabinoid acids do have anti-inflammatory effects and also decrease motility of the GI tract.[7] An investigation of the effects of α-pinene at very high doses (10 mg/kg) also demonstrated up to 50% protection against gastric mucosa ulceration in mice.[8] The entourage effect between terpenes and cannabinoids that might yield efficacy at lower doses is just beginning to be investigated.

THC also slows the rate of gastric emptying and small intestinal transit in mice and in rats as well as inhibiting gastric acid secretion.[9] In humans, THC at a dose used for preventing chemotherapy-induced nausea and vomiting delayed gastric emptying in volunteers who were experienced cannabis users.[10] This may be useful for hypermotility conditions. Cannabis also increases mucus secretion in the gastric mucosa. Cannabis extract given at 5, 10 and 20 mg/kg THC inhibited the development of gastric mucosal damage in rats in a dose-dependent manner. Note the very high concentration here, not likely to be used in humans. The authors concluded:

> Cannabis administered systemically exerts gastric mucosal protective effects against mucosal damage evoked by stimulation of gastric acid secretion, acidified aspirin or ethanol. These effects of cannabis are likely to involve inhibition of gastric acid and pepsin secretion, increased mucus, decreased oxidative stress and inflammation in gastric mucosa.[11]

Few studies have looked at the role of cannabinoids on esophageal function. In animals, lower esophageal sphincter pressure and swallowing were significantly reduced by THC administration. In a human study, 10 mg of THC reduced transient lower esophageal sphincter relaxations, while 20 mg THC led to nausea and vomiting, again a dose-dependent likely biphasic response.[12] But, cannabinoid receptor antagonists had no influence on esophageal peristalsis. A case report of improved symptoms in a person with dysphagia using cannabis was included in a review.[13] CBD has been studied in its role in reducing intestinal inflammation, but not really in upper GI disorders. As it has antispasmodic properties as well, it might be useful in esophageal spasm or dysphagia. This has not yet been studied, but there is a 2015 patent recorded for this purpose, which states, "The present invention relates to the use of an association of Δ9-tetrahydrocannabinolic acid (THC) and cannabidiol (CBD) for the treatment of achalasia or at least one of the symptoms thereof."[14]

There seem to be a difference in effects between acute and chronic dosing of cannabinoids. So, in fact, the results can be paradoxical depending on chronicity and dose. This may be relevant in the cannabinoid hyperemesis syndrome (see Chapter 38). Also, the patient's actual condition is relevant to treatment. If digestive problems are caused by low stomach acid, or if a patient is taking an acid-blocker drug to treat an ulcer, they no longer have high acid, and THC would not help, it may hurt. This may account for the fact that few patients actually use cannabis to treat upper GI problems, yet for some, especially with motility or spasm issues, it is helpful.

PATIENT REPORTS

To move on to patient results from my practice, the patients ranged in age from the teens to the elderly. Patients with upper GI issues encompassed so many types, such as ulcers, gastroparesis, reflux, esophageal strictures, to name but a few, that generalization is not useful. Reflux was a more common co-presenting symptom in the elderly, for which the benefits of cannabis were discovered only as they used it for other more pressing conditions, such as osteoarthritis. Here are a few illustrative case reports.

Patient 1: This is a 31-year-old male with complaints of gastroparesis and GI pain since his teens. He had been using cannabis daily by smoking. He also had constipation issues. He was on no medications. He used cannabis, first by smoking, then switched to vaporizing 4×/day, to help with appetite, pain and to stimulate bowels. Upon a 2-week tolerance break, he reported stomach burning resumed, and was relieved again with cannabis use. This patient ultimately found a method to treat his symptoms that has been working for the past several years. He says that immediately after dabbing he has bowel movements, and that he thinks using cannabis concentrate above 80% THC creates an artificial, and short lived, nerve stimulus, similar to a gastric pacemaker. He has very little pain with this change in bowel habits and more regular function.

Pearls: It is rare to treat patients with gastroparesis as a primary complaint. Cannabis should be considered in gastroparesis, including as a complication of diabetes as well as after bariatric surgery. Cannabis can improve decreased stomach emptying, even though it may slow intestinal transit time, and may provide a neurogenic stimulus to the bowel.

Patient 2: This is a 75-year-old female who initially presented with complaints of a "digestive disorder." She was not new to cannabis, but only used it rarely, a few times a week. Her medications included episodic low doses of Ativan or Vicodin as needed for GI pain. She had tried Lomotil and Donnatal in the past for diarrhea. Over the next year, she switched from smoking to using a vaporizer, and increased cannabis use to recover from a hip replacement. New esophageal spasms had appeared. Upon my advice, she increased cannabis use to at least 2x/day by vaporization, which did seem to relieve the esophageal spasm. We were working on increasing usage to 4x/day at our last visit. She preferred to grow her own, so CBD-rich strains were not as accessible, although I did suggest a CBD/THC 1:1 mix.

Pearls: As expected, THC did alleviate esophageal spasm. We would expect the 1:1 mix to be just as effective. Having access to seeds or clones for CBD-rich strains continues to be a limiting factor for home gardeners, even for elderly patients who actually prefer to limit psychoactive effects. It's available now in dispensaries, but some elderly patients don't have the funds to buy the cannabis they need.

Patient 3: This is a 15-year-old female with complaints of reflux, abdominal pain, anxiety and depression. She had been using cannabis by smoking for about 1 year. She thought she might have food sensitivities. I advised a food allergy test and continued cannabis as needed for mood, seeking strains with D-linalool and D-limonene preferably by vaporizing. At our next visit, she continued to have mood complaints as well as increased GI distress throughout, including vomiting in the mornings and abdominal bloating. She had switched to using a water pipe only used in the evenings. She was newly diagnosed with gastritis. An endoscopy had revealed fungal overgrowth in her esophagus for which she was taking antifungal medication. She was also taking Zoloft. I advised adding a CBD-rich tincture for daytime use as well as continued cannabis, especially strains with β-myrcene and D-limonene, as these both have antifungal properties. We did not have another follow-up.

Pearls: This case brings up the added benefit that cannabis has for antifungal action while at the same time acting as an antiemetic, mood stabilizer and bringing pain relief. It also demonstrates the uncommon instance of asking a teen to use more cannabis to offer increased benefit. So often with teens, we try to ensure minimal effective dose. In this case as her symptoms were progressing, she needed more cannabis, especially with the option of adding daytime CBD.

Patient 4: This is a 13-year-old male brought in by his parents for complaints of severe GI pain associated with reflux and nausea for 3 years and insomnia. The pain was throughout the gastric and intestinal tract, and associated with dietary choices.

He was sensitive to many foods, which he was avoiding, but had chronic pain. I advised a CBD-rich tincture to be titrated up to moderately high doses, up to 20 mg 3x/day. He never reached that level, saying he "felt out of it" on a CBD/THC 20:1 tincture. The next year as his symptoms continued, we tried a lower dose with more THC, a CBD/THC 2:1 tincture. He did find relief using a 1:1 vape pen and/or tincture. By this time, he was 16 years old. At our last visit, he was using cannabis only 2x/week, mostly a 1:1 mouth spray, now only for nausea. The severe GI pain was long gone, allied with discrimination with food choices.

Pearls: CBD-rich products were widely available when I saw this patient. We were immediately able to start with a CBD-rich mix, which is common in therapy with children. We slowly advanced to a CBD/THC 1:1 mix, demonstrating a rare case of needing to increase the THC content, which is indicated for greater pain relief. As this young man related, higher doses of CBD can be sedating or dissociative. Too much THC is not preferable in children. Finding the right ratio and right dosage was critical to efficacy.

CANNABIS THERAPY SUMMARY

The actions of cannabis for upper GI disorders are rarely reported and we know little about what to expect clinically. Here we see that THC-rich cannabis in acute high-potency doses, such as by dabbing, was remarkably effective in stimulating GI motility in a patient with gastroparesis. Because THC is a cannabinoid agonist, it is expected to affect motility, pain, reflux and possibly stomach acid as well. As with all cannabinoid receptor agents, the dose is expected to be biphasic, with most effective use seeming to occur at low to moderate, rather than high doses, such as that achieved by inhalation of even a few puffs of cannabis. The limited research seems to support this conclusion, as evidenced by the study given previously where 10 mg of THC promoted esophageal sphincter relaxation, likely to reduce reflux, while 20 mg of THC caused nausea and vomiting. Of course, this would be evident in those patients who have not yet reached tolerance. Several of my patients reported alleviation of GERD with a few puffs of a THC-rich cultivar before bed, by vaporization or by smoking. As far as esophageal spasm is concerned, both THC and CBD are expected to be effective, as they are both antispasmodic, likely dosed as usual for muscle spasm, that is, on average 10 mg doses (see Chapter 37). In such cases a CBD/THC combination would be expected to bring the best results with the least psychoactivity. One of my patients report relaxation of esophageal strictures by only 5 mg of CBD by tincture, although she did say it was difficult to swallow. More research needs to be done on the effects of CBD for upper GI disorders. Both neutral cannabinoids and cannabinoid acids would bring relief from inflammation, which would apply to gastritis and/or inflammatory GI pain.

REFERENCES

1. Massa F, Storr M, Lutz B. The endocannabinoid system in the physiology and pathophysiology of the gastrointestinal tract. *J Mol Med (Berl)*. 2005;83(12):944–954.

2. Izzo AA, Coutts AA. Cannabinoids and the digestive tract. *Handb Exp Pharmacol.* 2005;168:573–598.
3. Abdel-Salam O. Gastric acid inhibitory and gastric protective effects of cannabis and cannabinoids. *Asian Pac J Trop Med.* 2016;9(5):413–419.
4. Nalin DR, Levine MM, Rhead J, et al. Cannabis, hypochlorhydra, and cholera. *Lancet.* 1978;312(8095):859–862.
5. Kinsey SG, Cole EC. Acute D(9)-tetrahydrocannabinol blocks gastric hemorrhages induced by the nonsteroidal anti-inflammatory drug diclofenac sodium in mice. *Eur J Pharmacol.* 2013;715(1–3):111–116.
6. Wallace JL, Flannigan KL, McKnight W, et al. Pro-resolution, protective and anti-nociceptive effects of cannabis extract in the rat gastrointestinal tract. *J Physiol Pharmacol.* 2013;64(2):167–175.
7. Cluny NL, Naylor RJ, Whittle BA, Javid FA. The effects of cannabidiolic acid and cannabidiol on contractility of the gastrointestinal tract of Suncus murinus. *Arch Pharm Res.* 2011;34(9):1509–1517.
8. Pinheiro Mde A, Magalhães RM, Torres DM, et al. Gastroprotective effect of alpha-pinene and its correlation with antiulcerogenic activity of essential oils obtained from Hyptis species. *Pharmacogn Mag.* 2015;11(41):123–130.
9. Hornby PJ, Prouty SM. Involvement of cannabinoid receptors in gut motility and visceral perception. *Br J Pharmacol.* 2004;141(8):1335–1345.
10. Aviello G, Romano B, Izzo AA. Cannabinoids and gastrointestinal motility: animal and human studies. *Eur Rev Med Pharmacol Sci.* 2008;12(Supp 1):81–93.
11. Abdel-Salam OME, Salama RAA, El-Denshary EE, et al. Effect of Cannabis sativa extract on gastric acid secretion, oxidative stress and gastric mucosal integrity in rats. *Comp Clin Pathol.* 2015;24:1417–1434.
12. Beaumont H, Jensen J, Carlsson A, et al. Effect of delta9-tetrahydrocannabinol, a cannabinoid receptor agonist, on the triggering of transient lower oesophageal sphincter relaxations in dogs and humans. *Br J Pharmacol.* 2009;156(1):153–162.
13. Gotfried J, Kataria R, Schey R. The role of cannabinoids on esophageal function: what we know thus far. *Cannabis Cannabinoid Res.* 2017;2(1):252–258.
14. Luquiens A. Use of cannabis for the treatment of achalasia. 2015. https://patents.google.com/patent/WO2015198209A1/en Accessed March 10, 2020.

29 Glaucoma, Corneal Edema

GLAUCOMA, CORNEAL EDEMA AND CANNABIS

Cannabis use for any reason, either recreationally or medicinally, does affect eye pressure. It's important to understand its effect on glaucoma, whether it is used therapeutically for this condition or for other reasons. It may be acting to lower eye pressure in glaucoma or glaucoma suspect patients unbeknownst to them and if withdrawn, or used intermittently, they would lose protection. As early as 1971, during an investigation of its effects in healthy cannabis users, it was observed that cannabis reduces intraocular pressure (IOP). It was found that some derivatives of cannabis lowered the intraocular IOP when taken intravenously, by smoking or orally, but not by topical application to the eye.[1] Cannabis is also neuroprotective for the retina and other nerve pathways relating to the eye.[2,3] Cannabinoid receptors (CB1-type) have been detected in the human retina.[4] Clinically, while exogenous cannabinoids may prove therapeutic for neurotoxicity affecting the eye, this has not been proven, but the lowering of ocular pressure by cannabinoids has long been established. Anecdotally in humans and supported by animal studies, cannabis decreases intraocular pressure by an average 25–30%.

The signaling pathways of both CB1 and CB2 involve differential changes in aqueous humor outflow and IOP of the trabecular meshwork.[5] Cannabinoids not only act through the CB1 pathway but also activate cyclooxygenase (COX)-2, enhancing the outflow of aqueous humor and reducing IOP.[6] Non-psychotropic cannabinoids as well as some non-cannabinoid constituents of the hemp plant also decrease intraocular pressure. The mechanism of action to lower IOP is not fully elucidated but is thought to involve a CB1 receptor-mediated mechanism.[7,8] Cannabinoid receptors present in corneal epithelium also function to decrease inflammation and pain.[9] Topical administration of THC and CBD in mice showed dose-dependent results. The corneal antinociceptive and anti-inflammatory effects of CBD were independent of CB1 or CB2 and are thought to act at 5-HT1A receptors.[10]

It has generally been thought that a drawback to using cannabis to treat glaucoma was that it required constant inhalation, as often as every 3 hours and the side effects significantly outweighed the benefits.[11,12] Other methods of administration have been investigated. Early animal studies showed that eyedrops containing THC caused a reduction in IOP with 0.05% and 0.1% topical solutions of THC. This was not effective when administered to six subjects with primary open-angle glaucoma.[13] Cannabis extracts containing a low dose of THC or CBD administered via a sublingual spray were investigated to see if they could provide longer lasting effects. It was found that 2 hours after sublingual treatment with 5 mg of THC, the IOP was 4 mmHg lower. CBD up to high doses (40 mg) did not show IOP-lowering effects.[14]

DOI: 10.1201/9781003098201-40

CBD has been found to be without effect on IOP in most studies. Three of four studies that have tested CBD for effects on IOP have reported no effect, but the fourth actually reported an increase in IOP. The question of whether CBD is effective, synergistic or problematic was further confirmed in a recent study in animals. Effects of topically applied THC and CBD showed opposing effects. A single topical application of THC lowered IOP substantially (~28%) for 8 hours in male mice. This effect was shown to be due to combined activation of CB1 and GPR18 receptors and was sex-dependent, being stronger in male mice. CBD was found to have two opposing effects on ocular pressure, one of which involved antagonism of the lowering effect by THC.[15] The most significant use of cannabis for glaucoma has been in combination with prescription eyedrops, as the effects seem to be additive. We know that that they operate most likely by different or possibly synergistic mechanisms. Prescription eyedrops can alter intraocular pressure by acting on different circulation routes of the aqueous humor. A non-psychoactive extract of cannabis was tested in combination with timolol eye-drops in patients with high IOP in 1980.[16] They found that the effects of the two medications were complementary and were even effective in some cases where other medications had failed.

The development of functional cannabinoid eyedrops is of interest. In a review of cannabinoid effects on the eye, it is noted that "The discovery of ocular cannabinoid receptors implied an explanation for the induction of hypotension by topical cannabinoid applications, and has stimulated a new phase of ophthalmic cannabinoid research."[17] Canasol eyedrops for glaucoma treatment have been developed and sold in Jamaica for some time. It is unclear whether they are currently available. The physician who developed them has published data on a small subject sample, which appears to show maximal effects for 2 hours, then a decrease.[18] The potential effects of cannabinoid acids on eye pressure are reflected in a report of CBGA eyedrops being tested, so perhaps an application for cannabinoid acids will arise.[19] More testing needs to be done to determine how and when cannabinoids are indicated not only in the treatment of glaucoma, but in other inflammatory and neurodegenerative diseases of the eye, especially those avenues that do not result in psychoactive effects.

PATIENT REPORTS

To move on to patient results from my practice, most of my patients with glaucoma aged 60–70s. I saw the greatest benefit with an appropriate dose of THC. CBD was generally not as effective. Many patients used cannabis to replace one of two or three prescribed eyedrops to reduce the itchiness, redness or discomfort caused by these multiple medications. With patients who use cannabis to treat glaucoma, it seems that inhalation every 3 hours is not required for long-lasting eye pressure reduction. Here are a few illustrative case reports.

Patient 1: This is a 70-year-old female who required three different eyedrop medications that poorly controlled her glaucoma: timolol, Lumigan and dorzolamide. Her ocular pressures averaged 15 and 20. She was enquiring about cannabis because the drops bothered her eyes and interfered with her vision. She had never used cannabis before and was apprehensive, not wanting to feel "stoned." Our first tactic was to use an overnight dose of 10 mg THC in an edible so that she would sleep through the unwanted side effects, that is, disorientation. She said she couldn't find the product we agreed upon and got THCA instead, which she took in the a.m. Hoping for the best, she discontinued the dorzolamide and her eyes felt immediately better. I then advised her to switch to a CBD/THC 1:1 mix and use 5 mg 2x/day and 10 mg at night. On this regimen, her eye pressures remained 16 and 19, with minimal effects of being "stoned."

Pearls: It is interesting that this patient inadvertently used THCA, a cannabinoid acid, which may or may not have helped. In this case, cannabis replaced one of three eyedrops. She did this by using an appropriate THC dose even with CBD added. For those who want less psychoactivity, a 1:1 mix may be useful.

Patient 2: This is a 62-year-old male with long-standing glaucoma with a 45-year history of cannabis use. He presented on no eyedrops, but was using a half a cannabis cookie daily. His cannabis use prior to the edible was mainly by smoking. He reported and his medical records substantiated that his eye pressures had been 29 and 24 in the past, going to 24 and 14 with the cookie, a reduction of 4–10 points. His eye pressures remained stable over the next 2 years on the half cookie daily. The dosage was not known, as he was growing his own medicine and his cookie was not tested.

Pearls: Anecdotal reports from patients such as this one teaches us that consistent, adequate dose of long-lasting medicine is effective for eye pressure control. Edibles may be better than smoking for glaucoma control.

Patient 3: This is a 65-year-old female with narrow angle glaucoma. Her eye pressures were adequately controlled by two eyedrop medications, brimonidine and latanoprost, averaging 12 and 15. She was new to cannabis use. I advised an overnight tincture with CBD/THC 1:1. The next visit she reported using a tincture nightly that was 4:1. She was wary of the THC. I advised her to increase her dose to at least 2x/day. She reported doing so at a dose of approximately 5 mg, that's only 1 mg of THC 2x/day. Unexpectedly, her eye pressures were now measuring 7 and 8. She remained on her prescribed eyedrops throughout.

Pearls: This is one of the rare cases where a low dose of THC brought such good results, and presumably the CBD did not negate the effect. In a sensitive patient, a "microdose" may be enough to get the results we want. Or, possibly, less cannabis is required to act in concert with other prescribed eyedrops, than used alone.

Patient 4: This is a 53-year-old female with multiple reasons for using cannabis, including glaucoma. She also was treating PTSD, insomnia, migraine and nausea. She had been using cannabis for 30 years, but not daily, and then by smoking 1–2x/day. She was recently diagnosed with glaucoma. She then started taking 1 drop of latanoprost at bedtime. She reported that her eye pressures were up to 21–23. When she used cannabis daily, smoked 3–4x, her pressures went down to 15–16 one year, 13–14 another year. It suited her to increase her cannabis use rather than add another eyedrop medication because of her other diagnoses. During the 5 years that we worked together, she discontinued Valium 10 mg at night, which she had been taking to sleep for 5 years, she stopped Tylenol with codeine 4–6/day and carisoprodol, 3x/day. She continued to smoke cannabis 4x/day.

Pearls: This was not primarily a glaucoma case, yet it does illustrate the effectiveness of inhalation of THC at a frequency of several times/day. I rarely advise smoking as a therapeutic regimen, but in patients that are going to do it anyway, it's not surprising that the eye pressure is lowered. I believe that 1–2×/day is probably not a high-enough dose in non-naive users, but it should be studied further.

Patient 5: This is a 68-year-old male with "pre-glaucoma." He was already a medical cannabis patient, smoking 3–4×/day, regularly, for multiple joint pains. His eye pressures were in the 22–25 mm range. Over the next few years as I followed this patient, he continued to vaporize cannabis 3–4×/day, while his eye pressures decreased from 22–25 to 16–18. His usage increased in the last year to include 50 mg of oil before bed, upon which his pressures decreased even further. He was no longer considered to be a glaucoma suspect.

Pearls: This is a case where cannabis used for one purpose, that is, joint pain, was affecting another condition, glaucoma. Apparently, the dose of the cannabis was relevant to how much of an eye pressure reduction this patient achieved, here. This patient may have developed a tolerance on high-dose oil in the evenings, yet increasing his dose was associated with more pressure reduction. As in any dosage consideration, tolerance is to be considered at moderate to higher levels.

CORNEAL EDEMA – FUCH'S DYSTROPHY

Patient 1: This is a 67-year-old female who had Fuch's dystrophy of the eye, with corneal thickening, eye edema and pain. She was about to consider corneal transplants. She was new to cannabis use. I advised a CBD/THC 1:1 tincture at a dose of 5 mg 3×/day. After 2 months, she reported decreased pain and better night vision. She deferred the corneal transplant option.

Pearls: Cannabis seems to be useful for corneal edema and has previously been shown to decrease corneal pain and inflammation. Its use for eye disorders other than glaucoma has not been publicized, but here is a clear example of success.

CANNABIS THERAPY SUMMARY

The complaint of the American Academy of Ophthalmology regarding cannabis use in eyes is that you'd have to smoke it throughout the day and night to achieve ongoing protection, especially for eye pressure.[11] The use of edibles or tinctures with longer duration of effects is therefore preferred. The curious thing is that many of my patients used cannabis overnight, and not during the day. So at the time when their eye pressures were measured, they were effectively unmedicated. We might have expected the effect to have worn off, but at least in some, more chronic users, this is not the case. Does this mean that the effects of cannabis can be sustained on eye pressures for a period following significant blood levels? We don't know how long the effect is good for. It would be a good thing to study. But clearly, the notion that the medicine has to be on board 24 hours/day is not accurate. As far as the dosage needed is concerned, it may be an individualized response, with naive users needing as low a dose as 1 mg of THC 2×/day, or some combined CBD/THC effect being effective. Other patients I've had used a CBD/THC mix of 15 mg 2×/day with good results. Cannabis for other eye disorders such as pain and inflammation should not be disregarded, especially in the event that eyedrops become available.

REFERENCES

1. Hepler RS, Frank IR. Marihuana smoking and intraocular pressure. *JAMA*. 1971;217:1392.
2. Yazulla S. Endocannabinoids in the retina: from marijuana to neuroprotection. *Prog Retin Eye Res*. 2008;27(5):501–526.
3. Crandall J, Matragoon S, Khalifa YM, et al. Neuroprotective and intraocular pressure-lowering effects of (–)Delta 9-tetrahydrocannabinol in a rat model of glaucoma. *Ophthalmic Res*. 2007;39:69–75.
4. Adelli GR, Bhagav P, Taskar P, et al. Development of a Δ9-tetrahydrocannabinol amino acid-dicarboxylate prodrug with improved ocular bioavailability. *Invest Ophthalmol Vis Sci*. 2017;58(4):2167–2179.
5. Green K. The ocular effects of cannabinoids. *Curr Top Eye Res*. 1979;1:175–215.
6. Panahi Y, Manayi A, Nikan M, Vazirian M. The arguments for and against cannabinoids application in glaucomatous retinopathy. *Biomed Pharmacother*. 2017;86:620–627.
7. Tomida I, Pertwee RG, Azuara-Blanco A. Cannabinoids and glaucoma. *Br J Ophthalmol*. 2004;88(5):708–713.
8. Oltmanns MH, Samudre SS, Castillo IG, et al. Topical WIN55212–2 alleviates intraocular hypertension in rats through a CB1 receptor mediated mechanism of action. *J Ocul Pharmacol Ther*. 2008;24:104–115.
9. Iribarne M, Torbidoni V, Julián K, et al. Cannabinoid receptors in conjunctival epithelium: identification and functional properties. *Invest Ophthalmol Vis Sci*. 2008;49(10):4535–4544.
10. Thapa D, Cairns EA, Szczesniak A. The cannabinoids Δ8THC, CBD, and HU-308 act via distinct receptors to reduce corneal pain and inflammation. *Cannabis Cannabinoid Res*. 2018;3(1):11–20.
11. American Academy of Ophthalmology. Complementary therapy assessment marijuana in the treatment of glaucoma. 2006. www.aao.org/complimentary-therapy-assessment/marijuana-in-treatment-of-glaucoma Accessed February 25, 2020.
12. Green K. Marijuana smoking vs cannabinoids for glaucoma therapy. *Arch Ophthalmol*. 1998;116(11):1433–1437.
13. Merritt JC, Perry DD, Russell DN, Jones BF. Topical delta 9-tetrahydrocannabinol and aqueous dynamics in glaucoma. *J Clin Pharmacol*. 1981;21(8–9 Suppl):467S71S.
14. Tomida I, Azuara-Blanco A, House H, et al. Effect of sublingual application of cannabinoids on intraocular pressure: a pilot study. *J Glaucoma*. 2006;15(5):349–353.
15. Miller S, Daily L, Leishman E, Bradshaw H, Straiker A. D9-tetrahydrocannabinol and cannabidiol differentially regulate intraocular pressure. *IOVS*. 2018;59(15):5904–5911.
16. West ME, Lockhart AB. The treatment of glaucoma using a nonpsychoactive preparation of cannabis sativa. *West Indian Med J*. 1978;27(1):16–25.
17. Järvinen T, Pate DW, Laine K. Cannabinoids in the treatment of glaucoma. *Pharmacol Ther*. 2002:95(2):203–220.
18. West M. The use of certain cannabis derivatives (Canasol) in glaucoma. https://pdfs.semanticscholar.org/9ee1/b623969c375c27989deed13f6f31a7cd738e.pdf Accessed February 25, 2020.
19. Fingeret M. 2018. Cannabinoid nanoparticles, hydrogel combo bolster glaucoma drops. www.aoa.org/news/clinical-eye-care/glaucoma-cannabinoid-np-drop Accessed February 25, 2020.

30 Harm Reduction

HARM REDUCTION AND CANNABIS

The term "harm reduction" in the current context is about 30 years old, and was first introduced as part of drug abuse treatment and policy. "Harm reduction is a set of ideas and interventions that seek to reduce the harms associated with both drug use and ineffective, racialized drug policies."[1] This strategy includes the substitution of a safer drug for one that is more dangerous. That is where medical cannabis comes in. Although it is inappropriately deemed a "drug" and historically considered a drug of abuse itself, applied as a botanical medicine, it is infinitely less dangerous than many substances for which it can be a replacement, notably, alcohol, tobacco or even prescription drugs. In fact, cannabis has been shown to be effective in replacing multiple medications that might pose a polypharmacy risk. When comparing cannabis to harmful substances, a recent risk assessment measuring MOE (the MOE defined as ratio between toxicological threshold and estimated human intake) on a population scale found tobacco in the risk category, alcohol in the high-risk category with an MOE <10, while all other agents (opiates, cocaine, amphetamine-type stimulants, ecstasy, and benzodiazepines) had MOEs > 100, and cannabis had an MOE >10,000.[2]

A review of prescriptions written for older consumers, those enrolled in Medicare Part D, looked at prescriptions written for a multitude of conditions for which cannabis might be helpful, including anxiety, depression, glaucoma, nausea, pain, psychosis, seizures, sleep disorders and spasticity. They found fewer prescriptions were written in states where a medical marijuana law was in effect for all of the study condition categories except glaucoma. This projects not only less prescription drug use but also an economic savings as well. "National overall reductions in Medicare program and enrollee spending when states implemented medical marijuana laws were estimated to be $165.2 million per year in 2013."[3] There has been much interest recently in reducing the harm of opiod use with cannabis as a substitute (see Chapter 40). "Prescribing cannabis in place of opioids for neuropathic pain may reduce the morbidity and mortality rates associated with prescription pain medications and may be an effective harm reduction strategy."[4] But, beyond opiate reduction, cannabis can help patients reduce many types of pharmaceuticals, that is, for mood disorders, for insomnia, for immune disorders, to name but a few. As summarized by a pro-cannabis advocacy group, the National Organization for the Reform of Marijuana Laws (NORML):

> Cannabinoids have a relatively unique safety record, particularly when compared to other therapeutically active substances. Most significantly, the consumption of cannabinoids – regardless of quantity or potency – cannot induce a fatal overdose because, unlike alcohol or opiates, they do not act as central nervous system depressants.[5]

DOI: 10.1201/9781003098201-41

Since the time that cannabis has been approved as a medical option by several states, there have been multiple demographic surveys providing information on patients' use of cannabis as a harm reduction agent.[6-11] This has been mostly a patient-centric movement, not one supported or advised by the ambient health care system. Again, an opportunity to learn from our patients. An early report of cannabis as a harm reduction agent was put forth in 2004 by Dr. Tod Mikuria in California, as a substitute for alcohol.[6] Over 90 patients reported benefit, indicating that "for at least a subset of alcoholics, cannabis use is associated with reduced drinking." In a study of patients from a dispensary in California (N = 350), 40% used it as a substitute for alcohol, 26% as a substitute for illicit drugs and 66% as a substitute for prescription drugs. The reasons given for substituting were less adverse side effects (65%), better symptom management (57%) and less withdrawal potential (34%).[7] In a large survey of dispensary patrons in Washington state (N = 2,774), 46% used cannabis as a substitute for prescription drugs. The most common classes of drugs substituted were narcotics/opioids (35.8%), anxiolytics/benzodiazepines (13.6%) and antidepressants (12.7%). The odds of reporting substituting were 4.6 times greater among medical cannabis users compared with non-medical users. Increased age of respondents was also a defining factor, with a 16.9 odds ratio in the 51–65-year age group.[8] And in a recent large study of medical cannabis patients (N = 2,032) in Canada, a total of 1,730 specific prescription drugs were substituted, 35.3% opioids, 21.5% antidepressants, 10.9% non-opioid pain medications, 8.6% anti-seizure medications, 8.1% muscle relaxants/sleep aids, 4.3% benzodiazepines, 3.4% stimulants, 1.4% antiemetics and 1% antipsychotics. This patient population was on the average 40 years old, as was the case for most of the earlier survey populations, in general. Common reasons for cannabis use were 51.2% a safer alternative than prescriptions, 39.7% fewer adverse side effects, 19.5% better symptom management and 11.4% fewer withdrawal symptoms. As far as alcohol substitution is concerned, of the 515 respondents who substituted cannabis for alcohol, 30.9% said they stopped completely, while 36.7% reported reducing by at least 75%.[9]

As is well known, tobacco cessation is a very challenging outcome to achieve. Anecdotally, cannabis can help. In the Canadian study (previous one), of the 406 participants who substituted cannabis for tobacco, 50.7% said they stopped using it completely (100% substitution) and 13.8% reported reducing their use by 75%. Those who substituted for tobacco were far more likely to smoke cannabis as their primary method of use (66% vs. 48% of those who did not).[9] An interesting development was found for tobacco cessation in a study using CBD. Smokers were given inhalers with placebo or CBD for 1 week. Those treated with CBD reduced the number of cigarettes smoked by 40% during treatment, from about 95 to 55 per week. The authors hypothesize that CBD may be acting as weak CB1 allosteric antagonist, citing studies with rimonabant (a CB1 antagonist), in which, a daily 20 mg dose increased the chances of quitting (nicotine) approximately 1.5-fold. Alternatively, CBD acting as a FAAH inhibitor, thereby also decreasing cannabinoid agonism, may be similar to a study in rats where nicotine reinforcement was also lessened by a FAAH inhibitor.[12] In a following study of the effect of CBD on tobacco cravings during overnight abstinence, a single 800 mg dose of pure CBD was given to smokers with a 10-year smoking history. Tobacco craving was not reduced, but the salience and pleasantness of cigarette cues were.[13] It is unlikely that a one-time dose of anything is sufficient to antagonize an addiction of this length. Furthermore, often continuing an inhalation practice is useful to diminish a smoking habit. These are all divergent theories, especially in that smoking THC-rich cannabis, a cannabinoid agonist, has traditionally been the route that most patients have used to decrease tobacco use. It could be that the act of smoking itself with a CBD-rich strain might prove most effective for tobacco substitution.

PATIENT REPORTS

To move on to patient results from my practice, there are many types of harm reduction possible with cannabis, so the typical patient profile is hard to generalize. Those dealing with alcohol reduction tended to be older, in their 50s and 60s. Those using it for tobacco reduction were somewhat younger in their 30–50s. All patients who replace pharmaceuticals with cannabis can be considered to display a form of harm reduction, but this was most apparent in the elderly population and on multiple medications. Patients who historically admitted to use of hard drugs that they replaced with cannabis were younger in their 20s and 30s. A separate chapter is dedicated to opiate reduction with cannabis (see Chapter 40). Here are a few illustrative case reports.

Patient 1: This is a 55-year-old female who had been using cannabis to replace alcohol and help sleep. She reported having 5 drinks/day for several years. She started having "the shakes," and then began daily cannabis use. She had previously used cannabis episodically for 16 years. By smoking 3–4×/day, she was able to stop the alcohol completely. She also increased exercise and began a healthy diet. As of our last visit, she was off alcohol for 4 years, and continued to smoke a THC-rich cannabis.

Pearls: This is typical of cannabis substitution for alcohol, requiring steady, daily use. The problem is that her cannabis use remained increased for the years we worked together. The next step would be to diminish the daily cannabis, which may not happen for a while. It is the essence of harm reduction to replace a substance for a less harmful one, yet they both are a form of dependence.

Patient 2: This is a 54-year-old male who had been smoking cannabis for 40 years. He also had a long history of drinking beer, which had escalated to 12 beers/day by his report. When he had a seizure due to alcohol abuse and dehydration, he wanted help in decreasing the alcohol. He wasn't ready to quit. He was prescribed a benzodiazepine for a time to help with alcohol withdrawal. At our next annual visit, he was down to 9 beers/day, then 3 beers/day, still having the occasional tremor. By the third year, he was down to one beer/day. His cannabis use changed from smoking to edibles, and as of our last visit, not daily.

Pearls: This is another scenario of harm reduction in using cannabis to reduce alcohol. Was it central to his reduction? We don't know, because he'd been using both for many years. Of note is a change in habit from smoking to edibles. Sometimes the habit of smoking and drinking can be more of a trigger than help. It's good to consider alternative delivery systems.

Patient 3: This is a 56-year-old male who has been using cannabis to replace alcohol. For the prior 3 years he had a binge-drinking problem following a divorce. He now vaporizes cannabis 1–2x/daily after work. He continued to have anxiety and rapid heartbeat associated with ongoing stress and anxiety post-divorce. His only medication was Toprol to regulate heart rate. He first presented to me during his first year off alcohol. We added a CBD-rich tincture every morning to help with anxiety and he continued to vaporize an indica at night. Over the next several years, his anxiety improved, he continued to avoid alcohol, but did admit to a rare beer, and felt more stable.

Pearls: This case portrays the value of CBD in managing the anxiety that often accompanies alcohol cessation. Patients often need to be educated about the value of CBD for anxiety control. In the previous cases, the patients relied on primarily THC-rich cannabis because they sought an altered mood, as this patient did in the evenings. A regimen involving both is useful and extends the range of symptom control. Furthermore, CBD may be useful in reducing cravings.

Patient 4: This is a 47-year-old male who used cannabis for many reasons, including mood management for PTSD, bipolar disorder and anxiety, and to stop tobacco. He had been using cannabis for 20 years, mostly by smoking 2x/day. To stop tobacco, he used a nicotine patch and increased his cannabis usage to 1 joint 3x/day. He was successful in stopping tobacco. He did then decrease cannabis use for a time, but at our last visit reported an increase in use to 3 joints/day.

Pearls: Some patients find smoking something other than tobacco does help them quit, just to be able to continue to smoke. Others find they are more successful if they switch to vaporizing cannabis, and yet others finally get off smoke, off vaporizing and continue with edibles. It appears, however, that mood stabilization may have been impaired off tobacco, as often happens for a time. It would have been better if he sought my advice during the transition, turning more to the addition of CBD than increasing the THC-rich smoking.

Patient 5: This is a 35-year-old female who presented with chronic cystitis, irritable bowel and nocturia leading to sleep problems. She had been using cannabis for 2 years, by smoking 3–4x/day. She was also trying to stop tobacco and was on a nicotine patch. We discussed dietary changes and strategies to use cannabis to replace tobacco. She also revealed ongoing anxiety. I encouraged her to try smoking a CBD-rich strain, which she did not do. Over the next 3 years, she struggled with tobacco cessation, saying that cannabis helped her not to smoke cigarettes, but she was still using a nicotine patch. At our last visit, she was smoking more cannabis, up to 5 joints/day, but was off the patch. During this time, she had a pregnancy and delivered a healthy child.

Pearls: This case is an example of risk management. The patient was determined to be off tobacco during pregnancy, and she did this by smoking a level of THC-rich cannabis that I would not advise. There is much debate about the safety of such cannabis during pregnancy, yet there is no debate about the risks of smoking tobacco. Tobacco does more harm. I would have much preferred that she smoked less cannabis with a higher CBD ratio, but she did not follow my advice.

CANNABIS THERAPY SUMMARY

This chapter focused upon demonstration of cannabis replacing typical "drugs of abuse," as listed in reports by the National Institute of Drug Abuse (NIDA), or in the National Survey on Drug Use and Health (NSDUH) produced by the US Department of Health Substance Abuse and Mental Health Services Administration (SAMHSA), such as alcohol and tobacco. Ironically marijuana is listed as the most prevalent "drug of abuse" by these agencies. To embrace the concept of cannabis as a harm reduction agent, a paradigm shift must occur in the classically trained clinician's outlook as it has been occurring for consumers globally who are reaping the benefits of medicinal cannabis. That is not to say that issues of overuse or dependence are not to be considered, because, as we have seen, often the replacement of one addictive habit by a less harmful one may result in a similar sort of dependence. In the case of cannabis, however, not only is use of this substance less harmful physiologically than alcohol or tobacco, but weaning off of it is a much easier process, because it is not physiologically addictive. Psychologically, a dependence or a "crutch" often requires counseling and/or more positive lifestyle choices, and these should be encouraged whenever appropriate. It is the clinician's role to facilitate not only the replacement of a harmful practice with a less harmful one, but to coach the patient until they arrive at a therapeutic minimally effective dose of this botanical medicine. As has been presented previously, it is almost always easier to reduce herbal dosage than that of a drug due to the synergistic mechanisms of the botanical compound, in this case cannabis, working to restore homeostasis in the patient's chemistry (see Chapter 2). Illustrations of cannabis reducing prescription medicine usage is found in case reports throughout most of the clinical chapters in Part III. The concept of harm reduction can be applied to these examples as well, especially as regard other potentially harmful drugs such as benzodiazepines, opiates or stimulants, and in the case of polypharmacy and in reduction of drug adverse effects. This can be as seemingly inconsequential as the reduction of eyedrops in glaucoma patients, thus reducing itching and burning, or as significant as reduction of opiate dosage which I've seen reduce from 300 mg/day of oxycodone to none. Even in cases where non-harmful drugs are involved, just the reduction of adverse effects of these drugs is a form of harm reduction. Of course, as always in cannabis therapy, we seek to choose the composition of product and dosage that brings the best benefit/risk ratio, which often involves the incorporation of CBD if THC is being used, the consideration of cannabinoid acids and the use of non-psychoactive delivery systems.

REFERENCES

1. Harm reduction. Drug Policy Alliance website. www.drugpolicy.org/issues/harm-reduction Accessed March 10, 2020.
2. Lachenmeier DW, Rehm J. Comparative risk assessment of alcohol, tobacco, cannabis and other illicit drugs using the margin of exposure approach. *Sci Rep.* 2015;5:8126.
3. Bradford AC, Bradford WD. Medical marijuana laws reduce prescription medication use in Medicare part D. *Health Aff (Millwood).* 2016;35(7):1230–1236.
4. Colleen M. Prescribing cannabis for harm reduction. *Harm Reduct J.* 2012;9:1.

5. Armentno P. Marijuana: a primer. NORML website. https://norml.org/aboutmarijuana/marijuana-a-primer Accessed March 16, 2020.
6. Mikuriya TH. Cannabis as a substitute for alcohol: a harm-reduction approach. *J Cannabis Ther*. 2004;4(1):79–93.
7. Reiman A. Cannabis as a substitute for alcohol and other drugs. *Harm Reduct J*. 2009;6:35.
8. Corroon Jr JM, Mischley LK, Sexton M. Cannabis as a substitute for prescription drugs: a cross-sectional study. *J Pain Res*. 2017;10:989–998.
9. Lucas P, Baron EP, Jikome N. Medical cannabis patterns of use and substitution for opioids & other pharmaceutical drugs, alcohol, tobacco, and illicit substances: results from a cross-sectional survey of authorized patients. *Harm Reduct J*. 2019;16:9.
10. Nunberg H, Kilmer B, Pacula RL, Burgdorf JR. An analysis of applicants presenting to a medical marijuana specialty practice in California. *J Drug Policy Anal*. 2011;4(1):1.
11. Perron BE, Bohnert K, Perone AK, Bonn-Miller MO, Ilgen M. Use of prescription pain medications among medical cannabis patients: comparisons of pain levels, functioning, and patterns of alcohol and other drug use. *J Stud Alcohol Drugs*. 2015;76(3):406–413.
12. Morgan CJA, Das RK, Joye A, Curran V, Kamboj SK. Cannabidiol reduces cigarette consumption in tobacco smokers: preliminary findings. *Addict Behav*. 2013;38(9):2433–2436.
13. Hindocha C, Freeman TP, Grabski M. Cannabidiol reverses attentional bias to cigarette cues in a human experimental model of tobacco withdrawal. *Addiction*. 2018;113(9):1696–1705.

31 Headache, Migraine

HEADACHE, MIGRAINE AND CANNABIS

The pathophysiology of headaches is complex, and made more challenging to review when looking at such a broad category of disorders. The three main types of headaches include tension headaches (the most common), migraine headaches (including cluster headaches), for which many patients seek cannabis use, and medication overuse headaches. Most headaches involve overactivation of the trigeminovascular pathway. While migraine and cluster headaches are thought to arise from brain in areas such as the hypothalamus, brain stem, or cortex. Tension-type headaches can not only originate in the central nervous system but may also arise from myofascial tissue.[1]

Cannabis has long been known as a botanical medicine that could relieve headache.[2,3] A review of the pathophysiology involved and what is known about the effect of cannabis and cannabinoids has been published.[3,4] Research into the involvement of cannabinoids into these areas of the brain confirm endocannabinoid regulation.[1,5-6] CB1 receptors are abundant in areas of the brain and brain stem involved with migraine pathophysiology. Activation of CB1 receptors in the PAG (periaqueductal gray) and RVM (rostral ventral medulla) inhibit GABAergic and glutamatergic transmission in modulating pain. Cannabinoids' action on migraine may be similar to that of triptans, which are suspected to inhibit GABAergic and glutamatergic signaling in the PAG. One theory is that that triptans may help to break migraines by activating the brain's endocannabinoid system.[3]

The pathogenesis of migraine is thought to include altered serotonin levels. Endocannabinoids also interact with serotonergic neurons in the brain stem dorsal raphe to modulate pain mechanisms. Studies show cannabinoid agonism at 5-HT1A receptors and an antagonism at 5-HT2A receptors. Cannabinoids have been shown to inhibit 5HT release from platelets during a migraine, thereby lowering serotonin release. Cannabinoid dose, specifically THC, may be a factor while the action of CBD, if any, is not documented.[7-9] The status of cranial vessel vasodilation during migraine is a delicate matter, likely dependent on local levels of endocannabinoids. Anandamide has been found to both reduce and cause a dose-dependent dural vessel dilation. Concentration of endo- and exogenous cannabinoids could determine whether a vasodilatory or vasoconstrictive effect results.[1,10] One theory of headache pathogenesis is a clinical endocannabinoid deficiency syndrome, supported by the finding that lowered endocannabinoid levels are found in the cerebrospinal fluid of migraine headache patients.[10] Cannabis and cannabinoids as headache medicine shows promise theoretically and in clinical practice. "Modulation of the endocannabinoid system through agonism or antagonism of its receptors, targeting its metabolic pathways, or combining cannabinoids with other analgesics for synergistic effects, may provide the foundation for many new classes of medications."[3]

DOI: 10.1201/9781003098201-42

There have been a lack of studies using cannabinoids or cannabis to actually treat headaches. There are as yet no placebo-controlled studies of cannabis for headache. In a study of the effect of THC on rat migraine-like symptoms, they found that THC has a dose and time dependent anti-migraine effect. Action at CB1 receptors occurred when 0.32 mg/kg but not 1.0 mg/kg of THC was administered immediately after migraine induction, but not 90 minutes later.[11] One report showed nabilone (0.5 mg/day) was slightly better than ibuprofen for migraine and medication overuse headache.[12] A case report documented dronabinol effectiveness for cluster headache.[13] Another reported THC and CBD at high doses – 200 mg/day, used as prophylaxis, helped migraine but not cluster headache.[14] A survey of 113 patients with chronic cluster headaches in France found that 26% regularly consumed cannabis.[15] Several surveys that confirm many patients are using cannabis to treat headache and migraine. A recent survey of medical cannabis patients in Canada, 25% related that they used it to treat headache.[14] One report of data collection from patients with migraine in Colorado found great efficacy for decreased frequency and pain. Ninety percent of patients with migraine used cannabis for both treatment and prophylaxis of migraine headache, with frequency decreasing from 10.4 to 4.6 headaches per month.[16] Of course, cannabis has other entourage compounds besides cannabinoids, which yet again, seem to be the key to action at lower doses. The review survey in Canada found that pain patients, including migraine patients, preferred a THC-rich strain with β-caryophyllene an anti-inflammatory and β-myrcene a muscle relaxant.[14]

Patients report that if cannabis is taken at the onset of the headache, the headache will not progress. Other patients report that the severity of the headache is lessened significantly. And some patients report that their migraines occur with less frequency as they state they have less stress and better sleep with cannabis use. Stress and sleep deprivation are two common triggers of migraines; if these causes are reduced, the frequency of migraines are also reduced. For many patients, the nausea and vomiting associated with migraine headaches are eliminated with the use of cannabis. Cannabis can also provide relief from muscle cramps that can accompany migraine (particularly of the neck and shoulders), and as in tension headaches.

PATIENT REPORTS

To move on to patient results from my practice, patients with headaches are generally in the mid-adult range, in their 40s and 50s, although in rare cases were younger. Headaches, especially migraine headaches, are common reasons for which patients seek the help of cannabis. Often the primary medicines used for migraines, triptans, are not safe to take as often as is needed, so cannabis provides an effective alternative. Patients also often present with headaches associated with neck tension for which cannabis may be effective if used only topically. Here are a few illustrative case reports.

MIGRAINE

Patient 1: This is a 56-year-old female with a history of migraine, neck pain and insomnia. At our first visit, she reported 4–12 migraines/month for the past 20 years.

She also had chronic neck tension at the back of the head palpable on exam. She was new to cannabis use. Her medications included lorazepam up to 6 mg qhs, and Imitrex 9–15 times/month as needed for headache. I advised her to smoke or vaporize a THC-rich strain of cannabis at the start of each headache, which pretty much was able to replace Imitrex over the next year to rare use, only three times for headaches not controlled by cannabis. Her neck tension was better as well. She was thrilled at the relief from headaches. Next, we focused more on helping her sleep with a goal to weaning the lorazepam. This happened over the next year. She found that using a small amount of sativa in the evenings was good for her mood, and she was able to sleep naturally after it wore off. Ultimately, she switched to a vaporizer, used in the evenings, and experienced an average of 1 migraine per year.

Pearls: This is a not uncommon case of cannabis being as effective as a triptan, yet paving the way for amelioration of symptoms to a much-reduced incidence of headache over time. Perhaps better sleep contributed to improvement as well, and the muscle-relaxing properties of cannabis alleviating neck tension.

Patient 2: This is a 53-year-old female with a 15-year history of migraines, which she described as severe. Her headaches averaged 1x/week, which she treated with Imitrex, Vicodin and Diclofenac. She had tried cannabis edibles that helped somewhat after the headache. She also tried acupuncture, chiropractic and Botox, all with little success. I advised vaporizing a THC-rich strain at the start of the headaches. She reported that this did help with the severity of the headaches, no longer using Vicodin, but although they did not progress, they still initiated. She was also using a CBD-rich tincture daily. Over the next year, she noted increasing neck stiffness, headache onset at increased levels, 5x/week, yet cannabis continued to reduce the severity of headache by vaporizing and using edibles.

Pearls: Sometimes the result of using cannabis for migraines can be that the severity is reduced, but not the incidence. The triggers in this case may not have changed, requiring the need for ongoing therapeutic management. This patient found some relief using it, albeit not a cure.

Patient 3: This is a 24-year-old female with chronic migraine, about 2x/week, after a head injury several years earlier, including a neck fracture and jaw dysfunction. This is a case of structural head/neck alignment issues contributing to migraine. On exam her jaw was tight and jutted forward. She was getting chiropractic adjustments. She also complained of insomnia and anxiety for which she was taking Klonapin 1 mg, not daily. I advised vaporizing a THC-rich cannabis at the start of headache and an indica chocolate before bed. She couldn't tolerate the chocolate saying edibles caused nausea, but found vaporizing a CBD/THC mix effective for headaches and anxiety, varying from a 20:1 to a 1:1 ratio. She also vaporized indica for sleep. After 2 years, the migraines decreased to an average of 2x/month, and Klonapin was discontinued.

Pearls: While mostly CBD is not usually helpful for migraines, a mix of CBD and THC can be an effective strategy for those uncomfortable with psychoactive effects, especially with concomitant anxiety. This is another example of the dual role of cannabis in alleviating insomnia and reducing migraine.

Patient 4: This is a 52-year-old female with a long history of migraines, about 4x/month. She also had neck pain and had C6–C7 fusion 3 years prior. She took

Imitrex as needed to treat the migraines, as well as smoking cannabis a few times/ week for the past few years. She was also taking nortriptyline 50 mg/day. I advised vaporizing at the start of the headache. Over the next 2 years, the frequency of migraines decreased to 1–2 episodes/month. After that, the patient tried to reduce nortriptyline without success. During this time, she added an edible 20 mg/day. We decided to reduce edible dosage, continue to vaporize as needed and add topical for neck tension.

Pearls: Consideration of the tension component in many cases of migraine leads to a simple intervention in which topical cannabis can be very helpful. Sometimes patients achieve benefit from applying topical to the temples as well.

CLUSTER HEADACHE

Patient 1: This is a 35-year-old male with a 21-year history of episodic cluster headaches. They often lasted up to 1 month, 4 times/year. He's tried cannabis for it before and thought it may help. His standard treatment included supplemental oxygen, Zomig and oxycodone as needed for pain. Because little is known about cannabis therapy for cluster headache, I recommended prevention with a low daily dose of CBD/THC 1:1, 5 mg 3×/day and vaping a THC-rich strain at the start of the headache. This strategy apparently worked, as he reported no cluster headache episodes in the next year. He found that using a CBD/THC mix usually only at night was really useful, allowing discontinuance of Zomig and oxycodone. He finally settled upon a "grain of rice" dose of a high potency CBD/THC 1:1 oil brought the best results, with no headache at all in the last 5 years.

Pearls: In a previous case study report, dronabinol was effective at terminating a cluster headache. Here, it seems that a CBD/THC 1:1 mix can be prophylactic if used regularly. How much CBD and THC are needed in what ratios should be studied. It's only one patient here, but indications are positive for cannabis treating a typically treatment-resistant cluster headache.

CANNABIS THERAPY SUMMARY

It is generally found that the best strategy for treating migraine headaches is a quick acting dose of THC-rich cannabis, preferably by inhalation or possibly by sublingual application. In most of the migraine patients, I've seen this helps to reduce frequency, severity and duration. It doesn't work in all cases, however. Eliminating ongoing triggers, improving sleep and reducing stress are all strategies that must still be incorporated. In a patient vestibular migraine for which traditional migraine medications such as triptans had been no help, the patient was leery of using THC due to the potential for increased dizziness. We tried a CBD/THC mix for nighttime use to help with sleep, but we were not able to achieve an appropriate dose. Headaches continued unabated. I have seen little success with patients using CBD-rich cannabis in preventing the progression of migraines. The options for tension headaches are greater as CBD, THC and β-myrcene are all muscle relaxant. The use of topicals at the site of tension is often helpful. There are even some patients who have found that topicals can reduce the severity of migraine headaches if applied to the temples.

What is truly encouraging is the cessation of cluster headaches by a moderate amount of a CBD/THC 1:1 mix, such as in the patient who was plagued with them for 5 months out of every year, then was headache free for 5 years (presumably ongoing) with no other medications. In some cases, such a mix is therapeutic for headaches in general, including migraines, providing a less psychoactive option, especially for daytime use.

REFERENCES

1. Baron EP. Comprehensive review of medicinal marijuana, cannabinoids, and therapeutic implications in medicine and headache: what a long strange trip it's been. *Headache.* 2015;55:885–916.
2. Lochte BC, Beletsky A, Samuel NK, Grant I. The use of cannabis for headache disorders. *Cannabis Cannabinoid Res.* 2017;2(1):61–71.
3. Lichtman AH, Cook SA, Martin BR. Investigation of brain sites mediating cannabinoid action: evidence supporting periaqueductal gray involvement. *J Pharmacol Exp Ther.* 1996;276: 585–593.
4. Russo E. Cannabis for migraine treatment: the once and future prescription? An historical and scientific review. *Pain.* 1998;76:3–8.
5. Papanastassiou AM, et al. Local application of the cannabinoid receptor agonist, WIN 55,212–2, to spinal trigeminal nucleus caudalis differentially affects nociceptive and non-nociceptive neurons. *Pain.* 2004;107:267–275.
6. Leimuranta P, Khiroug L, Giniatullin R. Emerging role of (endo)cannabinoids in migraine. *Front Pharmacol.* 2018;9:420.
7. Volfe Z, Dvilansky A, Nathan I. Cannabinoids block release of serotonin from platelets induced by plasma from migraine patients. *Int J Clin Pharm Res.* 1985;4:243–246.
8. Velenovská M, Fisar Z. Effect of cannabinoids on platelet serotonin uptake. *Addict Biol.* 2007;12(2):158–166.
9. Rossi C, Pini LA, Cupini ML, Calabresi P, Sarchielli P. Endocannabinoids in platelets of chronic migraine patients and medication-overuse headache patients: relation with serotonin levels. *Eur J Clin Pharmacol.* 2008;64(1):1–8.
10. Russo EB. Clinical endocannabinoid deficiency reconsidered: current research supports the theory in migraine, fibromyalgia, irritable bowel, and other treatment-resistant syndromes. *Cannabis Cannabinoid Res.* 2016;1:154–165.
11. Kandasamy R, Dawson CT, Craft RM, Morgan MM. Anti-migraine effect of Δ9-tetrahydrocannabinol in the female rat. *Eur J Pharmacol.* 2017;818:271–277.
12. Pini LA, Guerzoni S, Cainazzo MM, et al. Nabilone for the treatment of medication overuse headache: results of a preliminary doubleblind, active-controlled, randomized trial. *J Headache Pain.* 2012;13:677–684.
13. Robbins MS, Tarshish S, Solomon S, Grosberg BM. 2009. Cluster attacks responsive to recreational cannabis and dronabinol. *Headache.* 49(6):914–916.
14. Baron EP, Lucas P, Eades J, Hogue O. Patterns of medicinal cannabis use, strain analysis, and substitution effect among patients with migraine, headache, arthritis, and chronic pain in a medicinal cannabis cohort. *J Headache Pain.* 2018;9:37.
15. Donnet A, Lanteri-Minet M, Guegan-Massardier E, et al. Chronic cluster headache: a French clinical descriptive study. *J Neurol Neurosurg Psychiatry.* 2007;78:1354–1358.
16. Rhyne DN, Anderson SL, Gedde M, Borgelt LM. Effects of medical marijuana on migraine headache frequency in an adult population. *Pharmacotherapy.* 2016;36(5):505–510.

32 Human Immunodeficiency Virus, Acquired Immune Deficiency Syndrome

HUMAN IMMUNODEFICIENCY VIRUS, ACQUIRED IMMUNE DEFICIENCY SYNDROME AND CANNABIS

Patients with human immunodeficiency virus (HIV) or acquired immune deficiency syndrome (AIDS) are challenged by multiple symptoms such as fatigue, malaise, anorexia, nausea, depression and pain. HIV infection is commonly treated with strong antiviral drugs, which, in themselves, have many undesirable side effects such as nausea, diarrhea, loss of appetite and cachexia. The effectiveness of cannabis for treating symptoms related to HIV/AIDS is widely recognized. As far back as 1999, a review by the Institute of Medicine concluded, "Cannabinoids could be beneficial for a variety of effects, such as increased appetite, while reducing the nausea and vomiting caused by protease inhibitors and the pain and anxiety associated with AIDS."[1]

Its value as an antiemetic and analgesic has been proven in numerous studies (see Chapter 38). Dronabinol (synthetic THC) has been approved by the US Food and Drug Administration since 1992 as an antiemetic and appetite stimulant for patients with AIDS. The initial dose of dronabinol is 2.5 mg 2x/day. Its efficacy as an appetite stimulant is not impressive, and weight gain may not be evident (see Chapter 14). In some studies weight gain in some participants was modest at 3.2 kg, yet still some participants showed weight loss, similar to the placebo group.[2] Another study comparing dronabinol and cannabis in HIV patients showed increased weight in both groups. Over the 21-day study period, the placebo recipients gained 1.1 kg, while the participants in the cannabis and dronabinol groups gained a median of 3.0 kg and 3.2 kg, respectively.[3] Patients with HIV often prefer to use cannabis, likely due to its multiple effects, not only for appetite, but for mood and pain management. In addition, cannabis may facilitate, ART (antiretroviral therapy) adherence for patients with nausea.[4]

Over 30% of patients with HIV/AIDS have concomitant neuropathic pain, many as a result of ART therapies. There is no approved treatment for such pain that is satisfactory for a majority of patients. In a 2007 study, smoked cannabis 3x/day was found to be effective to treat HIV neuropathy, reducing daily pain by 34% versus 17% with placebo.[5] In a subsequent study using the same low-potency cannabis (1–8% THC), 46% of participants achieved at least 30% reduction in pain versus 18% in placebo, smoked 4x/day. They also found improvement in mood, physical

DOI: 10.1201/9781003098201-43

disability and quality of life.[6] Current potencies of THC-rich cannabis available in dispensaries can be up to 20% by weight, so adjustments in dose and delivery need to be calculated with commonly available products. Also, neuropathic pain studies indicate that CBD/THC mixtures may be more effective for overall quality of life (see Chapter 39). Thus far cannabis use in HIV-infected individuals has been reported for unspecified compositions of cannabis strains, and these mostly by smoking or vaporization. Combinations including CBD have yet to be reported. In a proposed study protocol, the efficacy of a CBD/THC mix of cannabis by oral delivery is being studied. HIV participants with an undetectable viral load for at least 3 years will receive CBD/THC in a 1:1 ratio or a 9:1 ratio by capsule daily for 12 weeks to assess safety, tolerability and effect on immune activation.[7] Another trial in progress proposes to study vaporized cannabis with three different CBD/THC ratios: high THC, high CBD or an equivalent mix. For some reason not immediately apparent, they predict that the highest CBD dose will provide the greatest pain reduction (results not yet available).[8]

As the mechanism of cannabinoid action has become more well-understood, the possible immunomodulatory and anti-inflammatory action of both THC and CBD have been proposed as disease-modifying agents for HIV infection. A recently realized potential benefit of cannabis use in HIV patients is to reduce viral load. Measurement of peripheral blood mononuclear cells (PBMCs) from HIV-infected individuals with heavy cannabis use versus non-use showed cannabis use was associated with decreased frequencies of activated T cells and inflammatory antigen-presenting cells.[9] Several studies have shown a lower viral load among "heavy" cannabis users (usually meaning at least daily use).[10,11] Other studies have not confirmed this effect, but its action as an immunomodulatory agent affecting CD4 and CD8 counts were confirmed.[3,12] An in vitro study of HIV-infected cells showed that cannabinoid activation of CB2 inhibits HIV infection by altering CD4+ T cell actin dynamics. Selective CB2 activation blocked both cell-free and cell-associated viral infection, reducing the frequency of infected cells by 30–60%.[13] The potential anticancer effect of cannabinoids was studied in patients with Kaposi's sarcoma (KSHV). They found CBD reduced proliferation in the virus-infected cells by 79% of the controls. They propose that CBD preferentially inhibits the proliferation of KSHV-infected endothelium and induces apoptosis in KSHV-infected cells.[14] One author proposed, "Cannabinoids may represent a feasible method to reduce immune activation and enhance immune profile. This, in turn, may hasten the progression of non-opportunistic complications associated with HIV."[7]

Estimates of the number of AIDS patients using cannabis range from about 20% to 40%. Reported benefits from a 2003 survey in the United States include relief of anxiety and/or depression (57%), improved appetite (53%), increased pleasure (33%) and relief of pain (28%).[15] HIV patients in a survey in the UK noted using cannabis to improve appetite (97%), for muscle pain (94%), nausea (93%), anxiety (93%), nerve pain (90%), depression (86%) and paresthesias (85%). Many (47%) also reported associated memory deterioration.[16] In a more recent survey in Canada, almost all HIV cannabis users, 98%, stated its primary benefit was recreational, for euphoria. Average consumption was by smoking, 18 grams/month, which was similar to use prior to the HIV diagnosis.[11] Another Canadian survey of HIV-hepatitis C coinfected individuals reported that 53% had smoked cannabis in the past 6 months.[7] This seems to indicate that continuing smoked cannabis was a stabilizing factor for HIV patients. This is perhaps the most significant aspect of cannabis use in HIV/AIDS patients to continue a medicine that has already been useful. I would challenge the classification of the antidepressant, euphoric effect in someone with a chronic debilitating disease as "recreational," rather than an ongoing therapeutic benefit.

PATIENT REPORTS

To move on to patient results from my practice, in earlier years I saw more patients with HIV as it was one of the few well-documented reasons for medical cannabis use. I do not currently have access to those records, although I have included one case here. In my recent patient population, HIV/AIDS was a rare diagnosis for cannabis use, although that may be a reflection of the community I practiced in rather than its efficacy. Here are a few illustrative case reports.

Patient 1: This is a 59-year-old female who I had seen for several years prior for HIV complaints, such as low appetite secondary to the multiple HIV medications she was taking. She had been using cannabis for 10 years by smoking or vaporizing. She was also prescribed Marinol 5 mg in the morning for nausea. She smoked an indica strain most nights to help with sleep. She consulted me for 5 years, during which time her HIV, medications and cannabis usage remained the same.

Pearls: This case illustrates a modest use of cannabis for the common reasons for which most HIV/AIDS patients claim benefit, appetite, nausea and sleep. It is also a rare case of concomitant cannabis use with a pharmaceutical cannabinoid. Marinol is rarely prescribed, but it is approved for HIV anorexia.

Patient 2: This is a 45-year-old male with a 20-year history of AIDS who stated he has "full blown AIDS." He's been on retroviral medications for many years with resultant nausea and anorexia. He stated that cannabis helps him to regain an appetite, deal with the stress of a serious chronic debilitating illness, and deal with constant leg pain. When questioned about the cause/nature of his leg pain, he relates daily leg spasms, sometimes to where he can't walk, of unknown origin. He was somewhat despondent and in despair about his health. Upon further discussion, the patient revealed that he had recently been diagnosed with syphilis, probably in late stage, and that is the most likely cause of his leg spasms and pain. He was on multiple retroviral medications, an antidepressant, Seroquel for sleep, Marinol 2×/day, as well as an inhaler and an antifungal medicine. He had a wasted appearance, appeared frail and was emotionally labile. His cannabis usage was high, smoking several times a day, up to ½ ounce per week. We discussed options for a tolerance break to achieve improved pain control.

Pearls: This is a report of a patient seen a while ago at which time tinctures, capsules and readily available vaporizers were not stocked in dispensaries. In fact, this patient should have switched to a non-smoked method, because he required daily inhaler treatment for his lungs. He was most likely treating neuropathic pain due to syphilis, although we cannot rule out a contribution by HIV. For severe pain, we often see patients using greater amounts of cannabis. CBD-rich products were not available at this time.

Patient 3: This is a 58-year-old male who I had seen for several years prior for complaints of low back pain, who was also treating long-term HIV infection. He had been using cannabis for over 10 years. He was on several HIV medications, which were working well to keep his condition stable. In addition, he took oxycodone up to 40 mg/day for pain. He noted that cannabis helped him maintain a stable mood, but was aware that he was using as well for help with low back pain. We worked together for 6 years, during which time his HIV remained stable, and his oxycodone usage decreased from 40 mg/day to 10 mg/day. This was facilitated by a switch from smoking 2–3x/day to added vaporizing up to 3x/day as needed for pain.

Pearls: As this case illustrates, HIV/AIDS patients often have multiple medical issues, here – severe low back pain. The primary benefit of cannabis may have been the reduction in oxycodone dose demonstrating the effectiveness of inhalation 6x/day for analgesic coverage.

Patient 4: This is a 47-year-old male with a long history of being HIV positive and treated successfully with Atripla. He had a 30-year history of cannabis use. He said it helped with anxiety, sleep and appetite. He had modest use, smoking or vaporizing rarely, but mostly using an edible before bed. Over the next 4 years, his health remained stable while on a drug-holiday off Atripla and cannabis use switched to vaporizing indica before bed. He was planning to resume HIV medication in the near future.

Pearls: Here we again see the common complaints for which HIV/AIDS patients claim benefit from cannabis – nausea, appetite, sleep and in this case, anxiety. It is interesting to speculate whether cannabis usage can affect the length of time that a patient can successfully take a drug holiday (a rare event) from ART. The scant research on the subject implies that heavy, but not occasional usage can reduce levels of immune-activating cells in subjects with HIV infection.

CANNABIS THERAPY SUMMARY

The use of cannabis for HIV/AIDS is one of the most long-standing conditions for which patients have been approved for medical cannabis, and one of the few conditions that reviews, such as the IOM report of 1999, have indicated evidence for cannabis and cannabinoid therapeutic efficacy. This is contributed to, in part, by the approval of dronabinol in 1992 for HIV-related anorexia. The practice of using cannabis for this condition, therefore, dates back to times when few delivery methods were available, resulting in a preponderance of smoking in the HIV population. In fact, smoking has been the delivery method employed in human clinical studies. This later was expanded to vaporization in subsequent studies. Even to this date over half of HIV/AIDS patient prefer smoking. The benefits of THC-rich cannabis delivered in several acute, short-acting doses is a widespread strategy for appetite stimulation and mood enhancement, not unique to this cohort. I would encourage the use of vaporization as the best method to promote these effects, yet smoking is a long-held practice in HIV/AIDS patients. It is important to address tolerance in heavy cannabis users, especially with THC-rich cannabis, as paradoxical effects may occur depending on the dose. As regards appetite, for example, cannabis can be an effective stimulant when used at low to moderate doses, but higher chronic use can result in a dependence upon cannabis to elicit a normal hunger response (see Chapter 14). There is no data about the efficacy of more recently available CBD/THC mixed cultivars, although some CBD may be useful to mitigate the psychoactive effects of THC, especially in cases of concomitant anxiety. More research needs to be done on enhancement of mood by appropriate cultivar selection, such as with the inclusion of D-limonene as uplifting and D-linalool for relaxation. The hypothesis that cannabis may prove to be a disease-modifying agent by decreasing viral load and potentially reduce the need for ART is just beginning to be investigated, although human trials on this question have not yet been initiated.

REFERENCES

1. Joy JE, Watson SJ Jr, Benson JA Jr, eds. Institute of Medicine. *Marijuana and Medicine: Assessing the Science Base*. Washington, DC: National Academies Press (US); 1999.
2. Badowski ME, Perez SE. Clinical utility of dronabinol in the treatment of weight loss associated with HIV and AIDS. *HIV AIDS (Auckl)*. 2016;8:37–45.
3. Abrams DI, Hilton JF, Leiser RJ, et al. Short-term effects of cannabinoids in patients with HIV-1 infection: a randomized, placebo-controlled clinical trial. *Ann Intern Med*. 2003;139(4):258–266.
4. De Jong BC, Prentiss D, McFarland W, Machekano R, Israelski DM. Marijuana use and its association with adherence to antiretroviral therapy among HIV-infected persons with moderate to severe nausea. *J Acquir Immune Defic Syndr*. 2005;38:43–46.
5. Abrams DI, Jay CA, Shade SB, et al. Cannabis in painful HIV-associated sensory neuropathy. *Neurology*. 2007;68:515–521.
6. Ellis RJ, Toperoff W, Vaida F, et al. Smoked medicinal cannabis for neuropathic pain in HIV: a randomized, cross-over clinical trial. *Neuropsychopharmacology*. 2009;34(3): 672–680.
7. Costiniuk CT, Saneei Z, Routy J, et al. Oral cannabinoids in people living with HIV on effective antiretroviral therapy: CTN PT028 – study protocol for a pilot randomised trial to assess safety, tolerability and effect on immune activation. *BMJ Open*. 2019;9: e024793.
8. University of California San Diego. Effect of cannabis administration and endocannabinoids on HIV neuropathic pain primary study – phase 2. https://clinicaltrials.gov/ct2/show/NCT03099005 Accessed March 13, 2020.
9. Manuzak JA, Gott TM, Kirkwood JS, et al. Heavy cannabis use associated with reduction in activated and inflammatory immune cell frequencies in antiretroviral therapy-treated human immunodeficiency virus-infected individuals. *Clin Infect Dis*. 2018;66(12):1872–1882.
10. Milloy MJ, Marshall B, Kerr T, et al. High-intensity cannabis use associated with lower plasma human immunodeficiency virus-1 RNA viral load among recently infected people who use injection drugs. *Drug Alcohol Rev*. 2015;34:135–140.
11. Harris GE, Dupuis LR, Mugford G, et al. Patterns and correlates of cannabis use among individuals with HIV/AIDS in maritime Canada. *Can J Infect Dis Med Microbiol*. 2014;25(1):e1–e7.
12. Okafor CN, Zhou Z, Burrell II LE, et al. Marijuana use and viral suppression in persons receiving medical care for HIV-infection. *Am J Drug Alcohol Abuse*. 2017;43:103–110.
13. Costantino CM, Gupta A, Yewdall AW, et al. Cannabinoid receptor 2-mediated attenuation of CXCR4-tropic HIV infection in primary CD4+ T cells. *PLoS One*. 2012;7(3): e33961.

14. Maor Y, Yu J, Kuzontkoski PM, et al. Cannabidiol inhibits growth and induces programmed cell death in Kaposi sarcoma-associated herpesvirus-infected endothelium. *Genes Cancer.* 2012;3(7–8):512–520.
15. Prentiss D, Power R, Balmas G, Tzuang G, Israelski DM. Patterns of marijuana use among patients with HIV/AIDS followed in a public health care setting. *J Acquir Immune Defic Syndr.* 2004;35(1):38–45.
16. Woolridge E, Barton S, Samuel J, et al. Cannabis use in HIV for pain and other medical symptoms. *J Pain Sym Man.* 2005;29(4):358–367.

33 Insomnia

INSOMNIA AND CANNABIS

Insomnia is a common complaint. Almost 50% of the adult population in the United States experiences insomnia with high rates of dissatisfaction (50%) over the effectiveness and potential side effects of conventional pharmaceutical medications. Medical cannabis patients routinely report that its use improves sleep. In a survey of patients who presented to medical cannabis evaluation clinics in California, 71% stated that they were using cannabis to improve sleep, with 14% reporting that it was the main symptom for which they were seeking care.[1] Many patients were told to use over-the-counter sleep aids or had been given prescription for sleeping pills. Patients report that these don't work in the long term or leave long-lasting effects that cause a hangover the next day. Paradoxically, much of the literature about cannabis and sleep lists sleep disturbance during cannabis withdrawal as a major deterrent to its use, stating that this can last up to 45 days.[2] In most cases, however, the withdrawal syndrome from daily cannabis use lasts closer to 2 weeks. In comparison to ongoing insomnia after discontinuing zolpidem, and/or when the sleeping medicine no longer works, cannabis often presents the lesser problem. In fact, a common regimen I prescribe is 5 nights/week on cannabis and 2 nights/week on a sleeping medication, to prevent tolerance effects from each.

The literature is full of conflicting reports about the exact effects of cannabinoids on sleep.[3,4] Early studies of cannabis and sleep in the 1970s showed that THC reduced sleep latency (the time it takes to fall asleep) in normal and insomniac subjects, and caused some suppression of slow wave sleep (SWS). THC changes the nature of sleep. It can cause a mild decrease in rapid eye movement (REM) sleep in low doses, increase deep sleep or total sleep time at first, an effect that may diminish with tolerance, and decrease both REM and deep sleep at high doses. A corollary effect of decrease in dreams, including nightmares, has been a benefit for some patients with PTSD.

As far as specific roles for cannabinoids are concerned, we know that the endocannabinoid system regulates the circadian sleep–wake cycle. Anandamide modulates sleep and a sleep-inducing adenosine receptor reactivity may be involved.[5] On the other hand, other authors suggest that chronic use of cannabis, referring to its THC content, which downregulates endocannabinoid activity, may disrupt sleep in the long term.[6] THC stabilized respiratory patterns during all sleep stages and reduced sleep apnea in a dose-dependent fashion in rats.[7] THC, 0.1, 1.0 or 10.0 mg/kg was tested. They found that the only change in sleep architecture was a decrease in REM sleep expression at the highest dose. Of course, 10 mg/kg is higher than would be used clinically. In a review of THC dosing, they concluded:

> Oral THC has not shown consistent effects on nighttime sleep latency or duration with single 1.5–30 mg dose, 20–40 mg daily for up to 14 days, or 210 mg daily for 16 days.

DOI: 10.1201/9781003098201-44

Interpretation is limited by small sample sizes (2–10 subjects per study) and heterogeneity in degree of cannabis use at the time of study.[8]

It's no surprise that inconsistent results were found with such a wide range of dosing in the earlier studies. We now know that cannabinoids exhibit biphasic effects, and optimum dose matters, not only empirically, but in relation to the patient's tolerance.

A review of hundreds of articles on cannabis' effect on sleep concluded that the quality of studies was poor:

> There was little consistency in the results of the six studies with objective sleep measures. A total of five studies employed subjective measures of sleep, the most consistently reported impact of administering cannabis on sleep was a decrease to sleep latency.[3]

The highest rating, 84.4%, was found in a study of low doses of THC and CBD, relevant to clinical use, summarized next. A study of the effect of CBD mixed with THC by use of cannabis extracts was instructive. Clinically relevant doses of either 15 mg THC, 5 mg THC plus 5 mg CBD, or 15 mg THC plus 15 mg CBD were given by oromucosal spray. THC decreased latency and REM sleep, but the next day memory was impaired and subjects felt sleepy. THC 5 mg plus CBD 5 mg, decreased stage 3 sleep. THC 15 mg plus CBD 15 mg also decreased stage 3 sleep, and also increased awake activity. The authors concluded that 15 mg of CBD might be alerting.[9] Another recent review concluded: "Recent research has demonstrated that the type of cannabinoids (THC, CBD), ratio of cannabinoids, dosage, timing of administration, and route of administration all play a critical role in outcomes."[10]

The effects of CBD are equally as varied. CBD has sedative and anxiolytic properties depending on the dose. No significant effects on sleep were found with an anxiolytic dose of CBD in the sleep cycle of healthy volunteers. In an early report of subjects with insomnia, acute use of a high CBD dose (160 mg/day) was associated with an increase in total sleep time and less frequent awakenings.[11] In a review of the effects of CBD on sleep, in one study, 200 mg caused no effect, in another, 10 mg 2x/day might have caused somnolence, and higher doses produced variable results. CBD can also be a wake-inducing agent. CBD injected into specific wake-related areas in rat brains during the lights-on period increased wakefulness and decreased SWS and REM sleep.[12] Clearly, CBD also exhibits a biphasic, dose-dependent effect on sleep. In studies of Sativex, an extract with approximately 1:1 CBD/THC, they found that Sativex had little effect on sleep hours, but improved sleep quality. Studies of Sativex in patients with pain also confirmed improved sleep quality.[13] Patients with insomnia using various mixed CBD/THC strains noted a sleep symptom severity reduction of 4.5 points on a 0–10-point scale. According to their data, it looks like a 1:2 mix of CBD/THC produced good results for sleep. They noted the strains and found, as expected, indica to be better than sativa.[14] The important effects of terpene composition in cultivars, such as β-myrcene which is sedating, has not been adequately studied.

PATIENT REPORTS

To move on to patient results from my practice, insomnia was a very common complaint among those seeking medical cannabis advice. Patients were all ages, from the teens through the 90s. Even if patients didn't come in with insomnia as a primary complaint, upward of 40–50%, as parallels the prevalence of insomnia in the general population, found that cannabis helped their insomnia. Not all causes of insomnia were the same, nor was the patient's tolerance for "indicas" that are THC-rich. Here are a few illustrative case reports.

Patient 1: This is a 65-year-old male who consulted me about depression and insomnia. He was grieving over the death of his wife 2 years earlier. He was doing counseling for grief and depression. He had previously been taking Lexapro for 15 years, lithium carbonate for 1 year and lorazepam 2 mg at night for 6 months. He had been using a small amount of cannabis for 45 years. He was also on 60 mg of Armour thyroid, which turned out to be too high a dose, and caused tremors, which he said the cannabis helped. He was smoking sativa once in the daytime and not using cannabis at night. He said falling asleep was really a challenge, and then he slept for only 1 hour at a time, and that the lorazepam was not enough help. His doctor had recently added Sonata for sleep, which he used occasionally. He preferred to use natural medicines, so we began with several supplements: L-tryptophan, Kavanace, plus 10 mg of indica chocolate all at night. At the same time, he weaned the Lexapro and lorazepam. All of the aforementioned was not enough to give him good sleep, although he was able to reduce to 0.5 mg of lorazepam by 1 year later. Nothing was working! I suggested adding CBN, but this did not happen as it was hard to find in his area. Over the next 2 years, his depression improved, but sleep still proved elusive. He was now taking daytime sativa by tincture and smoking, and nighttime indica by tincture. The counseling continued, the pharmaceuticals were gone and eventually his cannabis use reduced to vaporizing sativa a few times/day. After 4 years he reported that he was again happy, sleep was improving and he used no supplements or cannabis at night.

Pearls: This is a case of situationally induced insomnia that was significant. Really, the cannabis was not enough of a sedative, nor were the supplements or even the benzodiazepine. He did not want to become dependent on a sleeping pill, so he chose to tough it out, resolve the underlying mood disorder and eventually better sleep resumed. Cannabis facilitated three different goals: it helped him to move through his grief, get off of multiple medications and supported sleep somewhat. This reminds us always to tend to underlying disorders while attempting to treat symptoms.

Patient 2: This is a 66-year-old male who had insomnia secondary to his use of Prograf, which he had been on for the past 12 years following a liver transplant. He was prescribed temazepam 0.5 mg to use for sleep, but he preferred cannabis. He smoked only 2 puffs in the evening, which did help him sleep. He also had mild asthma, using Dulera inhaled 2x/day. I advised switching off smoking to vaporizing or tincture. He found a CBD/THC 2:1 tincture that helped to relax him at night, so he could fall asleep. He also tried vaporizing indica, but ended up primarily using the tincture, which worked well.

Pearls: This is a case where a relaxant, rather than a sedative was called for, and here we find the benefits of a CBD-dominant strain for sleep. Although CBD is not sedating at low doses, in combination with some THC it provides a non-alerting relaxant. It is of note that this particular strain, Harlequin, was not considered to be an indica. With other patients using a CBD/THC mix before bed, we achieved good results with another strain, Cannatonic, which is considered to be an indica, but hard to find in tincture form.

Patient 3: This is a 41-year-old male with significant low back pain, insomnia and anxiety. He had previously been on opiates for pain, and Klonapin for anxiety but was now off. He had a 20-year history of cannabis use, and was smoking or vaporizing several times a day as well as edible use before bed. Initially, we tried to lower his cannabis intake by using topical for back pain. That was not successful. Then he tried smoking less and using an edible during the day, while smoking indica before bed. We spoke about his tolerance being too high and he needed to lower his dose, or switch to a CBD/THC edible for daytime use. This he did. But he started to resume edible use before bed, and he got up to 60 mg/cannabinoids/day, at which point his tolerance was again high, and effectiveness went down. He again switched to smoking indica before bed, but he was awaking at 2–3 a.m. We again reviewed a tolerance break protocol, this time getting off edibles all together and smoking only once before bed. He was to use alternative sleep aids as needed during this time. That worked, and allowed him to eventually sleep well by smoking once before bed, and sometimes again if he awoke.

Pearls: This is a not uncommon result of using cannabis edibles daily, especially twice daily, that tolerance becomes an issue, and a tolerance break was crucial. I've used multiple strategies with patients, such as using cannabis 5 nights/week and alternative sleep aids 2 nights/week, or introducing CBD as earlier to replace some of the THC, and returning to lesser levels of cannabis by smoking an appropriate strain, that is, an indica, to aid sleep at a lower THC level.

Patient 4: This is a 60-year-old male with insomnia, osteoarthritis and hypertension. He was not new to cannabis use, smoking it occasionally. His medications included amlodipine and losartan. He used only cannabis for sleep, which so far hasn't worked very well. His history revealed he was drinking 8 cups of coffee/day and only 2 cups of water. He was likely dehydrated, which contributed to hypertension. In addition, the excessive caffeine he was ingesting daily would preclude good sleep even with the help of cannabis. I advised him to decrease caffeine, increase water and smoke indica before bed nightly. His sleep improved, and he was down to 3 cups of coffee/day. He had not yet increased his water. I advised him to continue to decrease caffeine and increase water, including cannabis use nightly.

Pearls: What do you do when cannabis as medicine doesn't work? Well, a thorough history is just as important in cannabis medicine as in all other disciplines. This patient's problem was due to caffeine intake, it needed adjustment. It's unfortunate that neither his primary care physician nor his cardiologist provided this advice, but I'm glad I could help him rebalance with a holistic approach. Cannabis alone is often not enough.

Patient 5: This is a 68-year-old male with disturbed sleep due to an enlarged prostate. He'd been using cannabis for his adult life, approximately 40 years, but more recently to help with sleep. He reported using half of a cookie at night, the dosage was not specified. He reported previous nocturia waking him five times a night, to only once/night with the cannabis edible. His only medication was a statin. This continued for several years, after which he started taking Terasozin, which added no benefit, and was ultimately stopped. After 4 years on cannabis therapy, he was still waking only once/night.

Pearls: Benign prostatic hypertrophy (BPH) is a common complaint in elderly male patients, estimated to occur in 70% of those in this patient's age range. While I have not documented this condition in many of such patients in my cannabis practice, it is likely that those taking an edible for overnight relief, either due to insomnia or pain, or other conditions, has likely helped nocturia as well. It would be worthwhile to study how much of this benefit is due to the sleep-inducing properties of cannabis versus the anti-inflammatory properties of cannabis. In the latter case, even using CBD-rich cannabis during the day might bring improvement.

Patient 6: This is a 70-year-old male who was referred by his primary care physician for cannabis advice to help with sleep. He had been using cannabis for 40 years, currently smoking or vaporizing before bed. He reported using ½ g of cannabis/day. He was also taking zolpidem 10–20 mg every night, an untenable high dose. I advised an indica tincture, something to last through the night and to begin to wean zolpidem. He initially said the "edible" made him feel drugged. The next year his doctor switched him off zolpidem and on to 100 mg of Trazodone, and he was using a 20 mg capsule of indica. Finally, he got off Trazodone and was using a 30 mg edible. Now it was time to start weaning back the cannabis, after using it for 3 years to replace sleeping pills. He did this, and was able to revert to a few puffs before bed as he'd been doing all along.

Pearls: This is a classic example of how cannabis, if used correctly, can substitute for a pharmaceutical medication, in this case, sleeping pills. Patients with significant sleep disorders are often taking pharmaceutical sleep aids at the time that they present for a cannabis consultation. Weaning sleeping pills is a common part of cannabis therapeutic use. Often this involves modulating the cannabis dose as the medication is slowly withdrawn. In fact, a 20-mg dose of zolpidem is extremely high and the patient's own physician practiced a form of harm reduction in switching him to 100 mg of Trazodone.

CANNABIS THERAPY SUMMARY

Patients who use cannabis for insomnia often can reduce or eliminate their previous sleeping medicines, with fewer side effects. Many pharmaceuticals that are used to help insomnia may also cause insomnia as they are withdrawn, or skipped. Cannabis does not create the same sort of dependence; you can use it as needed. In my practice of clinical cannabis, the issue was not if cannabis was the perfect sleep aid, because it's not, but it was less harmful than long-term dependence on zolpidem, benzodiazepines or other sleep aids. A patient's tolerance to cannabis, the dose of THC, the dose of CBD and the presence of sedating terpenes such as β-myrcene all contribute to the efficacy of cannabis as a sleep-inducing agent. It's important to use cannabis in a long-acting form, such as capsules, edibles or tincture if you find you're waking up in the middle of the night. Indica strains are best used as sedatives. Preparations containing the cannabinoid CBN, even in small amounts, such as 5 mg, are also effective. Since it was found that 10 mg of CBD can be alerting, in most cases I advise keeping the CBD dose below this level, best used in combination with an indica THC. This propensity reverses at high doses of CBD, perhaps 50 mg or greater, which is likely to be sedating. The exception to this caveat for CBD is when insomnia is exacerbated by anxiety, or caused by menopausal hot flashes or nocturia, in which case a low dose of CBD can reduce the cause of insomnia and prove an effective sleep aid on its own, especially if used at 10 mg doses or less, potentially with daytime use as well. As far as THC is concerned, 5–10 mg delivered in an edible can be enough, especially in the case of a patient with no tolerance. In chronic uses, unfortunately tolerance can develop and higher amounts of THC may be required. In these cases, a tolerance break is the best strategy, even if it means using a pharmaceutical for several nights/week during the tolerance break, or even regularly to avoid tolerance in severe cases. I've seen several patients with severe insomnia titrate up to 60 mg of a cannabis edible before bed to relieve insomnia. In these cases, aside from a tolerance break, switching to CBN provides a good strategy. CBN is sedating even at low doses and should be considered in all cases of insomnia, although it is not always readily available. Lastly, as we have seen, a good history to address ongoing causes of insomnia, such as excess caffeine, is required for success.

REFERENCES

1. Nunberg H, Kilmer B, Pacula RL, Burgdorf J. An analysis of applicants presenting to a medical marijuana specialty practice in California. *J Drug Policy Anal.* 2011;4(1):1–16.
2. Angarita GA, Emadi N, Hodges S, Morgan PT. Sleep abnormalities associated with alcohol, cannabis, cocaine, and opiate use: a comprehensive review. *Addict Sci Clin Pract.* 2016;11:9.
3. Gates PJ, Albertella L, Copeland J. The effects of cannabinoid administration on sleep: a systematic review of human studies. *Sleep Med Rev.* 2014;18(6):477–487.
4. Ferguson G, Ware MA. Review article: sleep, pain and cannabis. *J Sleep Disord Ther.* 2015;4:2.
5. Murillo Rodriquez E. The role of the CB1 receptor in the regulation of sleep. *Prog Neuropsychopharmacol Biol Psychiatry.* 2008;32(6):1420–1427.
6. Maple KE, McDaniel KA, Shollenbarger SG, Lisdahl KM. Dose-dependent cannabis use, depressive symptoms, and FAAH genotype predict sleep quality in emerging adults: a pilot study. *Am J Drug Alcohol Abuse.* 2016;42(4):431–440.
7. Carley DW, Paviovic S, Janelidze M, Radulovacki M. Functional role for cannabinoids in respiratory stability during sleep. *Sleep.* 2002;25(4):391–398.
8. Gorelik DA, Goodwin RS, Schwilke E, et al. Around-the-clock oral THC effects on sleep in male chronic daily cannabis. *Am J Addict.* 2013;22(5):510–514.
9. Nicholson AN, Turner C, Stone BM, Robson PJ. Effect of delta-9-tetrahydrocannabinol and cannabidiol on nocturnal sleep and early-morning behavior in young adults. *J Clin Psychopharmacol.* 2004;24(3):305–313.
10. Babson KA, Sottile J, Morabito D. Cannabis, cannabinoids, and sleep: a review of the literature. *Curr Psychiatry Rep.* 2017;19:23.

11. Linares IMP, Guimaraes FS, Eckeli A, et al. No acute effects of cannabidiol on the sleep-wake cycle of healthy subjects: a randomized, double-blind, placebo-controlled, crossover study. *Front Pharmacol.* 2018;9:315.

12. Murillo-Rodríguez E, Millán-Aldaco D, Palomero-Rivero M, Mechoulam R, Drucker-Colín R. The nonpsychoactive Cannabis constituent cannabidiol is a wake-inducing agent. *Behav Neurosci.* 2008;122(6):1378–1382.

13. Russo E, Guy GW, Robson PJ. Cannabis, pain, and sleep: lessons from therapeutic clinical trials of Sativex, a cannabis-based medicine. *Chem Biodivers.* 2007;4(8):1729–1743.

14. Vigil JM, Stith SS, Diviant JP, et al. 2018. Effectiveness of raw, natural medical cannabis flower for treating insomnia under naturalistic conditions. *Medicines (Basel).* 2018;5(3):75.

34 Intestinal Disorders

INTESTINAL DISORDERS AND CANNABIS

Cannabis has several physiological effects that make it a good choice of medicine for inflammatory bowel disease (IBD). It is an anti-inflammatory, immune modulator, muscle relaxant, including the smooth muscle of the intestine, it slows GI motility and, importantly, can alleviate stress. Inflammatory bowel disorder is one of the few areas in which human studies with cannabis have been done. Surveys of cannabis use in IBD patients in Spain, the United States and Canada have found that approximately 10–16% of patients currently use cannabis, and up to 50% have tried cannabis to relieve IBD symptoms.[1] Other intestinal disorders that benefit from cannabis, but have not been as fully investigated, include abdominal, intestinal and anal pain.

The gastrointestinal (GI) tract houses 80% of the immune system, and is rich in cannabinoid receptors. The endocannabinoid system (ECS) plays many roles in the GI tract.[2] These include regulation of motility, visceral sensation, inflammation, pain and satiety.[3] The ECS is also involved centrally in the modulation of stress, with endocannabinoid signaling modulating the activity of hypothalamic-pituitary-adrenal pathways. There is increasing evidence that the ECS also modulates chronic stress-associated increases in abdominal pain.[4] Endocannabinoid levels, specifically anandamide (AEA), have been found to be both reduced and increased in IBD patients.[5] Examination of colonic mucosa in UC patients showed both upregulation of CB1 and reduction of AEA as a result of decreased synthesis and increased degradation.[6] CB1 receptors in the gut have been found on epithelial cells, smooth muscle cells, inflammatory/immune cells and in neurons. CB2 receptors are found on enteric neurons, and also expressed by immune and epithelial cells in the GI tract. In vivo studies have shown that cannabinoids reduce GI transit in rodents through activation of CB1, but not CB2, receptors.[7] CB2 receptors in the GI tract were shown to regulate abnormal motility, modulate intestinal inflammation and to limit visceral sensitivity and pain.[8] It has been proposed that a CB2-specific agonist would accomplish many essential functions while limiting psychoactivity. So far, no such agent has been identified, but CBD has emerged as a non-psychoactive alternative.

In a rat model of colitis, both THC and CBD showed a dose–response bell-shaped curve for parameters indicating improvement in colonic injury. Both cannabinoids were effective for motility and injury repair, although by different mechanisms. Only THC improved the function of cholinergic neurons. A CBD/THC 1:1 combination gave similar results as THC alone.[9] CBD normalized motility in mice treated with CBD 1–10 mg/kg, and was thought to involve cannabinoid CB1 receptors and fatty acid amide hydrolase (FAAH) modulation.[10] In a similar study, CBD, 5 mg/kg, was shown to act through independent mechanisms. CBD did not increase colon endocannabinoid levels and, in fact, significantly decreased them. Nor did it change FAAH mRNA expression. Rather, CBD reduced reactive oxygen species production

DOI: 10.1201/9781003098201-45

and lipid peroxidation. Studies on intestinal epithelial cells suggest that CBD prevents oxidative stress, which may be one of the underlying factors leading to mucosal protection.[11] CBD is also known to act as a GPR55 antagonist, inhibiting GI inflammation by activation of enteric glial cells.[5] In an investigation of the effect of a standardized cannabis sativa extract with a high content of CBD on mucosal inflammation and hypermotility in mouse intestinal inflammation, they showed that CBD by oral gavage decreased the extent of the damage. It also reduced intestinal hypermotility. Under the same experimental conditions, pure CBD did not ameliorate colitis, but it did reduce hypermotility.[12] A cannabis ethanolic extract dose-dependently reduced the severity of experimental colitis.[13] What's interesting here is that the authors did not describe heating their ethanolic cannabis extract. Possibly they were actually testing a THCA-rich extract, and not THC. In fact, cannabinoid acids do have anti-inflammatory effects and also decrease motility of the GI tract.[14]

In human studies, dronabinol 7.5 mg was associated with relaxation of the colon and eased post-eating cramping in human volunteers.[15] In a survey of 100 patients with ulcerative colitis (UC) and 191 patients with Crohn's disease, they found that 50% had tried cannabis for relief of pain, appetite and dissatisfaction with conventional treatment.[16] In a retrospective study of cannabis use in Crohn's disease patients using an average of 2.4 joints/day, they found that 21/30 subjects improved significantly after treatment, and had less need for prescription drugs and less surgical intervention.[17] This same group conducted a double-blind, placebo-controlled study on patients with active Crohn's disease. They showed that 8-week treatment with THC-rich cannabis was associated with a significant decrease of 100 points in Crohn's Disease Activity Index scores. Of note, cannabis was not able to reduce the steroid dose for those patients taking them.[18] One opinion on the use of cannabis for IBD states, "This should be followed by larger trials confirming these results and by trials establishing the involved mechanisms to open a promising direction for future treatment of IBD."[19]

A review of cannabis use with ulcerative colitis found two studies, one using CBD and one with smoked THC. They concluded that, "No firm conclusions regarding the efficacy and safety of cannabis or cannabidiol in adults with active UC can be drawn. There is no evidence for cannabis or cannabinoid use for maintenance of remission in UC."[20] A recent review of cannabis use and IBD summarized statistics and analyzed published studies. The authors relayed the concern "that cannabis may simply be masking symptoms without affecting intestinal inflammation, and its use in human trials has failed to provide objective evidence of therapeutic efficacy on endoscopy, biopsy, and inflammatory marker levels."[1] Despite multiple reviewers finding insubstantial evidence on a large enough scale for the benefits of cannabis use in IBD, patients using medical cannabis for the relief of ulcerative colitis and Crohn's disease report that it relieves painful cramps and increases their appetite.

PATIENT REPORTS

To move on to patient results from my practice, they were of all ages, from teens, to adults, to the elderly. The primary complaints encompassed irritable bowel syndrome (IBS) to more complex immune-mediated disease such as ulcerative colitis or Crohn's disease. Patients used cannabis for relief from a range of abdominal or intestinal pain. Here are a few illustrative case reports.

Patient 1: This is a 40-year-old male patient with a history of ulcerative colitis. He had been using cannabis for 26 years, as a medical patient for several years, smoking one joint/day. He was also taking sulfasalazine, slippery elm and fish oil daily. He reported that he can feel immediate relief with cannabis. He had annual flare-ups during which time he used more cannabis. For the next 2 years, I advised using cannabis in suppository form, which he was unable to find. Then I instructed him in how to make his own suppositories. He declined to do that. We then discussed using a CBD/THC 1:1 tincture to be used twice daily, which he did try. He continued to smoke daily and added the tincture. Flare-ups continued annually.

Pearls: I have no way of knowing how much cannabis was helping his condition, or not, because he'd been on the same regimen for as long as he had the disease. At our last visit, with the tincture added, he did say he was more functional, able to surf again after 1 year of incapacitating symptoms. I would have liked to see the effect of suppositories, but these are hard to find.

Patient 2: This is a 36-year-old female with abdominal cramping, diarrhea and gas for 1 year, with a provisional diagnosis of colitis. She was treating her symptoms with homeopathic remedies. She had tried vaporizing cannabis rarely. I advised a CBD-rich tincture as she preferred to avoid the feeling of being "high." I also referred her to a gastroenterologist for evaluation of possible ulcerative colitis. She declined to do this. Her condition continued over the next year while she used three methods of cannabis delivery: vaporizing as needed, a CBD/THC 1:1 mouth spray and a 20:1 tincture not regularly. I again advised her to use the tincture one to times daily. Finally, by the third year, she was taking 10 mg of a CBD/THC 4:1 tincture 2×/day and had added raw juiced cannabis as often as she could obtain it. She was feeling much improved. Her colitis symptoms were almost gone over the next 3 years that she consulted me. She was still doing homeopathy and changed to a less stressful job.

Pearls: This patient was doing a host of treatments for colitis, so it's difficult to know the role cannabis played. I have heard from other patients that raw cannabis, providing cannabinoid acids, can be useful for chronic inflammatory conditions, and has been documented as useful for colitis in animal studies. In fact, her colitis resolved.

Patient 3: This is a 75-year-old female with multiple medical conditions, including liver cancer, s/p resection 2 years earlier, a long history of IBS with small bowel obstruction secondary to abdominal adhesions, joint pains and fibromyalgia. She was on several medications, including a diclofenac patch, sertraline, blood pressure medications and Synthroid. She was new to cannabis use. I advised a CBD-rich tincture 2×/day and topical for joint pain. She understood that she was using cannabis for her joint pain and did not directly relate to it also treating the IBS. She was compliant and used 10 mg of a 20:1 tincture two to three times daily for almost 2 years, as well as the topical. She then stopped using the tincture, reporting that her IBS continued to flare about once/week, so it wasn't helping. Unfortunately, about the time she stopped the tincture, she then had a second episode of abdominal adhesions, which may or may not have had any relation to this discontinuance.

Pearls: Especially with elderly cannabis naive patients, a full explanation of the potential effects of cannabis as well as an entreaty to follow-up if they feel it's not working is crucial. I'm glad she followed my advice for 2 years, yet I did not specifically say, "Your risk for recurrent adhesions is greater off the cannabis," but I believe this may have been the case. Pain is the primary sign by which patients rate the success of therapy. The anti-inflammatory action of cannabis will not only affect intestinal pain, but acts upon the abdominal cavity as well, possibly reducing adhesions.

Patient 4: This is a 38-year-old male first seen for psoriasis and "digestive problems." He had been using cannabis for 25 years, mostly by smoking it several times a day. He had ongoing peri-umbilical pain, frequent vomiting and weight loss. He had already been advised to treat his psoriatic plaques with topical cannabis, which was helping. He was on no medications. Over the next few years, his digestive complaints improved with changes in diet and increased exercise. Even the psoriasis seemed to be gone. Then his symptoms escalated, to small intestine perforation, resection and partial colectomy and diagnosis of Crohn's disease. All this with daily smoked cannabis, about 2–4x/day. He was started on Stelara and loperamide. I advised adding daily multiple dosing of a CBD/THC tincture. The patient declined to continue this due to cost, and his unfamiliarity with CBD. We compromised on a THC-rich capsule overnight, which increased his dose above daily smoking.

Pearls: Studies would indicate that cannabis should have been somewhat protective against a severe Crohn's outbreak. First of all, clearly it is not absolutely protective, and second, perhaps chronic cannabis use actually delayed the onset of the Crohn's diagnosis, and was, therefore, protective. He was 40 years old at diagnosis, while most are diagnosed by age 30. As often with younger patients used to a "lifetime" of smoking cannabis, it's really hard to change habits. While it was easy to add topical to this patient's regimen, adding CBD didn't carry the same incentive.

Patient 5: This is a 29-year-old male who presented with rectal and anal pain, hemorrhoids, abdominal pain, intermittent diarrhea and multiple mood issues, including anger, ADHD and alcohol abuse. He was already using cannabis medicinally, with a 15-year history of cannabis use. He was smoking 2–3x/day. He had recently been hospitalized for abdominal pain. He reported alcohol abuse in the past, but stopped 1 year ago. He said that smoking cannabis helped him stay off alcohol. His diet was poor, with excessive caffeine. I advised him to try to switch to some vaporizing, reduce his caffeine and eat healthier. At our next visit, he reported decreased abdominal pain with dietary changes, but was now experiencing rectal/anal tension associated with constipation. His colonoscopy was normal except for hemorrhoids. I advised cannabis suppositories, but they were hard to find, and he did not use them. He did add some cannabis edibles to his regimen. By our third visit, he revealed that he was a veteran, and was awaiting counseling from the VA. In fact, he said that cannabis really helped him manage his mood, and he preferred sativa strains.

Pearls: This patient was not officially diagnosed with IBS, nor with PTSD, but it's likely that his intestinal symptoms were associated with stress as well as poor self-care habits. While cannabis suppositories would have been very useful for anal pain and hemorrhoids, he really needed a more holistic approach, including dietary advice, counseling, a supportive environment in addition to cannabis. Sometimes patients fall through the cracks. Even though I was not his primary provider, several suggestions that I made were useful for him. Even as a cannabis specialist, other suggestions during a patient interaction bring us closer to the goal of improved health.

CANNABIS THERAPY SUMMARY

Intestinal conditions may be treated by a range of cannabis products. Both THC and CBD are anti-inflammatory and antispasmodic, so the choice here would depend upon the patient's preference for psychoactivity, or not, keeping in mind that THC also provides appetite stimulation and may provide added benefit for Crohn's disease patients who are often undernourished. A higher percentage CBD would be appropriate in IBS patients who may also be experiencing anxiety. There is also the option of inclusion of cannabinoid acids, for their anti-inflammatory effect by ingestion of unheated tinctures and/or raw juiced cannabis. Lastly, for inflammatory bowel disorders, if choosing a cultivar, selection of ones high in β-caryophyllene provides added anti-inflammatory effects and may increase the potency of the cannabis used. Ingestion of cannabis is a good way to take it in for intestinal disorders, as the medicine is delivered directly to the digestive tract. For example, encapsulated cannabis is released directly into the small intestine after the capsule is digested, providing long-lasting action up to 8 hours. Typical dosing might start at 10 mg of cannabinoids 3×/day. With inhalation, we see that some patients choose a 3–4×/day regimen, possibly for mood and/or appetite stimulation. For ulcerative colitis, rectal suppositories would provide focused delivery to the affected area, again increasing the effectiveness of the dose, possibly allowing for lower dosing. Several of my patients used such delivery to treat conditions such as rectal fissures or anal pain. Suppository dose could be 10–25 mg of THC, CBD or a combination, depending upon what is available. Remember that this delivery method is not expected to be as psychoactive as oral dosing, so 25 mg of THC used overnight would not be disorienting yet may help with sleep. As with all chronic conditions, continuance of cannabis therapy should be used preventatively, and not just reserved for flare-ups.

REFERENCES

1. Ahmed W, Katz S. Therapeutic use of cannabis in inflammatory bowel disease. *Gastroenterol Hepatol (NY)*. 2016;12(11):668–679.
2. Massa F, Storr M, Lutz B. The endocannabinoid system in the physiology and pathophysiology of the gastrointestinal tract. *J Mol Med (Berl)*. 2005;83(12):944–954.
3. Izzo AA, Coutts AA. Cannabinoids and the digestive tract. *Handb Exp Pharmacol*. 2005;168:573–598.
4. Sharkey KA, Wiley JW. The role of the endocannabinoid system in the brain-gut axis. *Gastroenterology*. 2016;151(2):252–266.
5. Di Sabatino A, Battista N, Biancheri P, et al. The endogenous cannabinoid system in the gut of patients with inflammatory bowel disease. *Mucosal Immunol*. 2011;4(5):574–583.
6. Hasenoehrl C, Storr M, Schicho R. Cannabinoids for treating inflammatory bowel diseases: where are we and where do we go? *Expert Rev Gastroenterol Hepatol*. 2017;11(4):329–337.
7. Aviello G, Romano B, Izzo AA. Cannabinoids and gastrointestinal motility: animal and human studies. *Eur Rev Med Pharmacol Sci*. 2008;12(Suppl 1):81–93.

8. Wright KL, Duncan M, Sharkey KA. Cannabinoid CB2 receptors in the gastrointestinal tract: a regulatory system in states of inflammation. *Br J Pharmacol.* 2008;153:263–270.

9. Jamontt JM, Molleman A, Pertwee RG, Parsons ME. The effects of Δ9-tetrahydrocannabinol and cannabidiol alone and in combination on damage, inflammation and in vitro motility disturbances in rat colitis. *Br J Pharmacol.* 2010;160(3):712–723.

10. Capasso R, Borrelli F, Aviello G, et al. Cannabidiol, extracted from Cannabis sativa, selectively inhibits inflammatory hypermotility in mice. *Br J Pharmacol.* 2008;154:1001–1008.

11. Borelli F, Aviello G, Romano B, et al. Cannabidiol, a safe and non-psychotropic ingredient of the cannabis plant Cannabis sativa, is protective in a murine model of colitis. *J Mol Med (Berl).* 2009;87:1111–1121.

12. Pagano E, Capasso R, Piscitelli F, et al. An orally active cannabis extract with high content in cannabidiol attenuates chemically-induced intestinal inflammation and hypermotility in the mouse. *Front Pharmacol.* 2016;7:341.

13. Wallace JL, Flannigan KL, McKnight W, et al. Pro-resolution, protective and antinociceptive effects of cannabis extract in the rat gastrointestinal tract. *J Physiol Pharmacol.* 2013;64(2):167–175.

14. Cluny NL, Naylor RJ, Whittle BA, Javid FA. The effects of cannabidiolic acid and cannabidiol on contractility of the gastrointestinal tract of Suncus murinus. *Arch Pharm Res.* 2011;34(9):1509–1517.

15. Esfandyari T, Camilleri M, Busciglio I, et al. Effects of a cannabinoid receptor agonist on colonic motor and sensory functions in humans: a randomized, placebo-controlled study. *Am J Physiol Gastrointest Liver Physiol.* 2007;293:137–145.

16. Lal S, Prasad N, Ryana M, et al. Cannabis use amongst patients with inflammatory bowel disease. *Eur J Gastroenterol Hematol.* 2011;23(10):891–896.

17. Naftali T, Lev LB, Yablecovitch D, Half E, Konikoff FM. Treatment of Crohn's disease with cannabis: an observational study. *Isr Med Assoc J.* 2011;13(8):455–458.

18. Naftali T, Bar-Lev Schleider L, Dotan I, et al. Cannabis induces a clinical response in patients with Crohn's disease: a prospective placebo-controlled study. *Clin Gastroenterol Hepatol.* 2013;11(10):1276–1280.

19. Schicho R, Storr M. Cannabis finds Its way into treatment of Crohn's disease. *Pharmacology.* 2014;93:1–3.

20. Kafil TS, Nguyen TM, MacDonald JK, Chande N. 2018. Cannabis for the treatment of ulcerative colitis. *Cochrane Database Syst Rev.* 2018 Nov 8;11:CD012954.

35 Movement Disorders

MOVEMENT DISORDERS AND CANNABIS

There are many conditions that fall under the movement disorder category for which patients use cannabis medicinally. Some of these are reviewed under their own heading and are presented elsewhere (see Chapters 36 and 42). Here we review others, including Tourette's syndrome, dystonia, tremor and restless leg syndrome (RLS). The endocannabinoid system (ECS) modulates neurotransmission involved in motor function, particularly within the basal ganglia. We would expect a great impact by CB1 agonists such as THC. A review of the impact of the ECS and clinically relevant studies with cannabinoids suggests that cannabis can be very beneficial in movement disorders.[1,2]

Therapeutic approaches to treat tics and Tourette's syndrome have largely focused on behavioral therapy and psychotropic drugs with undesirable side effects, creating interest in cannabis as a replacement therapy. There have been several anecdotal reports of success with cannabinoids and cannabis. Two small controlled trials have investigated the effect of THC in Tourette's patients. One was a double-blind, single-dose crossover trial, and the other was a double-blind, parallel group study.[3,4] Both trials reported a positive effect from THC, but the improvements in tic frequency and severity were small. There was also a small improvement in concentration and visual perception.[5-7] A survey of the efficacy of cannabis versus THC in adults with Tourette's reported better results. In the cannabis group, 18 out of 19 patients experienced a decrease in total tic severity and impairment scores, as well as improvement in obsessive–compulsive symptoms, attention, impulsivity, anxiety, irritability, rage outbursts and sleep.[8] It appears that cannabis is a potentially more effective therapy than pure THC. A new double-blind, randomized, crossover pilot trial is in progress to compare the efficacy of three vaporized medical cannabis products with differing combinations of THC and CBD in adults with Tourette's syndrome.[9]

Cannabinoids have shown conflicting results for dystonias.[10] Some positive results were found in one study with CBD but not with nabilone.[11,12] One case of dystonia did show a 50% reduction of spasm in a patient with Meige syndrome at a CBD high dose of 400 mg/day.[13] Use of cannabis with varying CBD/THC ratios, as opposed to pure CBD, was more promising. In children with a complex motor disorder, CBD-enriched formulations with a CBD/THC ratio of 20:1 or 6:1 improved dystonia and other quality of life (QOL) indicators including sleep, mood, constipation and appetite. In the 20:1 group, both dystonia and QOL improved with an average THC dose of 3–7 mg/day, with a CBD dose of 90–160 mg/day. Improvements in QOL in the 6:1 group occurred with an average THC dose of 6–13 mg/day and a CBD dose of 38–81 mg/day.[14] These are relatively high doses, not likely to be used by patients without supervision. It could be that strain selection with differing terpene contents may be important in finding the most efficacious product for dystonias.

DOI: 10.1201/9781003098201-46

Tremor is a symptom of many conditions, each of which may have a somewhat different underlying physiology. There is limited research to guide the use of cannabis for tremor and even less understanding of how different types of tremor may or may not respond. In a study of cannabis effects on patients with Parkinson's disease, an improvement in multiple symptoms, including tremor 30 minutes after smoking cannabis in a clinic setting, was reported.[15] A case report of improvement in parkinsonian tremor is presented in Chapter 42. Although animal models suggest that cannabinoids may reduce multiple sclerosis (MS)-related tremor, a cannabis extract was not found to provide improvement in a human study.[16] Following studies of large numbers of multiple sclerosis patients with tremor yielded inconclusive results. Again, the exact strain selection, with terpene content, rather than simply the CBD/THC ratio, may be a determining factor. Patients with essential tremor have anecdotally reported benefits with the use of cannabis. A clinical trial of cannabis in an oral capsule is currently underway to investigate its effect on essential tremor.[17]

Restless leg syndrome is a movement disorder associated with sleep disturbance. Dopamine agonists are one of the pharmaceutical therapies indicated for this condition. We know that cannabinoids affect dopamine transmission, most likely through an indirect mechanism exerted through the modulation of GABA and glutamate neurotransmission or may directly activate TRPV1 receptors, which have been found in some dopaminergic pathways providing direct regulation of dopamine function.[18] There are currently no studies that have been directly done on cannabis and RLS. Anecdotal reports including a report of six patients using smoked cannabis for RLS all reported benefit.[19] A follow-up report of 12 patients with refractory RLS confirmed that all but one of the patients "admitted total relief of symptoms following cannabis smoking."[20] Patients who smoked (most likely a THC-rich strain) and used sublingual extracts of CBD found inhaling cannabis to be the more effective treatment option.

PATIENT REPORTS

To move on to patient results from my practice, I have represented here, an eclectic group of patients characterized by neurodegenerative disease, not given elsewhere. The Tourette's patients were generally youthful, in their teens or young adult. Dystonia occurred in a child and at older ages associated with significant neurodegenerative disease, and tremor was a condition of older adults. Of these, only Tourette's was commonly responsive to cannabis therapy, dystonia and tremor less so. Here are a few illustrative case reports.

TOURETTE'S SYNDROME

Patient 1: This is a 34-year-old male with Tourette's syndrome. He had been using cannabis medicinally to treat it for 6 years with success. He reported that the symptoms were worse in the evenings, for which he smoked cannabis or did an edible for relief. Twitching mouth movements and blinking all reduced. He said cannabis lets him "live a normal life." He was on no medications. He did admit to anger issues as well, which could come throughout the day. I suggested he use a small amount of cannabis during the day to see if it helped his mood. He began vaporizing, using it 3x/day, as needed, more so in the evenings. He had stopped smoking or edibles.

Pearls: This is common of Tourette's patients that symptoms are worse in the evenings. The fact that THC-rich cannabis is successful for Tourette's is as expected. Vaporization as a useful delivery method is evidenced here.

Patient 2: This is a 16-year-old male with Tourette's syndrome and OCD (obsessive compulsive disorder). He had been experiencing tics since age 5. He was on no medications, but treated his symptoms with meditation, martial arts and a high-protein diet. His primary discomfort was in posterior neck tension and tics. He reported that prior exposure to cannabis did help alleviate his tics. I recommended a CBD/THC tincture as needed to relax his neck and help the tics. He found that a 20:1 CBD/THC capsule stopped progression of the tics. He supplemented this therapy with vaping the same mix. The OCD was not significantly affected.

Pearls: It has commonly been thought that THC or THC-rich cannabis is successful for reducing tics. We don't have sufficient information to know about the effects of CBD for Tourette's syndrome. It could be that by relieving muscle tension, CBD is effective in this case, but that may not hold true for all cases, although the study in progress should help to answer that question.[9]

DYSTONIA

Patient 1: This is a 4-year-old male with a diagnosis of alternating hemiplegia of childhood. He had episodic bouts of dystonia, paralysis and seizures, but with a normal EEG. The paralytic episodes lasted 2–3 weeks/month, with 1 week in between. Mom reported that medications were not effective. He was new to cannabis use. We titrated up to 20 mg of a CBD-rich 20:1 tincture 2x/day. His weight was 40 lb, so this dose was 0.45 mg/kg/day. On this regimen, the episodes decreased to 3 days, occurring 4x/month. We then experimented with a CBD/THC 1:1, or 4:1 mouth spray for added relief during the episodes. Over the next year, we found the sprays brought no change. We ended up with a regimen of 25 mg of 20:1 tincture 2x/day and 20 mg of a 4:1 tincture in the evenings for sleep. He showed improved mood, no seizures and daily short episodes of hemiplegic paralysis lasting up to 1 hour. He was able to attend school and showed improved cognition. At our last follow-up, the patient had been switched to Epidiolex at a dose of 200 mg 2x/day and was now 100 lb. This translates to a dose of 1.8 mg/kg/day. Severe paralytic episodes were only occurring at 1–2x/month. He still used a 1:1 tincture as needed for dystonia relief.

Pearls: This is an extreme case of dystonia, associated with paralysis, which did show improvement on cannabis. This is especially promising, as medications were not effective. The inclusion of a small percentage of THC in the evening dose is typical of use for help with sleep. As has happened with several patients who have switched to Epidiolex, the dosage was increased about fourfold.

Patient 2: This is a 68-year-old male diagnosed with cortico-basal syndrome, which was rapidly progressing. He experienced dystonia and tremor of his arm and rigidity. He was on Sinemet 25/100, 3 tabs, 3x/day, clonazepam 1 mg 4x/day for muscle spasm and an antidepressant. He was new to cannabis use, but hoped it would help. He reported that alcohol helped the tremor. I advised a strong dose of a CBD/

THC tincture, up to 20 mg three times/day. He got up to 20 mg/day and saw no effects. He then switched to a THC-rich edible before bed, about a 15 mg dose, also with no effect. I suggested adding vaporized cannabis during the day every 3 hours with a CBD/THC mix, and continuing the edible at night. He declined to vaporize and continued to try low-dose CBD/THC edibles, 5 mg dose, but not regularly, also with no effect. He then gave up on using cannabis therapeutically.

Pearls: As is the case with progressive neurological disease, there is a limit to how much help cannabis can be with progression of the disease. It is unfortunate that 20 mg/day of cannabinoids in a cannabis extract was no help for this patient's dystonia. It would have been preferable for him to have attempted the multiple (3x/day) regimen I prescribed, as he was doing with clonazepam, but the patient was not hopeful. As we learn more, and can say what is required, with evidence-based data, perhaps our recommendations might hold more weight.

TREMOR

Patient 1: This is a 65-year-old male with essential tremor in his hands. He was also a post-polio patient, saying "he always had a shake." He had been using cannabis for 40 years, mostly by smoking 2x/day. He was prescribed propranolol as needed for tremor. He said cannabis worked better. In fact, over the next year, as he continued to smoke 3x/day, he stated he felt more relaxed, but there was no help with his tremor. He ended up continuing to smoke 2–3x/day, finally deciding that beer helped his tremor, and cannabis helped his mood.

Pearls: Cannabis did not help this patient in reducing essential tremor. We had no information on cultivar content as far as terpenes is concerned, and did not have the opportunity to experiment. The results with tremor have been inconclusive. We might postulate that dosage, chemotype and type of tremor all contribute to efficacy. More research is needed.

CANNABIS THERAPY SUMMARY

One might expect that THC-rich cannabis by its action as a CB1 agonist would be effective for movement disorders. Less is known about what to expect with CBD, although the study of children with complex motor disorder indicated efficacy. Of course, we don't know if the combination was more helpful than THC-rich cannabis alone as that was not tested. Anecdotally, several of my patients with Tourette's syndrome have reported relief from tics with THC-rich cannabis, mostly by smoking. What is also interesting is the patient who responded to CBD-rich therapy, but he also had an element of muscle tension that is relieved by THC. I think in such cases, the addition of CBD to a THC dose would not harm the outcome and may improve QOL, especially if anger or anxiety is co-diagnosed. As far as dystonia is concerned, it is unclear whether THC-rich cannabis will be useful. One patient I treated with cerebral palsy found no reduction in dystonias by vaporization plus a 50 mg edible dose daily. However, another patient with cervical dystonia reported relief from smoking 3x/day. CBD may provide a better alternative. It is likely that significant doses are required, based upon the sparse research in the literature and results from the cases given here, where low dose was not effective, but 0.5 mg/kg was. It is interesting to note that in the pediatric case in which 0.5 mg/kg/day was effective, the corresponding Epidiolex dose was increased fourfold, as is typically found when comparing cannabis to Epidiolex in seizure disorder cases. As far as tremor is concerned, most of my patients with essential tremor reported no help with cannabis. In contrast, there has been relief reported by patients with parkinsonian tremor using THC-rich cannabis. Many patients with RLS do report that cannabis can alleviate but not completely eliminate their symptoms, but this is from smoking that would wear off in a few hours anyway. More research needs to be done on the effects of cannabis delivered by longer-lasting oral methods in RLS patients.

REFERENCES

1. Kluger B, Triolo P, Jones W, Jankovic J. The therapeutic potential of cannabinoids for movement disorders. *Mov Disord.* 2015;30(3):313–327.
2. Peres FF, Lima AC, Hallak JEC, et al. Cannabidiol as a promising strategy to treat and prevent movement disorders? *Front Pharmacol.* 2018;9:482.
3. Müller-Vahl KR, Schneider U, Koblenz A, et al. Treatment of Tourette's syndrome with delta 9-tetrahydrocannabinol (THC): a randomized crossover trial. *Pharmacopsychiatry.* 2002;35(2):57–61.
4. Müller-Vahl KR, Schneider U, Prevedel H. Delta 9-tetrahydrocannabinol (THC) is effective in the treatment of tics in Tourette syndrome: a 6-week randomized trial. *J Clin Psychiatry.* 2003;64(4):459–465.
5. Müller-Vahl KR. Cannabinoids reduce symptoms of Tourette's syndrome. *Expert Opin Pharmacother.* 2003;4(10):1717–1725.
6. Müller-Vahl KR. Treatment of Tourette syndrome with cannabinoids. *Behav Neurol.* 2013;27(1):119–124.
7. Curtis A, Clarke CE, Rickards HE. Cannabinoids for Tourette's syndrome (Review). *Cochrane Database Syst Rev.* 2009 Oct 7;2009(4):CD006565.
8. Abi-Jaoude E, Chen L, Cheung P, Bhikram T, Sandor P. Preliminary evidence on cannabis effectiveness and tolerability for adults with Tourette syndrome. *J Neuropsychiatry Clin Neurosci.* 2017;29(4):391–400.
9. University Health Network, Toronto. Safety and efficacy of cannabis in Tourette syndrome. 2019. https://clinicaltrials.gov/ct2/show/NCT03247244 Accessed March 10, 2020.
10. Koppel BS. Cannabis in the treatment of dystonia, dyskinesias, and tics. *Neurotherapeutics.* 2015;12(4):788–792.
11. Consroe P, Sandyk R, Snider RS. Open label evaluation of cannabidiol in dystonic movement disorders. *Int J Neurosci.* 1986;30:277–282.
12. Fox SH, Kellett M, Moore AP, Crossman AR, Brotchie JM. Randomised, double-blind, placebo-controlled trial to assess the potential of cannabinoid receptor stimulation in the treatment of dystonia. *Mov Disord.* 2002;7(1):145–149.
13. Snider SR, Consroe P. Treatment of Meige's syndrome with cannabidiol. *Neurology.* 1984;34(Suppl):147.
14. Libzon S, Bar-Lev Schleider L, Saban N, et al. Medical cannabis for pediatric moderate to severe complex motor disorders. *J Child Neurol.* 2018;33(9):565–571.
15. Lotan I, Treves TA, Roditi Y, Djaldetti R. Cannabis (medical marijuana) treatment for motor and non-motor symptoms of Parkinson disease: an open-label observational study. *Clin Neuropharm.* 2014;37(2):41–44.

16. Fox P, Bain P, Glickman S, Carroll C, Zajicek J. The effect of cannabis on tremor in patients with multiple sclerosis. *Neurology.* 2004;62(7):1105–1109.
17. University of California San Diego. Trial of cannabis for essential tremor. 2019. https:// clinicaltrials.gov/ct2/show/NCT03805750 Accessed March 10, 2020.
18. Fernandez-Ruiz J, Hernandez M, Ramos JA. Cannabinoid–dopamine interaction in the pathophysiology and treatment of CNS disorders. *CNS Neurosci Ther.* 2010;16:e72–e91.
19. Megelin T, Ghorayeb I. Cannabis for restless legs syndrome. *Sleep Med.* 2017;36:182–183.
20. Ghorayeb I. More evidence of cannabis efficacy in restless legs syndrome. *Sleep Breath.* 2020;24(1):277–279.

36 Multiple Sclerosis, Amyotrophic Lateral Sclerosis

MULTIPLE SCLEROSIS AND CANNABIS

A good percentage of patients with multiple sclerosis (MS) try cannabis at one point in their disease, depending on its availability, with varying degrees of success. Recent studies have indicated that there is a wide acceptance of cannabis within the MS community, with 20–60% of patients currently using cannabis, and 50–90% would consider usage if it were legal and more research was in support of it.[1] Although current disease-modifying agents are useful in reducing relapses in some relapsing-remitting MS patients, their effectiveness in slowing disability progression is unclear. Cannabis may show promise in that regard, as well as relieving pain, spasticity, tremor, nocturia and improving general well-being in MS. Cannabis is a likely candidate to treat MS due to endocannabinoid involvement in protection against neurodegenerative changes arising from neuroinflammation. There is ample evidence that MS has immune as well as neurodegenerative pathogenesis.

An extensive review of the role of the endocannabinoid system in MS presents the results of relevant studies, summarized here. Studies in animal models of MS with experimental autoimmune encephalomyelitis may be interpreted as showing fluctuating levels of endocannabinoids at different phases of the disease. Treatment of these mice with cannabinoid agonists, including a high dose of THC, slows neurodegeneration and inhibits autoimmunity by a CB1 receptor mechanism. In humans, endocannabinoid levels are disparate as well. Anandamide levels have been found to be both elevated in the cerebrospinal fluid and in peripheral blood lymphocytes of MS patients and decreased in others.[2] This may indicate that not only the patient's endocannabinoid tone is relevant to the efficacy of cannabinoid therapy but also the stage of their disease, with early stages showing deficiency and later stages already upregulated.

A large study of 630 patients published in 2003 found no objective evidence of a treatment effect on muscle spasticity. However, significantly more participants taking either cannabis oil or THC reported subjective improvements in spasticity, spasms, sleep and pain, but not tremor or bladder symptoms. Walking times before and during treatment were measured. The group taking THC had improved walking time. There was no improvement on any other mobility test. Also, investigators noted there were fewer relapses in the cannabis treatment groups.[3] A following study of urinary symptoms in MS patients did show improvement with cannabis extracts. Patients' self-assessment of pain, spasticity and quality of sleep improved as well.[4] A later

DOI: 10.1201/9781003098201-47

study showed that cannabis was rated significantly more effective than placebo in relieving spasticity.[5] The implication of these results is that cannabis makes patients feel better, even if it doesn't show any objective improvement. More recently, studies using Sativex showed reduced spasticity and pain in MS patients. Treatment with standardized oral extract relieved muscle stiffness. The proportion of participants experiencing relief was almost twice as large in the treatment group as in the placebo group (29% vs. 16%), especially for muscle spasm. The authors concluded: "The study met its primary objective to demonstrate the superiority of CE (cannabis extract) over placebo in the treatment of muscle stiffness in MS."[6] Another inference from this study was that there was no evidence that THC had an effect on MS progression. Participants with less disability did show better scores, but they were not statistically significant. Improved efficacy for cannabis therapy in patients with less severe disease is a possibility that needs to be explored further. As one reviewer commented:

> More research will be needed to investigate these findings and patients will need to be selected at the lower end of the disability spectrum before meaningful conclusions on the neuroprotective ability of cannabinoids or endocannabinoids to slow the rate of disease progression in MS can be drawn.[2]

Similar results were found for nabiximols in an observational, prospective, multicenter, non-interventional study.[7] A further trial was done to test long-term and maximum-dose tolerability of Sativex, with benefit over 1 year with doses of up to 130 mg/day of THC and 120 mg/day of CBD.[8] These are high doses, patients are not likely to use without supervision. Lower doses, with inhalation as a mode of delivery, was also investigated. The efficacy of vaporized Sativex spray was evaluated in a retrospective observational study of MS patients from 2008 to 2012. This was reported to be effective for spasticity and pain in 80% of patients at a median dose of 5 (2–10) inhalations/day[9] (for further presentation of MS spasticity, see Chapter 37).

The American Academy of Neurology did a review and released a summary of the efficacy of cannabis for neurological conditions. They reached several conclusions: there is evidence for cannabis extract and synthetic THC for reducing patient-reported spasticity and pain; there is evidence for Sativex for improving patient-reported spasticity, pain and urinary frequency, but not bladder incontinence; there is insufficient evidence to assess the effectiveness of smoked cannabis for treating MS-related spasticity, pain, balance, posture and cognition.[10] In an additional report, they further elaborated upon the ineffectiveness of cannabis extract for short-term spasticity and tremor.[11] Perhaps one of the most significant contributions cannabis may provide in patients with this chronic disease is mood elevation that has not been adequately evaluated.

AMYOTROPHIC LATERAL SCLEROSIS AND CANNABIS

Amyotrophic lateral sclerosis (ALS) is neurodegenerative disease resulting in progressive muscle weakness with ensuing spasticity symptoms. There is still no good treatment or cure to modify the progression of ALS. Cannabinoids and/or cannabis may have therapeutic benefit for ALS, as for other neurodegenerative diseases.[14] It may be disease-modifying, that is, slow down the progression of the disease, but minimally it can help with symptom control, such as spasticity, excess salivary secretions, mood management and appetite.[2]

As with MS, the endocannabinoid system is thought to be involved.[12] Relevant studies are found summarized in an extensive review.[2] In a mouse model of ALS, increased levels of endocannabinoids were found. Treatment of these mice with Sativex showed only weak improvement in the progression of neurodegeneration and survival. The mechanism of action was thought to be by non-CB1 pathways, including activation of CB2 receptors. An animal study in dogs confirmed upregulation of CB2 receptors in the spinal cord in canine degenerative myelopathy.[13]

In a survey of 131 patients with ALS, those who were able to obtain cannabis found it preferable to prescription medication in managing their symptoms.[15] In a more recent study of 32 patients with ALS using Sativex, they found that moderate to severe spasticity was associated with a higher dose of self-titrated medicine. The average dose was approximately 30 mg/day.[16] Dosing is an important characteristic in interpreting any results. For example, in a study of ALS patients with "cramping," given a low dose of THC, 5 mg twice daily, no improvement in cramps, fasciculations, quality of life, quality of sleep, appetite or depression were noted.[17] As found for other neurodegenerative diseases, cannabis extracts seem to perform better than pure THC in management of this constellation of symptoms.

PATIENT REPORTS

To move on to patients results from my practice, patients with MS ranged in age from their 30s to 60s at the time of presentation. I've seen the entire range of products used in my patients' treatment of MS, with varying degrees of success. Some preferred CBD-rich, some preferred vaping a THC-rich strain, some used higher doses, especially when treating spasticity, and some discontinued use stating the effects were not significant enough. I have treated one patient with ALS. Here are a few illustrative case reports.

MULTIPLE SCLEROSIS

Patient 1: This is a 68-year-old male with a 30-year history of slow progressive MS. On presentation, he ambulated freely with no slurred speech. He has been treated with Copaxone for the past 12 years. He also suffered from trigeminal neuralgia. He had a 40-year history of using cannabis. He preferred to vaporize a THC-rich strain 4×/day. On increasing vaporizing to 6×/day, the trigeminal neuralgia resolved and he was able to discontinue Trileptal. The next year he took my advice to add CBD-rich cannabis, using a spray 3×/day, and he reported discontinuing Copaxone. The next year he switched to a CBD-rich 20:1 tincture, for a higher dose, approximately 10 mg 3×/day. His appearance, cognition, ambulation, speech and function have been stable over this period.

Pearls: THC-rich cannabis was his preferred product, being comfortable with it for 40 years. It took 2 years for him to add CBD in the dosage I recommended. At least we got there! The addition of CBD may have facilitated ease in discontinuing Copaxone. Ordinarily, a CBD/THC mix brings better results for this condition than either cannabinoid alone. Trigeminal neuralgia may have been helped by THC at sufficient dose.

Patient 2: This is a 59-year-old female with an 8-year history of MS. She had been on Avonex for 2 years, and cannabis for the past 3 years. Her preferred usage was by pipe, smoking a THC-rich strain frequently throughout the day. She ambulated with a walker, had no slurred speech or cognitive difficulties. She added a CBD/THC 2:1 tincture with a dose of 3–4 mg 3x/day. She discontinued Avonex as she believed "it wasn't doing any good." Ultimately, she switched to a CBD/THC 1:1 tincture with a dose of 10 mg only at night.

Pearls: This is an example of a patient who was able to switch from THC-rich to a CBD/THC mix, and from smoking to tincture. Her dosing ended up to be lower on this regimen than on THC alone (i.e., smoking 4–5x/day), yet it felt sufficient to her. Dosing at the lower end of the spectrum may be useful for some MS patients, perhaps due to cannabinoid biphasic effects, and/or the benefit of the two cannabinoids mixed brought better results at a lower dose.

Patient 3: This is a 50-year-old female with a 24-year history of MS. She was taking baclofen 2x/day and Rebif. She was able to ambulate on her own, had no slurred speech or cognitive difficulties. She was using a THC-rich tincture 2x/day and a tea ball with cannabis flower (providing mostly cannabinoid acids) at night. I advised adding CBD to her tincture. The next year her medications were the same, but she switched to smoking 2x/day and vaporizing 3x/day. Then she tried adding a CBD-rich tincture, but at a low dose 3–4 mg 2x/day. Her need for baclofen decreased and was now rarely using it. Unfortunately, the dose wasn't sufficient to replace baclofen, and by the next visit she was back on it. She stopped the CBD but continued to smoke or vaporize for a total of 5 doses/day.

Pearls: This patient saw no benefit in CBD, likely because she "didn't feel it." This is common with many MS patients that inhalation of a stimulating strain, THC-rich, not only improves mood, but alleviates fatigue. The continued need for baclofen for spasticity is also common in MS patients. It's challenging to be able to wean off of it, more often reducing the dose can be accomplished.

Patient 4: This is a 45-year-old female who had a 12-year history of MS. Her complaints on presentation included poor sleep, chronic pain in her leg and cervical spine, headache, nausea and fatigue. She was seeing a pain specialist for cervical pain after a cervical fusion, which led to further injury. Neck pain and headaches have been worse since. She has been taking methadone for 5 years, currently 60 mg 3x/day. She was also on Avonex, blood pressure medications, Effexor, Topamax for headache, an inhaler and Provigil, among other prn medications. She was not new to cannabis, but had no idea how to use it to her best advantage. I recommended vaporizing sativa frequently for energy, mood and pain relief. After a bout of pneumonia, she switched to a tincture that was CBD-rich on the advice of her delivery service. Unfortunately, this did not help her pain, or her sleep and her methadone dose remained the same. She then switched to a vape pen with a CBD/THC 1:1 mix during the day and a CBD-infused honey and indica edible before bed, which helped pain and sleep. She discontinued methadone in 1 year, concurrent with changing her pain medicine specialist. Cannabis was her only pain medicine.

Pearls: This is a complex case with multiple conditions. We need to bring in pain management here, opiate substitution, insomnia treatment, fatigue relief, as well as MS issues. What did we end up with that worked? A vape pen with a balanced 1:1 mix, and again both CBD and THC ingestibles before bed. In fact, just because someone has a primary chronic disease diagnosis does not alleviate the need to address as many symptoms as we can with cannabis medicine.

Patient 5: This is a 47-year-old female with MS. She had been confined to a wheel-chair for 15 years. She was on no medications at all, preferring a natural route. She was already a medical cannabis patient and was using an edible made from home-made cannabis butter 3x/day. She said it helped with spasticity, mood and sleep. The dosage was unknown. Over the next few years that I saw her, she was confined to a wheelchair, exhibited slurred speech and while she maintained her condition was stable, I noticed some irritability in her mood and new dystonia. She slowly added use of a bong a few times/day and reduced the edible dose. Lastly, she added raw juiced cannabis 1x/week. I advised her to use the raw form daily. We did not meet after this visit. It would have been good to know if the raw cannabis helped.

Pearls: This patient was a steadfast champion of the benefits of cannabis. I saw her for the entire time I was in private practice as a cannabis specialist. Every year she came in a wheelchair. Every year she was excited about her homegrown canna-bis. Every year she was hopeful. And she was always open to utilizing her cannabis medicine in new forms. I do believe cannabis was not only physiologically positive for her, but it provided empowerment over her condition, which is so needed and so valuable.

AMYOTROPHIC LATERAL SCLEROSIS

Patient 1: This is a 52-year-old female with a 6-month history of being diagnosed with Bulbar ALS. She was already using CBD derived from hemp oil before our first visit. She reported that "CBD helped slow the nerve symptoms and gave her more energy. It also lessened the fasciculations in her limbs." She was concerned that she was using the wrong kind and/or amount of CBD for best results. She could speak slowly with slurred speech, but communicated best by email. She had been taking hemp CBD oil, 8 drops of 24% oil (240 mg/ml = 60 mg dose) 2x/day for the past 6 months. Her only other medicine was guaifenesin for mucous. We discussed the benefits of cannabis-derived CBD versus hemp-derived CBD, which was all that was available in her county. She agreed to get it by mailed delivery service. She switched to a CBD/THC 20:1 tincture, but was only able to tolerate 12 drops 2x/day, that was about 6 mg, not 60 mg, before diarrhea onset! With time, she was able to tolerate a 10 mg dose 3x/day. Yet, as her disease progressed, she was feeling more fatigue and weakness. I advised her to add THC-rich sativa to her cannabis mix. She reported that it didn't help at all. Unfortunately, she purchased a THCA tincture, so she did not get relief from fatigue. By the time she was able to find a sativa tincture or sublingual mint, we were unable to follow-up. Communication was too difficult.

Pearls: Could the higher dose CBD from hemp have been a more useful product for her, or did we reach an equivalent dose with cannabis CBD? Was the entourage effect of cannabis such that 1/6th the dose was similarly effective? We were never able to achieve high doses with cannabis. Also, this case demonstrates the frustrations of working with long-distance patients, in places where products are not readily available. We were able to work together for 3 years, during which time her quality of life improved.

CANNABIS THERAPY SUMMARY

Due to the fact that MS can be relapsing and episodic, it is difficult to know what to attribute improvement to, as far as increased ambulation or decreased spasm is concerned. There may have been more impactful results with a form of MS that is slow-progressing. A pattern of preference in my patient population became clear. Many MS patients preferred THC-rich effect, especially by inhalation that has rapid onset, several times/day. This may be due to the stimulation contributing to a feeling of well-being. One patient said, "I can feel it immediately." Whereas the effect of CBD, especially in tincture, supplementing the muscle-relaxant properties of THC is not cognitively felt. The research done on Sativex indicates that a wide range of dosing was used – 10–50 mg/cannabinoids/day. I've also seen MS patients who use edibles for longer acting effects, but that is less common. The greatest use of edibles is in patients with pain or insomnia where long-acting effects are preferred.

The clinical use of cannabis for ALS has barely been investigated, although there are anecdotal reports of both THC- and CBD-rich products being useful for spasm reduction and to decrease salivary secretions. Much more research needs to be done about these different routes of delivery and dosing for these neurodegenerative conditions.

REFERENCES

1. Rudroff T, Honce JM. Cannabis and multiple sclerosis: the way forward. *Front Neurol.* 2017;8:299.
2. Pryce G, Baker D. Endocannabinoids in multiple sclerosis and amyotrophic lateral sclerosis. *Handb Exp Pharmacol.* 2015;231:213–231.
3. Zajicek J, Fox P, Sanders H, et al. Cannabinoids for treatment of spasticity and other symptoms related to multiple sclerosis (CAMS study): multicentre randomized placebo-controlled trial. *Lancet.* 2003;362:1517e26.
4. Brady CM, DasGupta R, Dalton C, et al. An open-label pilot study of cannabis-based extracts for bladder dysfunction in advanced multiple sclerosis. *Mult Scler.* 2004;10(4):425–433.
5. Collina C, Davies P, Mutibokoc IK, Ratcliffe S. Randomized controlled trial of cannabis-based medicine in spasticity caused by multiple sclerosis. *Eur J Neurol.* 2007;14:290–296.
6. Zajicek JP, Hobart JC, Slade A, Barnes D, Mattison PG. Multiple sclerosis and extract of cannabis: results of the MUSEC trial. *J Neurol Neurosurg Psychiatry.* 2012;83:1125–1132.
7. Flachenecker P, Henze T, Zettl UK. Nabiximols (THC/CBD oromucosal spray, Sativex) in clinical practice: results of a multicenter, non-interventional study (MOVE 2) in patients with multiple sclerosis spasticity. *Eur Neurol.* 2014;71(5–6):271–279.

8. Serpell MG, Notcutt W, Collin C. Sativex long-term use: an open-label trial in patients with spasticity due to multiple sclerosis. *J Neurol*. 2013;260(1):285–295.

9. Lorente Fernández L, Monte Boquet E, Pérez-Miralles F, et al. Clinical experiences with cannabinoids in spasticity management in multiple sclerosis. *Neurologia*. 2014;29(5):257–260.

10. Koppel BS, Brust JC, Fife T, et al. Report of the Guideline Development Subcommittee of the American Academy of Neurology. Systematic review: efficacy and safety of medical marijuana in selected neurologic disorders. *Neurology*. 2014;82:1556–1663.

11. Yadav V, Bever Jr C, Bowen J, et al. Summary of evidence-based guideline: complementary and alternative medicine in multiple sclerosis. *Neurology*. 2014;82(12):1083–1092.

12. Bedlack RS, Joyce N, Carter GT, Pagononi S, Karam C. Complementary and alternative therapies in ALS. *Neurol Clin*. 2015;33(4):909–936.

13. Fernández-Trapero M, Espejo-Porras F, Rodríguez-Cueto C, et al. Upregulation of CB2 receptors in reactive astrocytes in canine degenerative myelopathy, a disease model of amyotrophic lateral sclerosis. *Dis Model Mech*. 2017;10:551–558.

14. Carter GT, Abood ME, Aggarwal SK, Weiss MD. Cannabis and amyotrophic lateral sclerosis: hypothetical and practical applications, and a call for clinical trials. *Am J Hosp Palliat Care*. 2010;27(5):347–356.

15. Amtmann D, Weydt P, Johnson KL, Jensen MP, Carter GT. Survey of cannabis use in patients with amyotrophic lateral sclerosis. *Am J Hosp Palliat Care*. 2004;21:95–104.

16. Meyer T, Funke A, Münch C, et al. Real world experience of patients with amyotrophic lateral sclerosis (ALS) in the treatment of spasticity using tetrahydrocannabinol:cannabidiol (THC:CBD). *BMC Neurol*. 2019;19(1):222.

17. Weber M, Goldman B, Truniger S. Tetrahydrocannabinol (THC) for cramps in amyotrophic lateral sclerosis: a randomised, double-blind crossover trial. *J Neurol Neurosurg Psychiatry*. 2010;81:1135–1140.

37 Muscle Spasm, Spasticity

MUSCLE SPASM, SPASTICITY AND CANNABIS

The muscle-relaxant properties of cannabis are well-known by consumers, both medically and recreationally, and have long been noted in historical accounts. In fact, one of the components of "body relaxation" experienced by indica users is due to muscle relaxation and sedation most likely augmented by the inclusion of β-myrcene. Medical cannabis patients from California reported relief from muscle spasms as one of the most common reasons for using cannabis, 41%.[1] A survey of 1,248 respondents in Washington state who used cannabis reported that 7.5% found they were able to substitute for muscle relaxants.[2] Although there are many anecdotal reports of relief from muscle spasms using cannabis, modern research is surprisingly sparse.

The involvement of the endocannabinoid system in muscle contractility has been documented. It was previously thought that CB1 receptors are the main cannabinoid target to deliver an antispastic effect. In visceral smooth muscle, stimulation of both CB1 and CB2 receptors with anandamide (AEA) resulted in marked relaxation of contraction.[3] In a study done on heart tissue, AEA again decreased contractility in a dose-dependent manner.[4] The postulated mechanisms of action for antispasmodic compounds overlap with many of the systems in which cannabinoids have activity. These include:

> [I]nhibition of the response to the neurotransmitters 5-hydroxytryptamine (5-HT) or serotonin and acetylcholine . . . (i) capsaicin-sensitive neurons, (ii) the participation of vanilloid receptors, (iii) the activation of K+ ATP channels, (iv) the blockade of Na+ channels and muscarinic receptors, (v) the reduction of extracellular Ca^{2+}, or (vi) the blockade of Ca^{2+} channels.[5]

These mechanisms suggest that both THC and CBD may have antispasmodic activity.

Studies of the actions of cannabinoids on muscle function are lacking. In one case report, muscle spasm in the calves, secondary to a chemotherapy drug, was 100% resolved with cannabis, while baclofen and cyclobenzaprine were not successful. The patient used one joint 3–4 times/day.[6] This is a common clinical occurrence of muscle spasm being effectively treated. In contrast to the success cannabis seems to have on patients with common muscle spasm, its effect on spasticity is less impressive, but that is what most studies have focused on. Spasticity proceeds by a different mechanism than muscle spasm, although often, increased muscle spasm is the result.

> Spasticity can be defined from the pathophysiological perspective as a disordered sensorimotor control resulting from an upper motor neuron lesion, presenting as intermittent or sustained involuntary activation of muscles. It is perceived by the patients as continuous muscle stiffness, often associated with exacerbating spasms.[7]

DOI: 10.1201/9781003098201-48

An early study of the effect of THC on patients with spasticity showed that 10 mg caused a reduction in spasticity, but only effective in three out of eight patients in reducing tonic spasm.[8] THC was also found to be significantly better than codeine in reducing muscle spasm in a paraplegic patient.[9] A study using a THC analogue, nabilone, for spasticity in spinal cord injury subjects reported a small significant decrease on the Ashworth spasticity scale in the most involved muscle. Nabilone 0.5 mg was used one to two times a day for 4 weeks.[10] Most studies on cannabis and cannabinoids in treatment of spasticity have been done with multiple sclerosis (MS) patients, and most often with cannabis extracts.[11] Cannabis-extract capsules with a ratio of CBD/THC 0.9:2.5 were used to provide doses up to 15–30 mg THC, and were taken by subjects for 14 days. Improvements in spasm frequency and mobility were reported.[12] In another study, 40% of patients self-reported a benefit of 30% or more using a 1:1 cannabis extract (Sativex) over a period of 6 weeks, although changes in the scores on the Ashworth score did not support these reports.[13] Similar results were found in a study involving 337 patients with treatment-resistant spasticity.[14]

A pilot study of Sativex oromucosal spray in patients with MS showed the mean spasticity (0–10) NRS score decreased from 6 to 3.6. A small decrease in spasticity was noted, and the mean number of spasms/day decreased.[15] In the multiple sclerosis and cannabis extract (MUSEC) 12-week trial, the rate of relief from muscle stiffness was almost twice as high among those given the cannabis extract as those given the placebo, 30% relief versus 16%. In this case, up to 25 mg THC in the oral extract divided into 2 doses/day was used (about half the patients used less).[16] Explanation of all of the earlier studies and others regarding CBD/THC in treating spasticity in MS may be found in a comprehensive review.[7]

The results using smoked THC-rich cannabis were more significant. In a study of smoked cannabis by MS patients, a significant change in the Ashworth scale was found. A decrease of almost 3 points in a 10-point scale was achieved.[17] Studies with CBD-rich cannabis or pure CBD have not been done. Although CBD has anti-inflammatory, neuroprotective, anticonvulsant, antioxidant properties, its action as a muscle relaxant is weak compared with THC.[18] Animal studies have shown that both CBD and CBDA exhibit inhibitory actions on the smooth muscle of intestines through non-CB receptor pathways.[19]

Often topical application of cannabis is used for muscle relaxation, yet no study of peripheral action on muscle has been done. It has been shown that peripheral cannabinoid receptors are involved in anti-inflammatory and analgesic effects, so we know the receptors are there.[20] Not only cannabinoid agonists such as THC, but CBD is effective topically as well, but only assessed for inflammation and pain.[21] More investigation needs to be done into the internal and topical effects of cannabinoids on muscle spasm before we have a clearer picture. The earlier results suggest that THC would have the strongest effects in this regard.

PATIENT REPORTS

To move on to patient results from my practice, patients of all ages exhibit muscle spasm, and have reported benefit from topical if not internal cannabis use. Those represented here are in the adult category, 50–60s, reflective of my patient population and the severity of muscle spasm complaints. Cases of muscle spasm associated with menstruation were common, especially in younger adults, and are presented in Chapter 47. Many patients used cannabis for common muscle spasm, but these often were diagnosed as part of a pain syndrome of the affected area (see Chapters 21, 31 and 41). Outlined here are significant cases in which muscle spasm or spasticity was a primary diagnosis. Here are a few illustrative case reports.

Patient 1: This is a 65-year-old female who presented with "terrible muscle pain" and suspected polymyalgia rheumatica. Her only medication was prednisone 30 mg/day for the past 2 weeks. She was new to cannabis but hopeful it could help. She began to use a CBD-rich tincture each day, and an indica tincture each night. This continued for the next year, yet her prednisone dose only decreased from 20 mg to 15 mg/day. I advised her to use more cannabis, up to 15 mg of a CBD/THC 2:1 mix 2x/day, plus the indica at night. She was hesitant to add THC during the day, so she continued on the same regimen. Over the next few years, she was able to wean off the prednisone, and her muscle pain decreased. Her joints continued to deteriorate, and she underwent hip and knee replacement. She had stopped cannabis when she got off the prednisone, and was now wondering if topical could help with joint pain.

Pearls: This patient's reaction to cannabis is very representative of a common hesitant approach often seen in the elderly. To use as little as possible, with THC only as required, preferably at night. If she had increased her dose and THC content, she may have experienced less pain, and most likely a speedier course off prednisone. Although CBD-rich cannabis was likely helpful with the inflammation, she used only 5 mg once/day. Other patients with PMR showed better results with a more aggressive dosing schedule.

Patient 2: This is a 53-year-old male with complaints of muscle spasm in his legs and foot pain for over 10 years. He had been using cannabis for 20 years, mostly by smoking a few times/week to relieve the spasms. He was a dancer, still practicing, and he presumed the muscle spasms were from dancing. I advised adding topical to his regimen, especially over the anterior tibial area where the muscle tension was most pronounced. He continued on this regimen, using cannabis butter as topical, and rarely used as an edible. I suggested he massage the area with cannabis oil.

Pearls: Smoking cannabis can bring immediate relief to spasms, but this is a perfect case for topical application. Cannabis in butter form is not expected to be an effective topical as the butter is not the correct vehicle for transdermal delivery. Shea butter or cocoa butter, or in this case a cannabis-infused massage oil would have been a better choice.

Patient 3: This is a 55-year-old female with a 19-year history of MS. She complained of muscle spasm, pain and insomnia. She was using 10 mg of baclofen for muscle spasms 5x/day, Ambien 10 mg at night, Valium 5 mg 2x/day for relaxation and had recently switched from Tysabri to Ampyra. She used a wheelchair for motility, had no slurred speech or cognitive difficulties. Her cannabis usage for the past 6 years was smoked 5–8 puffs/day. After adding a CBD-rich tincture 3x/day, and continuing to smoke at night she presented the next year using a cane. Rituximab had also been added that year. By the following year, her baclofen usage was down to 10 mg 3x/day, Ambien was no longer nightly, but 2–3x/week.

Pearls: Smoking a THC-rich strain may have facilitated the decrease in baclofen, while the nightly indica smoked not only helps with sleep but also acts as a muscle relaxant. It generally takes high levels of THC to deal with significant MS spasticity.

Combination with CBD may have potentiated this lower dose of THC. Dosage and tolerance are a unique process for each individual, and self-titration encompasses a range of results.

Patient 4: This is a 33-year-old-female with secondary progressive MS. She had considerable spasticity, along with some nausea, depression and insomnia. She had been using cannabis for several years by smoking 2–3 x/day. Her medications included Tysabri, Toviaz, lansoprazole, Lexapro and a significant amount of baclofen – 20 mg every 4 hours. She ambulated by wheelchair. I suggested adding a CBD/THC 1:1 tincture 10 mg 3x/day to help with the spasticity. At our next visit, she was still smoking cannabis, but more often, and had added the cannabis tincture, plus vaping an indica before bed. The MS continued to progress leading to more pain in several joints and several hospitalizations. The baclofen dosage did not reduce.

Pearls: This is a case where increased quality of life, decreased pain and/or disease mitigation was not evident. Was the cannabis helping at all? Probably for nausea, sleep and mood. How much it may have been affecting spasticity and pain, the primary symptoms for which research has shown benefit was not measurable, since her condition worsened. She did not want to stop cannabis use, as she claimed it made her condition "more bearable." An objective analysis would not prove cannabis is therapeutic, but by subjective analysis it was.

Patient 5: This is a 62-year-old male who presented with low back pain and also complained of leg fasciculations for the past year, which were resistant to treatment thus far. He had a history of an L5-S1 herniated disc 5 years earlier. He had tried acupuncture and yoga, all of which helped, but were not enough. He complained of ongoing back pain for which he was already using cannabis, smoked or vaporized 4x/day. On exam he had a negative straight leg raise, het his anterior tibialis muscle continued to twitch 40 times/minute all around the clock. I advised trying topical on the leg. He also added an edible before bed. Presumably, the fasciculations came on as a delayed reaction the lumbar herniation. The back pain was helped by increasing the frequency of his cannabis use, the fasciculations were not. He developed anxiety related to his leg twitches. He said the cannabis helped his anxiety as well as pain. Over the course of 5 years that we worked together, the fasciculations did not decrease at all.

Pearls: Fasciculations are muscle contractions caused by the spontaneous firing of a motor unit. In this case THC-rich cannabis did nothing to abate that firing. While cannabis often works well for some types of muscle contractility, it cannot be assumed that it will repair significantly damaged neurons, and clearly here, did not.

CANNABIS THERAPY SUMMARY

Cannabis is remarkably effective for common muscle spasm, yet little scientific evidence exists because the research hasn't been done. There are hundreds of patients I've seen with muscle spasm – from low back pain, an overuse or sports injury or from a car accident who have reported much relief, especially with topical THC or CBD or both. In my own experience, after a significant whiplash injury from a car accident, nothing helped more that topically applied cannabis. My neck muscles immediately stopped seizing up so much. In fact, anti-inflammatory agents or analgesics are not as effective as they are not muscle relaxants, while cannabis serves all of these functions. Many of my patients have been able to eliminate chronic use of SOMA for low back pain just by using topical cannabis. Topical applications of cannabis can be applied to the affected area without causing psychoactive effects, and provide a safe, potent method of delivery. Spasticity treatment is of a different order. Widespread spasticity often requires internal use likely a high dosage, that is, up to 50 mg/cannabinoids/day, and even then, may not show improvement. More research needs to be done in evaluating the efficacy of CBD versus THC for muscle spasm and spasticity, but it may be that THC-rich cannabis is preferable. No research has been done on cultivar specificity for muscle spasm therapy, yet this may be an important component in the choice of cannabis medicine. It is important to recall that indica strains are most noted for muscle relaxation, and may be the best choice, in large part due to the antispasmodic effect of the terpene, β-myrcene.

REFERENCES

1. Nunberg H, Kilmer B, Pacula RL, Burgdorf JR. An analysis of applicants presenting to a medical marijuana specialty practice in California. *J Drug Policy Anal.* 2011;4(1):1.
2. Corroon Jr. JM, Mischley LK, Sexton M. Cannabis as a substitute for prescription drugs: a cross-sectional study. *J Pain Res.* 2017;10:989–998.
3. Bermudez AM, Visina JM, Walker LA. Differential effects of cannabinoid receptor stimulation in smooth muscle. *FASEB J.* 2017;31(Supp 1):690.4–690.4.
4. Bonz A, Laser M, Küllmer S, et al. Cannabinoids acting on CB1 receptors decrease contractile performance in human atrial muscle. *J Cardiovascular Pharmacol.* 2003;41(4):657–664.
5. Martínez-Pérez EF, Juárez ZN, Hernández LR, Bach H. Natural antispasmodics: source, stereochemical configuration, and biological activity. *BioMed Res Int.* 2018;2018:Article ID 3819714.
6. Yuan JT, Tello TL, Hultman C, et al. Medical marijuana for the treatment of vismodegib-related muscle spasm. *JAAD Case Rep.* 2017;3:438–440.
7. Zetti UK, Rommer P, Hipp P, Patejdl R. Evidence for the efficacy and effectiveness of THC-CBD oromucosal spray in symptom management of patients with spasticity due to multiple sclerosis. *Ther Adv Neurol Disord.* 2016;9(1):9–30.
8. Petro DJ, Ellenberger C. Treatment of human spasticity with delta 9-tetrahydrocannabinol. *J Clin Pharmacol.* 1981;21:413S–416S.
9. Maurer M, Henn V, Dittrich A, Hofmann A. Delta-9-tetrahydrocannabinol shows anti-spastic and analgesic effects in a single case double-blind trial. *Eur Arch Psychiat Clin Neurosci.* 1990;240:104.
10. Pooyania S, Ethans K, Szturm T, Casey A, Perry D. A randomized, double-blinded, crossover pilot study assessing the effect of nabilone on spasticity in persons with spinal cord injury. *Arch Phys Med Rehabil.* 2010;91(5):703–707.
11. Malfitano AM, Proto MC, Bifulco M. Cannabinoids in the management of spasticity associated with multiple sclerosis. *Neuropsychiatr Dis Treat.* 2008;4(5):847–853.
12. Vaney C, Heinzel-Gutenbrunner M, Jobin P, et al. Efficacy, safety and tolerability of an orally administered cannabis extract in the treatment of spasticity in patients with multiple sclerosis: a randomized, double-blind, placebo-controlled, crossover study. *Mult Scler.* 2004;10(4):417–424.

13. Collin C, Davies P, Mutibokoc IK, S. Ratcliffe S. Randomized controlled trial of cannabis-based medicine in spasticity caused by multiple sclerosis. *Eur J Neurol.* 2007;14:290–296.
14. Collin C, Ehler E, Waberzinek G, et al. A double-blind, randomized, placebo-controlled, parallel-group study of Sativex, in subjects with symptoms of spasticity due to multiple sclerosis. *Neurol Res.* 2010;32:451–459.
15. Rekand T. THC:CBD spray and MS spasticity symptoms: data from latest studies. *Eur Neurol.* 2014;71(Suppl 1):4–9.
16. Zajicek JP, Hobart JC, Slade A, Barnes D, Mattison PG. Multiple sclerosis and extract of cannabis: results of the MUSEC trial. *J Neurol Neurosurg Psychiatry.* 2012;83:1125–1132.
17. Corey-Bloom J, Wolfson T, Gamst A, et al. Smoked cannabis for spasticity in multiple sclerosis: a randomized, placebo-controlled trial. *CMAJ.* 2012;184(10):1143–1150.
18. Russo E., Guy G. A tale of two cannabinoids: the therapeutic rationale for combining tetrahydrocannabinol and cannabidiol. *Med Hypotheses.* 2006;66:234–246.
19. Cluny NL, Naylor RJ, Whittle BA, Javid FA. The effects of cannabidiolic acid and cannabidiol on contractility of the gastrointestinal tract of Suncus murinus. *Arch Pharm Res.* 2011;34(9):1509–1517.
20. Richardson J, Kilo S, Hargreaves K. Cannabinoids reduce hyperalgesia and inflammation via interaction with peripheral CB1 receptors. *Pain.* 1998;75(1):111–119.
21. Hammell DC, Zhang LP, Ma F, et al. Transdermal cannabidiol reduces inflammation and pain-related behaviours in a rat model of arthritis. *Eur J Pain.* 2016;20(6):936–948.

38 Nausea, Vomiting

NAUSEA, VOMITING AND CANNABIS

The endocannabinoid system and cannabinoids are involved in regulating nausea and vomiting in humans and other animals. Cannabis has been used since ancient times to treat nausea. Ineffective treatment of chemotherapy-induced nausea and vomiting (CINV) prompted the investigation of the anti-emetic properties of cannabinoids in the late 1970s and early 1980s. Δ9-Tetrahydrocannabinol (THC) is currently approved in the United States (since 1985) as dronabinol (Marinol), for treatment of chemotherapy-associated nausea and vomiting, and anorexia.[1,2] Cannabis has also been documented as effective treating nausea in HIV patients.[3] A review of cannabinoids use for CINV found studies using nabilone, dronabinol and intramuscular levonantradol. All studies comparing cannabinoids to standard anti-emetic drugs found cannabinoids slightly more effective. A range of 38–90% of patients stated they preferred cannabinoids.[4] Cannabis has since been shown to be effective for nausea caused by a multitude of reasons, including from a drug reaction not only to HIV antivirals but also in cases of hepatitis C treatment and/or from hepatitis itself, from food sensitivities, and from migraine-induced nausea. Paradoxically, many patients who experience cannabis tolerance and rely on cannabis for appetite stimulation report feeling nausea during the withdrawal period.

Endocannabinoids inhibit peripherally and centrally initiated vomiting through their actions on CB1 receptors. Lower endocannabinoid levels and reduced CB1 mRNA expression were found in subjects with motion sickness during simulated parabolic flight compared to normal subjects.[5] The action of cannabinoids (including THC) on CB1 receptors in the brain stem and/or on vagal pathways is proposed as one mechanism of action of reducing nausea and vomiting. CBD is thought to reduce nausea by interacting with serotonin receptors through another mechanism. In animals the effect of CBD on toxin-induced vomiting displays a biphasic response with lower doses, 5 mg/kg, producing an anti-emetic effect, whereas very high doses, 20–40 mg/kg, enhanced vomiting.[6] Cannabinoid acids also suppress nausea. In animal studies, both THC at 0.5 mg/kg and THCA at 0.05 and 0.5 mg/kg suppressed conditioned gaping, a measure of nausea, in a CB1 receptor-dependent mechanism.[7] CBDA at doses of 0.1 and 0.5 mg/kg reduced induced emesis in shrews and increased the latency of onset of emesis in response to motion at even lower doses. CBDA not only binds to transient receptor potential (TRP) cation channels, but like CBD, CBDA's suppression of nausea and vomiting was reversed by pretreatment with a 5-HT1A receptor antagonist.[8] In a following study, lower concentrations of CBDA were effective at suppressing conditioned gaping.[9] These results suggest that cannabinoid acids are more effective at lower doses than their corresponding non-acid forms, but that their action may be at the same receptors as their counterparts'. Of interest as well is the potential for synergistic treatment at multiple receptors by these different classes of cannabinoids.

DOI: 10.1201/9781003098201-49

Dronabinol, ondansetron or the combination was studied for delayed CINV in a 5-day, double-blind, placebo-controlled study. Absence of nausea was 71% with dronabinol, 64% with ondansetron and 15% with placebo, confirming the anti-emetic effect of synthetic THC.[10] CBD was shown to suppress nausea and vomiting within a limited dose range (in animal models).[6] Sativex (CBD/THC approx. 1:1) has been found to decrease CINV in preclinical trials. The mean number of daily sprays taken during the 4 days after chemotherapy was 4.81 in the CBM (cannabis-based medicine) group, adding up to approximately 25 mg of cannabinoids/day.[11] A more prevalent delivery method, smoked cannabis, was found to reduce nausea and also emesis at a level comparable to or slightly better than ondansetron.[12]

CYCLIC VOMITING SYNDROME VERSUS CANNABINOID HYPEREMESIS SYNDROME

The effect of cannabis on nausea and vomiting appears to be dose and chronicity-dependent. Cannabis is commonly used in therapeutically cyclic vomiting syndrome (CVS) due to its anti-emetic and anxiolytic properties. Cyclical vomiting syndrome is not necessarily associated with high levels of cannabis use. These patients often have comorbid depression, anxiety or migraine headaches.[13] Patients with cyclical vomiting as a symptom but do not have a history of high chronic cannabis use may benefit from cannabis therapy. This is not the case for another syndrome, the cannabinoid hyperemesis syndrome (CHS). CHS refers to cyclic episodes of nausea and vomiting, relieved by hot bathing and associated with chronic, subjectively determined high cannabis use.[14–16] Symptoms may resolve after cessation of cannabis use.

The distinction between these two diagnoses has been recently reviewed.[17] Ninety-five percent of CHS patients were found to use cannabis daily for 10 years before symptom onset. The pathogenesis of paradoxical hyperemetic symptoms of CHS remain unclear. A review of the subject summarizes:

> We speculate that the paradoxical effects of chronic cannabis may be caused by differential degrees of CB1R downregulation in genetically predisposed individuals. . . . Postmortem studies in humans also demonstrate CB1R downregulation in the human brain with chronic cannabis use compared to non-users.[5]

The etiology of CHS is thought to be activation of CB1 receptors that can reduce gastric emptying. CHS may represent a case of dysregulation of one's own endo-cannabinoid system due to excessive phytocannabinoid use. Abstinence from THC-rich cannabis resolves the condition. This definitely qualifies as an adverse effect (AE) of using cannabis. This AE can be milder and not result in vomiting, but may account for underlying nausea and lack of appetite upon discontinuance of cannabis by chronic users as found in a withdrawal syndrome.

PATIENT REPORTS

To move on to patient results from my practice, my patients ranged in age from teens to the elderly. Nausea and/or vomiting was often a complaint associated with other symptoms, such as gastrointestinal disorders, chemotherapy or anxiety. Cannabis was often a treatment of choice addressing these multiple conditions, so that improvement, not merely symptomatic treatment, could occur. Here are a few illustrative case reports.

Patient 1: This is a 16-year-old female with constant nausea along with celiac disease. She was thin, underweight due to low food intake and nutritional deficiency and her rigorous training as a dancer. She was new to cannabis use, referred by her physician for a trial of CBD. Her mother served as caregiver. This was a very pleasant young woman who denied low appetite, just difficulty finding enough to eat with nausea and celiac issues. I advised a CBD-rich product oromucosally, by mouth spray, lozenge or vapor pen. She settled upon CBD in a gummy 1–2x/day, which worked well to treat her chronic nausea. She was able to continue with school and dance practice, and maintained her weight. She also admitted to some anxiety. I did advise counseling, as there was some exacerbation with stress, but she declined to do so.

Pearls: We know that CBD is effective for nausea, and not disorienting, so appropriate for use in a minor. In this case, its help with anxiety as well as nausea was an effective therapy for this young woman. Some THC for appetite stimulation may be indicated in adult patients, but fortunately was not required in this case.

Patient 2: This is a 103-year-old female with complaints of chronic nausea, anxiety and tinnitus. She was taking a low dose of Benicar for hypertension and eyedrops following retinal surgery. She also took an anti-emetic syrup daily for nausea, which was not fully successful. She ambulated with a cane, was fully cognizant of her surroundings and spoke clearly and appropriately. She was brought in by her daughter who thought that CBD might help her nausea. On exam, her abdomen was extremely distended with increased bowel sounds. The daughter reported that a work-up on abdominal swelling had not yet been done. She was in remarkable condition for her age. I advised a CBD-rich product by mouth spray or lollipop or lozenge. She was successful in finding a lollipop and also used a cookie. The only mouth spray available was a CBD/THC 1:1 mix. She reported that the mouth spray reversed nausea within 10 minutes that lasted 4–6 hours. The family was quite pleased. She came in again the next year, at age 104. The daughter reported that an MRI of the abdomen was normal, and abdominal swelling was reduced, not gone. Her anxiety and nausea were improved. She continued to use daily cannabis in a CBD/THC 1:1 ratio, by mouth spray and cookies. Her blood pressure was stable off Benicar. This was my last visit with this remarkable elderly patient.

Pearls: In the elderly a CBD-rich product is usually well-tolerated, and as in the preceding case, served well to treat chronic nausea as well as anxiety. What is useful to note is that even a 1:1 mix was well-tolerated. The dosage here was low, only 2 puffs of a mouth spray, or a piece (less than ¼) of a cookie. The total dose of cannabinoids was likely less than 5 mg. This happened at a time when CBD/THC 20:1 products were not widely available, nor were hemp-derived products yet on the market.

Patient 3: This is a 60-year-old male who came in primarily for insomnia, but also experienced cyclical vomiting episodes 2–4x/year that lasted weeks, as well as chronic nausea and anxiety. He was already smoking cannabis to help with sleep, by bong, three to four times in the evening. He also had low back pain, having had three low back surgeries with a current right drop foot. He took Norco 10 mg 3×/day for pain. His other medications included Ambien 12.5 mg CR, Seroquel 25 mg, lorazepam 1 mg 4×/day, Flexeril, Compazine and Phenergan suppositories and Zofran as needed for nausea. It was hard to switch him from smoking to other forms of cannabis, but over the next few years, he did add CBD by concentrated oil 1 drop/day and an indica chocolate 10–15 mg at night. The cyclical vomiting was mostly gone. Norco, lorazepam, Flexeril, Seroquel and anti-nausea drugs all were rarely used. Ambien use reduced to 5 nights/week. At our last visit, he increased his use of CBD to 2×/day, continued to smoke sativa during the day and indica at night and was down to 2 nights/week of Ambien use. There was only one cyclical vomiting episode in the past 2 years, and nausea was mostly gone.

Pearls: The most outstanding facet of this case was how many medications this patient was able to eliminate. A little bit of instruction in how to use cannabis as a medicine went a long way. By using cannabis several times a day as well as adding CBD, we were able to manage almost all of this patient's symptoms. He was not diagnosed with cannabis hyperemesis syndrome, rather cyclical vomiting, but it is unclear if he would have been if that had been a more well-known diagnosis at the time. In either case, it was much improved, without the necessity of stopping cannabis.

Patient 4: This is a 65-year-old female patient who had multiple complaints, including low back pain, COPD, tremor, insomnia, nausea, hypertension and cyclical vomiting. The vomiting occurred at least 4×/month lasting 2 days. She attributed this symptom to a genetic mitochondrial disorder. Her medications included multiple inhalers, amitriptyline, Ativan and Lunesta. She was smoking cannabis by bong 3–4×/day for the past 5 years. I tried to persuade her to switch to a vaporizer as smoking was contraindicated with COPD. It took a few years, but she did eventually switch to a vape pen, still used 4×/day. Unfortunately, the cyclical vomiting remained the same. On follow-up after our last visit, she had been diagnosed with abdominal migraine, treated somewhat successfully with sumatriptan, now having less than 2 vomiting episodes /month.

Pearls: In contrast to the previous patient, none of this patient's symptoms improved, none of her medications were reduced, so was cannabis medicinal. It's hard to say because she presented already on a cannabis regimen. I don't know what her symptoms would have been off of it. At least she was able to discontinue smoking as delivery. Apparently, cannabis was not as effective as sumatriptan at relieving her abdominal migraine.

Patient 5: This is a 53-year-old female, currently using cannabis for insomnia with a new diagnosis of breast cancer. Her primary complaint while undergoing chemotherapy was nausea. She had a 20-year history of using cannabis, currently an indica edible every night for insomnia. She was taking no medications prior to the cancer diagnosis. She added cannabis by pipe, or vaporization to help nausea, which she said worked quite well, using a sativa 3–4×/day also to lift her mood. The only recommendation I had was to add a topical to the breast area to help repair the irradiated area.

Pearls: This is an example of the multifactorial application of cannabis as medicine. She was on no medicine for insomnia, no medicine for nausea, no medicine for mood and no medicine other than the cancer chemotherapy. The use of pure THC such as in dronabinol, approved for chemotherapy-induced nausea, does not achieve the multimodal effect of cannabis, able to treat all of these symptoms that often accompany a cancer diagnosis.

CANNABINOID HYPEREMESIS SYNDROME

Patient 1: This is a 31-year-old male with complaints of nausea and episodic vomiting. He had been using cannabis for 8 years, by smoking, about 1 gram/day. He had been having episodes of nausea and cyclical vomiting three to six times a year for the past 3 years. His physician determined that no GI disorder, heartburn or food allergy was at fault. His worst episode of vomiting came on unexpectedly, and lasted for almost 24 hours. He was away from home and reported using cannabis from a source different than usual. He went to the emergency room and they diagnosed him with cannabis hyperemesis syndrome (CHS) and was advised to reduce or stop cannabis use. He did relate that the vomiting decreased with hot showers especially with water directed to the chest/abdominal area. He stopped cannabis for 2 weeks, then resumed. At this point he came in for a consultation. He was stressed with staring a new business and was prone to dehydration from working outside in a hot climate. He was not convinced his symptoms were due to cannabis and did not wish to stop. His cannabis usage was not excessive, nevertheless, I advised a tolerance break regularly, 2–3 days/week, and to keep a CBD-rich mouth spray handy for nausea episodes. Over the next few years, he had three to four more episodes, even with reduced usage, at which point he discontinued cannabis for 1 year. At our last visit, he was smoking cannabis again, about ½ gram/day and had not had recurrence of the syndrome in the past year.

Pearls: The one recommended treatment for CHS is to stop cannabis. It's important to understand the rationale behind this. It is to reduce tolerance, restore endocannabinoid tone and thereby reset this paradoxical response. If that is the case, then resumption of cannabis use at a low level after these biochemical readjustments have occurred might be a possible option. The literature does not discuss the potential effects of stress on the manifestation of CHS. It is possible that a small amount of cannabis provides enough benefit in stress management to consider resumption of cannabis after a long tolerance break rather than discontinuance indefinitely.

CANNABIS THERAPY SUMMARY

There are so many choices to treat nausea and vomiting with cannabis. All forms of cannabinoids are effective, including THC, CBD and cannabinoid acids. It is no surprise that some of my patients found that raw cannabis juice helped nausea. The advantage of THC is that it can also stimulate appetite and promote weight gain if these are concomitant issues. For example, in several of my patients with nausea and appetite loss from chemotherapy, HIV or hepatitis C, they preferred inhaled THC-rich cannabis. The advantage of CBD or cannabinoid acids is that no psychoactivity is expected. Some good methods of delivery include inhalation or sublingual products to avoid loss of ingested medicine due to vomiting.[10,11] Rectal administration would also work, resulting in decreased psychoactivity compared with inhalation or sublingual methods if using THC-rich cannabis, but these products are limited in availability. Typical dosing for mild cases of nausea may range from 1–2 puffs of inhaled cannabis or 5–10 mg of cannabinoids by sublingual application, such as tincture, lozenge or mouth spray. For more severe cases of vomiting, inhalation or rectal dosing may be indicated. Special attention must be paid to the overuse of THC-rich cannabis, which can have paradoxical effects, whereby instead of treating nausea and vomiting, hyperemesis can occur such as in CHS. This is most often a result of cannabis use for other conditions, resulting in severe vomiting in a patient who has not had this complaint before. The treatment for this is abstention from cannabis to reset endocannabinoid homeostasis.

REFERENCES

1. Darmani NA. Mechanisms of broad-spectrum antiemetic efficacy of cannabinoids against chemotherapy-induced acute and delayed vomiting. *Pharmaceutical.* 2010;3:2930–2955.
2. Brafford May M, Glode AE. Dronabinol for chemotherapy-induced nausea and vomiting unresponsive to antiemetics. *Cancer Manag Res.* 2016;8:49–55.
3. Jong BC, Prentiss D, McFarland W, Machekano R, Israelski DM. Marijuana use and its association with adherence to antiretroviral therapy among HIV-infected persons with moderate to severe nausea. *J Acquir Immune Defic Syndr.* 2005;38(1):43–46.
4. Tramèr MR, Carroll D, Campbell FA, et al. Cannabinoids for control of chemotherapy induced nausea and vomiting: quantitative systematic review. *BMJ.* 2001;323:16–21.
5. Venkatesan T, Levinthal DJ, Li UK. Role of chronic cannabis use: cyclic vomiting syndrome vs cannabinoid hyperemesis syndrome. *Neurogastroenterol Motil.* 2019;31(Suppl 2):e13606.
6. Parker LA, Rock EM, Limebeer CL. Regulation of nausea and vomiting by cannabinoids. *Br J Pharmacol.* 2011;163(7):1411–1422.
7. Rock EM, Kopstick RL, Limebeer CL, Parker LA. Tetrahydrocannabinolic acid reduces nausea-induced conditioned gaping in rats and vomiting in Suncus murinus. *Br J Pharmacol.* 2013;170(3):641–648.
8. Bolognini D, Rock EM, Cluny NL, et al. Cannabidiolic acid prevents vomiting in Suncus murinus and nausea-induced behaviour in rats by enhancing 5-HT1A receptor activation. *Br J Pharmacol.* 2013;168(6):1456–1470.
9. Rock EM, Connolly C, Limebeer CL, Parker LA. Effect of combined oral doses of Δ(9)-tetrahydrocannabinol (THC) and cannabidiolic acid (CBDA) on acute and anticipatory nausea in rat models. *Psychopharmacology (Berl).* 2016;233(18):3353–3360.
10. Meiri E, Jhangiani H, Vredenburgh JJ, et al. Efficacy of dronabinol alone and in combination with ondansetron versus ondansetron alone for delayed chemotherapy-induced nausea and vomiting. *Curr Med Res Opin.* 2007;23:533–543.
11. Duran M, Pérez E, Abanades S, et al. Preliminary efficacy and safety of an oromucosal standardized cannabis extract in chemotherapy-induced nausea and vomiting. *Br J Clin Pharmacol.* 2010;70(5):656–663.
12. Söderpalm AH, Schuster A, de Wit H. Antiemetic efficacy of smoked marijuana: subjective and behavioral effects on nausea induced by syrup of ipecac. *Pharmacol Biochem Behav.* 2011;69(3–4):343–350.
13. Campos-Outcalt D, Janousek A, Rosales C. Arizona Department of Health Services Medical Marijuana Advisory Committee Report. The relationship between marijuana use

and Cyclical Vomiting Syndrome. 2013. https://azdhs.gov/documents/licensing/medical-marijuana/debilitating/cyclic-vomiting-syndrome.pdf Accessed March 10, 2020.

14. Galli JA, Sawaya RA, Friedenberg FK. Cannabinoid hyperemesis syndrome. *Curr Drug Abuse Rev.* 2011;4(4):241–249.

15. Chen J, McCarron RM. Cannabinoid hyperemesis syndrome: a result of chronic, heavy Cannabis use. *Curr Psych.* 2013;12(10):48–53.

16. Patterson DA, Smith E, Monahan M, et al. Cannabinoid hyperemesis and compulsive bathing: a case series and paradoxical pathophysiological explanation. *J Am Board Fam Med.* 2010;23:790–793.

39 Neuropathic Pain

NEUROPATHIC PAIN AND CANNABIS

The treatment of neuropathic pain is one of the therapeutic applications of cannabis that has been of marked interest, distinguishing it as one of the few areas of cannabis research that has culminated in clinical trials. Neuropathic pain results from damage to or dysfunction of the peripheral or central nervous system and often, but not always, results in altered sensation in the periphery. Peripheral neuropathy is a common condition that we treat in cannabis practice, especially in the elderly. A particularly painful and difficult to treat category of neuropathic pain, complex regional pain syndrome (CRPS), also responds to cannabis therapy. It is of importance to remember that neuropathy encompasses not only pain but also nerve dysfunction. Cannabis as a neuroprotectant, antioxidant and pain modulator is an appropriate medicine for neuropathy, offering the potential for nerve repair, not just pain management.

Several reviews have been published on the multifactorial potential mechanisms of action involved in this complex topic.[1,2] In brief review, endocannabinoids modulate neural conduction of pain by activation of cannabinoid receptors CB1 and CB2. CB1 receptors are located at multiple locations in the peripheral and central nervous system, whereas CB2 receptors are located on inflammatory cells (monocytes, B/T cells, mast cells). Activation of central CB1 receptors leads to reduced dorsal horn excitability and activates descending inhibitory pathways in the brain. The net result is a reduction in both pain and hyperalgesia. Activation of peripheral CB1 receptors results in a reduction in the release of pro-inflammatory terminal peptides and a reduction in terminal sensitivity. Activation of CB2 suppresses neuropathic pain mechanisms through non-neuronal mechanisms (i.e., microglia and astrocyte). These increase in response to peripheral nerve damage, regulate neuroimmune interactions and interfere with inflammatory hyperalgesia. It is useful to recall that of the major cannabinoids, THC is a cannabinoid agonist, while CBD acts primarily through non-CBr mechanisms.

Other cannabinoid sites of action include non-CB1/CB2 cannabinoid G protein-coupled receptors, peroxisome proliferator-activated receptors and transient receptor potential channels, among others.[3] Due to their receptor binding specificities, THC and CBD have different effects on pain. THC as a cannabinoid agonist has effects similar to endocannabinoid CBr agonism, to promote antinociception and inhibit neuronal excitability. The effect of CBD on pain is less well understood, and has not been documented as useful alone for neuropathic pain, but is effective for inflammatory pain. CBD might inhibit hyperalgesia and it might support endocannabinoid function by inhibiting degradation. In any case, both THC and CBD show promise in treating neuropathy, not limited to pain.

Several studies using smoked or vaporized cannabis confirmed neuropathic pain reduction. Smoked cannabis in HIV patients reduced daily neuropathic pain by 34%.

DOI: 10.1201/9781003098201-50

The findings were comparable to drugs used for chronic neuropathic pain.[4] The effects of smoked cannabis in HIV-associated distal sensory predominant polyneuropathy were studied. The results using cannabis ranging in potency between 6% and 8% THC showed a differential scale pain intensity decrease of 3.3 points.[5] The concept of finding the most effective dose was explored in a study of patients with chronic neuropathic pain from CRPS, peripheral neuropathy or focal nerve or spinal cord injury. Comparable pain reduction was found for the smoked higher dose (7% THC content by weight) or lower dose (3.5%) groups.[6] In a follow-up study, they took it a step further. Patients with central and peripheral neuropathic pain inhaled vaporized medium-dose (3.53%), low-dose (1.29%) or placebo cannabis. Low dose was found to be as effective a pain reliever as the medium.[7] In another study, they found the opposite effect, that the higher concentration was the most effective for pain reduction.[8] Cannabis with three different potencies of THC (2.5%, 6% and 9.4%) was administered in a single smoked inhalation three times daily. Similar results were found for patients with diabetic neuropathy, with vaporized cannabis of 3 strengths, the highest, 7% being the most effective.[9] This clearly shows the limitation of understanding the one dose for all approach. Another factor important in dose understanding is the severity of the condition as well as the subject's endocannabinoid tone.

Sativex has been approved in Great Britain for use in the treatment of neuropathic pain in multiple sclerosis, and proven effective for pain and spasticity.[10,11] Nabiximols have also been studied with diabetic peripheral neuropathy, chemotherapy-induced neuropathic pain and peripheral or central neuropathic pain. Neuropathic pain patients receiving Sativex experienced a 14% reduction in pain compared to placebo.[12] In a study of peripheral pain patients using a cannabis spray, 36% of patients in the cannabis spray treatment group achieved at least a 30% improvement in pain scores, compared to 20% in the placebo group.[13] These were self-titrated dosing studies with a great variance in sprays, from 4–18 sprays/day in one and an average of 14 in the other (range not given).

A review of published data concluded:

> Inhaled cannabis results in short term reductions in chronic neuropathic pain for one in every five to six patients treated. Dose dependency further supports the notion of cannabis effect on neuropathy, suggesting that inhaled cannabis may be about as potent as gabapentin.[14]

Another review was more cautious, saying, "Cannabis-based medicines probably increase the number of people achieving (neuropathic) pain relief of 30% or greater compared with placebo . . . [but] there is a lack of good evidence that any cannabis-derived product works for any chronic neuropathic pain."[15] The director of Center for Medicinal Cannabis Research that supported much of this research presented an ethical and practical viewpoint on the use of cannabis for painful peripheral neuropathy. "The data suggest, on balance, that cannabis may represent a reasonable alternative or adjunct to treatment of patients with serious painful peripheral neuropathy for whom other remedies have not provided fully satisfactory results."[16]

Most of the earlier studies showed approximately 15–30% reduction in pain using cannabis as compared to placebo, using a range of 5–125 mg of cannabinoid extract or inhalation 3–4x/day of cannabis that was not as strong as is commonly used by current patients. Because dosage is critical to analgesia effects, it's difficult to extrapolate to patient use, especially if tolerance has developed. Modulation of pain is a uniquely individual experience, not only as regard perception but also one's own endocannabinoid tone and tolerance to cannabis.

Patients often report that they achieve better control of neuropathic pain with cannabis than with many other medications and can often decrease or eliminate their need for Neurontin or Lyrica. Often neuropathic pain and neuropathy require ongoing, chronic administration of cannabis for best results, weeks or months of ongoing treatment. For example, post-herpetic neuralgia may last for months, but over time, with cannabis therapy the pain improves. How much of that is due to cannabis has yet to be determined, although positive effects were documented using a topical cannabinoid receptor agonist for post-herpetic neuralgia. Over half of the subjects noted a mean pain reduction of 87.8%.[17]

PATIENT REPORTS

To move on to patient results from my practice, I have seen adult patients with neuropathic pain of all ages. Although advanced chronic neuropathic pain usually was not a complaint until an older age, from the 60s through the 90s. The more severe cases, such as those involving CRPS, require a long time to see improvement, but it was possible. While all cases fall under the category of "neuropathic" pain, the more prevalent ones in my patient population, such as peripheral neuropathy and CRPS, are listed in their own section. Here are a few illustrative case reports.

NEUROPATHIC PAIN

Patient 1: This is a 73-year-old female with post-herpetic neuralgia for 11 years, also diagnosed with rheumatoid arthritis and lupus. Her medications included prednisone 2.5 mg 3x/week and a topical ketamine-gabapentin cream for thoracic neuralgia. She started using a CBD/THC 20:1 tincture erratically, not 3x/day as advised. By our next visit, she had been started on Oxycontin, and complained of ongoing low back and thoracic pain. She was finally taking 10 mg of tincture 3x/day and using topical cannabis, which she stated did help the pain.

Pearls: It's important to treat chronic neuropathic pain with a sufficient dose of cannabis. Here this was provided by internal doses of a CBD/THC tincture 3x/day plus added topical. This case demonstrates efficacy for CBD-rich cannabis, which is expected to help inflammatory and neuropathic pain. Of course, she used more THC, perhaps she would not have needed as much Oxycontin.

Patient 2: This is a 74-year-old female with pain from post-polio syndrome, which is not classified exactly as neuropathic pain, but nerve pain can be a component. She stated that she felt pain everywhere. Her right leg was weaker and shorter. She was already taking tramadol 100 mg 3x/day, which she didn't like due to side effects. She was on 900 mg of gabapentin/day. Her experience with cannabis consisted of using an edible chocolate, which made her sick. She started on a CBD/THC 1:1 tincture, which was dosed at 10 mg 3x/day. She reported immediate muscle relaxation, decreased pain, but the pain was still "everywhere." She also thought cannabis was helping to process body–mind interaction. I then advised weaning of the tramadol, doubling the dose of the tincture and remaining on gabapentin. We did not have another follow-up.

Pearls: I included this case because it is representative of other patients I've treated with post-polio syndrome. Cannabis seems to help most of these patients due to its multifactorial function for pain management, muscle relaxant and mood management.

Patient 3: This is a 57-year-old female with RSD of the arm, which was amputated at the elbow due to infection. She had multiple medical problems besides chronic neuropathic pain, including gastroparesis, brain trauma from a motor vehicle accident in the past, biliary cirrhosis and low back and neck pain. She had a C2–C7 spinal fusion. Her medications were numerous, the most relevant being gabapentin 2700 mg/day, oxycodone 15 mg 2×/day, fentanyl 25ug patch and Skelaxin 800 mg 2×/day. She had been using medicinal cannabis for several years, a few drops of concentrated oils day and night. Her dosage was relatively high, so dosing by oil was more economical. The daytime mix was CBD/THC 1:1, and the p.m. dose was CBD/THC 3:7 ratio. She was taking a total of 100 mg cannabinoids/day. She developed cauda equina syndrome over the next year with severe pain and increased her cannabis dose to 30 mg 3–4×/day plus 100 mg at night. I knew tolerance was an issue, but there seemed to be no good solution. I advised switching to a low dose of CBN, maybe 5–10 mg for sleep instead of the 100 mg of the CBD/THC mix. After lumbar surgery her pain improved, she did not find CBN and stayed on 200 mg of cannabinoids/day for the next year. We did discuss a 1 day/week tolerance break, but that did not happen. Her RSD and pain remained the same on this ongoing regimen.

Pearls: I could not tell how much cannabis was helping in pain management in this patient, because she was already using it at high doses when we met. She said it helped, and was afraid to miss even 1 day/week for a tolerance break. I was more supportive here than instructive, as nothing I said really made a difference in her use over the course of five visits in 3 years. I'm not sure the RSD showed any improvement, likely not. This is a complex case with multiple medical issues. Sometimes not getting worse is the best we can achieve.

Patient 4: This is a 59-year-old female with RSD in her arm of 20-year duration. She had a 20-year history of opiate use, then switched to tramadol for the past 3 years. She had had 20 nerve blocks over the past 20 years. She was taking baclofen 20 mg at night as well. She had used cannabis before, but not medicinally. I advised a CBD/THC 1:1 tincture to start, 10 mg 3×/day. This did help to reduce the nerve pain, plus we added topical for shoulder and neck pain, which helped. She was able to discontinue tramadol. .

Pearls: I prefer to use a CBD/THC 1:1 mix whenever the patient can tolerate it, as it seems to bring better results for pain management than products with a higher CBD ratio. This level, 30 mg cannabinoids/day is a great dose for ongoing therapy as tolerance is not as great an issue.

PERIPHERAL NEUROPATHY

Patient 1: This is a 60-year-old male with chronic pain in one knee and both feet diagnosed with peripheral polyneuropathy with pain, burning and numbness. The etiology of the neuropathy was unclear. He had been using cannabis for 5 years, mostly by smoking. He was tapering off Nucynta, which he'd been on for 6 months following a knee replacement surgery. He was also bipolar, and on Abilify and Latuda. By the next year, he was off the Nucynta, but had developed pedal edema, also of unknown cause, contributing to his extremity pain. He was on a diuretic. He reported a newly diagnosed bladder tumor and was awaiting surgery. His cannabis use was now by vaping with an indica tincture some nights. By the next year, his tumor had been removed, and he had done chemotherapy. His knee was post-surgical yet again he was in a wheelchair. His pedal edema persisted, as well as the peripheral neuropathy. His cannabis use remained the same. At our last visit, he was out of the wheelchair, but all conditions remained. He finally increased his cannabis dose, now taking 30 mg THC capsules one/day. I advised him to double that and/or to add a CBD/THC 1:1 capsule.

Pearls: Patients with peripheral neuropathy often do not initially understand the need for a therapeutic level of cannabis, especially if they've been smoking it. Here it took 3 years to reach a therapeutic dose. They feel the mental effects at a much lower dose than is required to treat the neuropathy.

Patient 2: This is an 81-year-old male with a long history of peripheral neuropathy causing pain and poor sleep. He reported no help with gabapentin, and was on no pain medicine. He swiftly became endeared to me as a client when he published an editorial in our local paper, which said in part:

> Since the first night I tried the drops, the swelling in my ankles and the peripheral neuropathy pain in my feet disappeared. And for the first time in many years, I sleep well every night and for as long as I wish.

He was so pleased, as his primary care physician and neurologist told him that "the neuropathy was progressive, incurable and untreatable." He started on a CBD/THC 20:1 tincture, about 5 mg 2×/day, and an edible cookie to sleep at night. He did notice pain relief the first year, but complained of the neuropathy progressing with time. When heel pain increased to a high enough level to impede walking, we added topical with not much effect. Over the 5 years we worked together, his tincture dosage increased to 10 mg 3×/day, with continued 10–20 mg THC at night. Cost was an issue. He was receiving a senior discount from the dispensary, but he could not afford to increase his cannabis dose.

Pearls: Peripheral neuropathy in the elderly is not an uncommon problem. In this patient, his diabetes was short-lived and had reversed with weight loss, but it likely contributed to his problem. I really wanted this patient to find enduring relief, but that was not the case. We often talked about the progressive nature of this disease, wondering if his symptoms might have been worse off cannabis. In other patients with less significant neuropathy, I have noticed longer-lasting pain relief.

CHRONIC REGIONAL PAIN SYNDROME

Patient 1: This is a 38-year-old female with a 7-year history of CRPS following unilateral limb injury and subsequent injuries in both feet and arms and a motor vehicle accident. She had had several nerve blocks, but was on no medication except Lidoderm topically. She experienced constant chronic burning pain in all extremities and her back. She was unable to tolerate much weight-bearing in her feet. She had already tried CBD-rich cannabis, a 20:1 CBD/THC mix which did not help. On a 1:1 CBD/THC mix by tincture she experienced paranoia; therefore, it had too much THC for her. She said the 8:1 mix did help somewhat. She was able to tolerate one drop of an 8:1 mix 3×/day, which wasn't enough to do anything. Over the next year, we slowly titrated her up to 5 mg of the 8:1 tincture 3×/day and 5 mg of a 1:1 tincture at night. Our goal was 50 mg/cannabinoids/day. After 6 more months, we reached 40 mg cannabinoids/day derived from these two ratios. The nerve pain was slowly lessening. She reported that if she missed one dose the pain increased. We began to talk about a tolerance reduction strategy, perhaps 1 day off per week. She was able to accomplish this, but the pain was debilitating on that day off, and worse in the cold. After a while she switched to using a cannabis oil concentrate instead of tincture, but continues on this 40 mg/day regimen. At our last meeting after 4 long years of recovery, she was walking over 1 mile/day and beginning to wean down her cannabis dose.

Pearls: CRPS is extremely difficult to reverse and takes much time, as does neuropathic pain reduction with cannabis. Moderate doses are required, hopefully at least 50 mg/day, which can be costly and produce tolerance. Lots of patience and trust that improvement is possible, albeit slow is required. Another not unusual facet exhibited by this patient is sensitivity to medications, including cannabis. Taking a year to titrate up to this moderate dose is much slower than ordinary.

Patient 2: This is a 53-year-old female with multiple diagnoses associated with chronic pain, the pain being due to CRPS, as well as depression, muscle spasms, insomnia, also asthma associated with scoliosis. She had a spinal fusion at a young age from C3–C6 and C7-T12 to correct scoliosis. She had previously been on opiates, Nucynta 100 mg 2×/day, but was switched to tramadol. She was also using several asthma inhalers. She was new to cannabis use. I advised she take a CBD/THC tincture in a 2:1 ratio twice/day and an indica tincture before bed. She ended up doing this at a dose of 20 mg 2×/day plus 15 mg before bed plus 5 mg of a sativa tincture in the a.m. That's an average of 60 mg of cannabinoids/day. She reported that this helped the nerve pain a lot. Due to financial reasons, she ended up switching to a CBD isolate available over the counter. She said she felt best taking 500–1,000 mg/day of this product during the day, and added 3 mg of THC by tincture to supplement it, still using the indica tincture before bed. It seemed to me she did not do as well on this regimen, complaining again of poor sleep, leg and back pain. We discussed a tolerance break and resumption of cannabis-derived CBD, so she could resume a lower dose. Ultimately, this patient moved to a non-cannabis approved state and had to stay on the CBD isolate.

Pearls: Whenever 50 mg of cannabis or more is used daily, tolerance, or at least levels close to saturation, may occur and a plateau may result. Here, the increase to hundreds of milligrams of CBD, while more readily available, definitely raises tolerance issues, and is not preferable. As expected, a small amount of THC added to CBD provides better neuropathic pain relief.

CANNABIS THERAPY SUMMARY

Cannabis has been repeatedly proven effective for neuropathic pain relief, but often only up to 30% in pain reduction. How much relief do we expect from cannabis in patients already on opiates and anti-epileptics with many years of chronic neuropathic pain? Probably not much. For chronic neuropathic pain, high doses of cannabinoids are often required, up to or more than 50 mg/day. It's preferable to have a goal of a CBD/THC ratio of 1:1, but due to psychoactivity this is not always possible. In many cases, CBD-rich dosing during the day, with a THC-rich indica before bed is a good resolution. This protocol has been applied effectively not only in the cases I have illustrated previously but also for patients with diabetic neuropathy. Some chronic neuropathic cases can reverse, when the condition is not progressive, but in most cases, slowing the progression of the disease and alleviation of some of the pain is the best we can do, and this may take a long period of time, not days or weeks, but up to years. For the conditions reviewed here, it is important to remember that we are dealing with neuropathy, not merely neuropathic pain. Both THC and CBD inhibit glutamate neurotoxicity, are neuroprotective and display antioxidant properties. I do like to include both CBD and THC as they are both useful for neuropathy, but THC may be more effective for analgesia. I've noticed more effective pain relief with acute cases of neuropathic pain, such as new onset shingles. Another patient with post-herpetic neuralgia on the face dutifully applied topical for monthly flare-ups with resolution of symptoms. If used three times/day internally and externally in these cases, it does facilitate resolution of symptoms, hopefully so the case does not become chronic. Often topical application proves useful as an adjunctive therapy for peripheral neuropathic pain, but internal consumption is required to address the neuropathy.

REFERENCES

1. Rahn EJ, Hohmann AG. Cannabinoids as pharmacotherapies for neuropathic pain: from the bench to the bedside. *Neurotherapeutics.* 2009;6(4):713–737.
2. Hill KP, Palastro MD, Johnson B, Ditre JW. Cannabis and pain: a clinical review. *Cannabis Cannabinoid Res.* 2017;2(1):96–104.
3. Vučković S, Srebro D, Vujović KS, Vučetić Č, Prostran M. Cannabinoids and pain: new insights from old molecules. *Front Pharmacol.* 2018;9:1259.
4. Abrams D, Jay CA, MD, Shade SB, et al. Cannabis in painful HIV-associated sensory neuropathy. *Neurology.* 2007;68:515–521.
5. Ellis RJ, Toperoff W, Vaida F, et al. Smoked medicinal cannabis for neuropathic pain in HIV: a randomized, cross-over clinical trial. *Neuropsychopharmacology.* 2009;34(3):672–680.
6. Wilsey B, Marcotte T, Tsodikov A, et al. A randomized, placebo-controlled, crossover trial of cannabis cigarettes in neuropathic pain. *J Pain.* 2008;9(6):506–521.
7. Wilsey B, Marcotte T Deutsch R, et al. Low-dose vaporized cannabis significantly improves neuropathic pain. *J Pain.* 2013;14(2):136–148.
8. Ware MA, Wang T, Shapiro S, et al. Smoked cannabis for chronic neuropathic pain: a randomized controlled trial. *CMAJ.* 2010;182(14):E694–E701.
9. Wallace MS, Marcotte TD, Umlauf A, et al. Efficacy of inhaled cannabis on painful diabetic neuropathy. *J Pain.* 2015;16:616–627.
10. Rog DJ, Nurmikko TJ, Friede T, Young CA. Randomized controlled trial of cannabis based medicine in central neuropathic pain due to multiple sclerosis. *Neurology.* 2005;65:812–819.
11. Rog DJ, Nurmikko TJ, Young CA. Oromucosal δ9-tetrahydrocannabinol/cannabidiol for neuropathic pain associated with multiple sclerosis: an uncontrolled, open-label, 2-year extension. *Clin Ther.* 2007;29:2068–2079.

12. Nurmikko TJ, Serpell MG, Hoggart B, et al. Sativex successfully treats neuropathic pain characterized by allodynia: a randomised, double-blind, placebo-controlled clinical trial. *Pain*. 2007;133:210–220.
13. Serpell M, Ratcliffe S, Hovorka J, et al. A double-blind, randomized, placebo-controlled, parallel group study of THC/CBD spray in peripheral neuropathic pain treatment. *Eur J Pain*. 2014;18:999–1012.
14. Andreae MH, et al. Cannabis for chronic neuropathic pain: a meta-analysis of individual patient data. *J Pain*. 2015;16(12):1121–1232.
15. Mücke M, Phillips T, Radbruch L, Petzke F, Häuser W. 2018. Cannabis-based medicines for chronic neuropathic pain in adults. *Cochrane Database Syst Rev*. 2018 Mar 7;3(3):CD012182.
16. Grant I. Medicinal cannabis and painful sensory neuropathy. *Virtual Mentor*. 2013;15(5):466–469.
17. Phan NQ, Siepmann D, Gralow I, Ständer S. Adjuvant topical therapy with a cannabinoid receptor agonist in facial postherpetic neuralgia. *J Dtsch Dermatol Ges*. 2010;8(2):88–91.

40 Opiate Substitution

OPIATE SUBSTITUTION AND CANNABIS

Opioid overuse for pain management has become a growing community health problem and has proven not tenable as a long-term strategy for patients. In some cases, the inability to continue on prescribed opiates has led to use of street drugs such as black market Oxycontin or heroin. Traditional opioid replacement therapies such as methadone or buprenorphine may not be readily available in all communities. Even conservative organizations such as the American Medical Association or state governments have considered cannabis to have a potential role in an opiate substitution program.[1-5] A comprehensive meta-analysis of the opioid sparing effect of cannabinoids concludes: "The potential for cannabinoids to reduce opioid dose requirements and extend the duration of effective analgesia should not be understated."[6] A survey of physicians regarding cannabis use as adjunct to opioid therapy revealed that 84% believed opioids had greater risks than cannabis. While 75% of primary care physicians would consider using cannabis as adjunct therapy, only 35% of pain specialists agreed.[7] There is yet much education to be done regarding the benefits of cannabis therapy in opiate substitution.

Cannabis replacement for opioids is a prevalent form of harm reduction (see Chapter 30). Using age-adjusted opioid analgesic overdose death rates, the states with legal medical cannabis laws have been shown to be associated with significantly lower state-level opioid overdose rates.[2] Cannabis is opioid-sparing in chronic pain patients. In a recent survey of 3,000 chronic pain medical cannabis patients, 81–97% preferred cannabis as an opioid alternative.[8] In a survey of patients' use of cannabis with opioid medications, 59% of participants self-reported they stopped using their medication completely (100% substitution) and a further 18% reduced their use to one quarter of previous levels. Participants who substituted for opioids used more cannabis per day as compared to substitution for other pharmaceuticals, were more likely to report extract/oral use as their primary delivery method and to use extracts on a daily basis.[9] In fact, clinically it does require sustained long-acting dosing of cannabis to substitute effectively for opiates. Studies of this topic have shown that cannabis can decrease opioid consumption and/or prevent opioid dose escalation, with decreases in opioid use by 50% or more in some cases.[10-12] The one study that was an outlier to these results was a 4-year survey of opiate and cannabis use with chronic non-cancer pain patients in Australia. They concluded that cannabis did not reduce opiod use. On closer examination of the study, the frequency of cannabis use in the past month for the duration of the study, that was recorded as "none" ranged from 86% to 91%, while only 3–6% used it daily or near daily. It implies that the great majority of those surveyed were occasional cannabis users. Furthermore, by the end of the survey, 60% said they would use it more frequently if they had access.[13] Clearly, there is a difference, as there should be, between recreational use with poor

DOI: 10.1201/9781003098201-51

access and having a cannabis medicinal protocol sufficient to counter the strong effects of daily opioid use.

Opioids and cannabinoids both provide antinociception through G-protein coupled mechanisms in the spinal cord, and act along parallel pathways. Many studies have explored synergistic interactions between them. Although the relationship between opioid and cannabinoid systems is becoming better established, the specific mechanisms of their interaction is complex and not fully elucidated. Endocannabinoid activity may be critical for endorphin regulation. Reviews of relevant animal research of cannabinoid synergy with opiates summarize potential mechanisms and conclusions.[14,15] Studies with cannabinoid receptors suggest CB1 and mu-opiate receptor involvement in synergy, as well as demonstrating that THC causes a release of endogenous opioids acting on delta and kappa opioid receptors. Synergy has also been shown in the reverse as well, with opioids amplifying the antinociception induced by THC. Amplification of analgesic effect of up to ten times using both has been documented. A review of cannabinoid opiod interaction proposes that "With cannabinoid/opioid therapy one may be able to produce long-term antinociceptive effects at doses devoid of substantial side effects, while preventing the neuronal biochemical changes that accompany tolerance."[16]

Studies of human subjects verified improved analgesia with THC and opiates.[17] In a study of chronic pain, patients on opiates used vaporized cannabis in a regulated setting for 5 days, and pain decreased by 27%. Pharmacokinetics for both substances were not changed compared to single use, and cannabis was found safe to use with opiates.[18] We know that cannabinoids can reduce chronic pain (see Chapter 25). There is evidence that THC does not appear to be as effective as a CBD/THC mix. Patients with intractable cancer pain already on high-dose opiates (271 mg of oral morphine equivalents/day) using cannabis extracts containing approximately a CBD/THC 1:1 mix had more significant pain reduction than those on THC alone. Patients were allowed to self-titrate a CBD/THC or THC extract, dosing by number of sprays/day for 2 weeks. The mean number of sprays/day taken by the CBD/THC group (9.26 = 48 mg of cannabinoids/day) was minimally higher than the THC group (8.47 = 44 mg of cannabinoids/day). There was no change in opiate use, but twice as many patients taking the mix showed a reduction of more than 30% from baseline pain when compared with placebo, while the THC group scores did not change in a statistically significant manner.[19] This study is instructive in several points. One, that 2 weeks may be an insufficient amount of time to register a decrease in opiate use, especially in severe pain patients with high opiate use. Two, that although cannabinoids can cause an average reduction of up to 30% in chronic pain, intractable severe pain in patients already on opiates cannot be managed by the doses employed here. And three, that the inclusion of CBD may be bringing an added component to decreasing pain scores, beyond analgesia and synergy with opiates attributed to THC. It would be convenient if CBD-dominant extracts accomplished the same results, but CBD synergism with opiates has not been substantiated, although it was found safe to use.[20] Animal studies do suggest a role for CBD in reducing opiate cravings. "Overall, CBD was found to have an impact on the intoxication and relapse phase of opioid addiction. Data on its effect during the withdrawal phase remain conflicting and vary based on co-administration of other cannabinoids such as THC."[21] The use of CBD to inhibit opioid craving, while using THC to amplify the analgesia obtained with opiates, has great therapeutic potential. Clinically, that is what we find.

Cannabis providing a therapeutic option for opiate users is not always how these results are represented. In a review critical of cannabis use, they concluded: "Those seeking treatment for opioid dependence, cannabis is consistently reported to be among the most frequently co-abused substances, along with benzodiazepines and cocaine. Estimates of cannabis use in this group have ranged anywhere from 20% to 95% of the population."[22] The question is, in an opioid-dependent population in treatment, does the 20–95% of patients who concurrently use cannabis mean they have a dual drug addiction, or is cannabis acting as an adjunctive medicine? Therein lies one of the ongoing challenges in interpreting published studies on this topic and how they are reported. During this time of transition and discernment, from cannabis being viewed as solely a "recreational" substance, to a medicine of utility, a change in bias encompassing relevant study design must be made. Researchers and clinicians need to be reminded that medicinal cannabis requires professional supervision for enhanced effectiveness, especially in complex medical conditions, such as those significant pain and/or with concurrent pharmaceutical prescription such as opiates.

PATIENT REPORTS

To move on to patient results from my practice, I have seen many hundreds of patients who tried to use cannabis to reduce their opiate usage. Most patients were in the mid-adult age range, although a surprising number of the elderly also had opiate dependence. Contrary to the survey results noted earlier, I would say that only about 20% of the patients who presented wanting to get off opiates were successful. Many were able to lower their dose, but completely getting off although possible, was not common. There are many patients I did not cover here, with poor outcomes for using cannabis as an opiate substitute. As far as patients being on a non-prescribed opiate, such as heroin, and wanting to switch to cannabis, or had done so in the past are concerned, this was rare in my patient population. We had little success with the few patients I've treated who had already been switched to suboxone, following a heroin addiction. Cannabis did not seem to make the suboxone wean move along any faster or easier. Here are a few illustrative case reports.

Patient 1: This is a 59-year-old male first seen for chronic low back pain due to a 10-year history of herniated discs. He recently started hydrocodone 5 mg 3×/day for the pain. He wanted to use cannabis to replace the Vicodin. He had no recent cannabis use. I advised vaporizing or tincture. By the next year, his pain was much increased throughout his back and pelvis. He had been diagnosed with stage IV lung cancer, with back and pelvis metastases. He had undergone radiation, was on chemotherapy and was using a THC-rich tincture during the day and an indica chocolate at night. His opiate use had progressed to Oxycontin 40 mg 2×/day. He continued to use cannabis for symptom control, for mood, sleep and appetite. At our next visit, he reported that he had totally gotten off the opiates, but resumed them again after a hip replacement surgery, then fracture, then redo, all in the past year. Now his usage was up to Oxycontin 80 mg 3×/day plus oxycodone 80 mg every 4 hours as needed. Over the next year, he continued to use cannabis as an adjunct medicine, while his opiate dose remained ongoing at Oxycontin 120 mg 3x/day. He said cannabis still did help with pain.

Pearls: This is a case of cannabis being used more for palliative care than for pain management. Originally the patient came in for pain management, but his pain evolved into too great a burden for cannabis alone to be effective. At this level, 360 mg/day of Oxycontin, it's good to know that a 10 mg dose of cannabis could have any effect at all, for mood, sleep etc.

Patient 2: This is an 89-year-old female with back and hip pain, mild dementia and pruritis. She was brought in by a caregiver, as she was not ambulating due to loss of balance and in a wheelchair. She had been on opiates for 3 years and was taking Oxycontin 20 mg/day, and oxycodone 5 mg prn, usually 2x/day. She was on five other medications, some for the pruritis. Her arms and chest were covered with a red rash that itched. Her liver function tests were normal. Her caregiver agreed to give her the cannabis I advised and proceed with the opiate wean. She ended up taking CBD/THC 20:1 10 mg 2x/day and CBD/THC 2:1 7.5 mg at night by capsule. By the following year, she was off all opiates, and switched to Tylenol 2x/day. Her rash and pruritis were gone.

Pearls: It's never too late, and you're never too old to benefit from cannabis, even at low doses. Is she doing better overall from having less medicine, no opiates, no Benadryl? Probably. Her itching is gone and she says her pain is okay. Perhaps the pruritis was a side effect of some of her medications, now reduced. Following the pill regimen managed by a caregiver is helpful in providing consistent pain medication, including cannabis, especially in the elderly.

Patient 3: This is a 55-year-old male with Stickler syndrome. His symptoms included blindness, joint pain and insomnia. His pain was not only physical, but emotional, as he was adjusting to advancing loss of vision. He was new to cannabis use. His pain was such that he was taking methadone 10 mg 3x/day for 15 years, which wasn't working as it had been previously. He also took 5 mg of Ambien to sleep for 3 years. I advised indica chocolate at night and a THC-rich tincture during the day. By the next year, he had built up to a high usage of cannabis, which was helping his pain. He took sativa honey during the day plus vaporizing throughout the day, and indica capsules for sleep. He said it helped his mood a lot as well. I advised a tolerance break, which he tried to do 1 day/week. By the next year, he was on 30–40 mg of cannabis 3x/day as well as methadone 10 mg 2x/day and Norco 10 mg 3x/day. He now wished to use cannabis to reduce his opiate dosage. I gave him a weaning protocol, but the problem was that his cannabis dosage was also high, so this would be a challenge. Unfortunately, that was our last visit.

Pearls: Chronic pain management is multifactorial, requiring mood adjustment, pain adjustment and symptom control. When opiates are involved, it is instructive to recall that they function not only to control pain, but they affect mood as well. Sometimes it's not the physical pain that keeps patients drawn to their effects, but the emotional pain as well. I believe this patient advanced to a high dosage of cannabis because it brought him much sought-after emotional release. Managing tolerance is not only imperative for opiates, but for cannabis as well. Unfortunately, not many patients understand the importance of tolerance management.

Patient 4: This is an 82-year-old male, who was a retired physician. He came in stating he would like to get off opiates, which he'd been on for 4 years. His pain was in his joints, due to advanced osteoarthritis. He already had a hip and knee replaced. He was using a walker due to leg weakness and poor balance. At our first visit, his MS Contin dose was 30 mg 2×/day, which he'd been on for the past 4 years, plus additional 5 mg Percocet, usually 4×/day. He was new to cannabis use. He started on a CBD/THC 2:1 tincture, about 7 mg 3×/day. On this regimen he was able to discontinue the Percocet and cut the MS Contin in half in 1 year. That's more than a 50% reduction. By the following year, he was off opiates entirely, a 100% reduction. Cannabis continued as his sole pain management medicine. He was also able to graduate off the walker with a knee brace for support.

Pearls: Here we have a compliant patient, who obviously understood what he wanted and what was involved as he had medical knowledge. But as a patient, he didn't know how to achieve his goal without help. Fortunately, even a low THC dose of cannabis was able to facilitate his opiate substitution. We wouldn't ordinarily expect 2 mg of THC with 5 mg of CBD, 3×/day (which is essentially what he was on) to be enough to meet his needs, but it was. Remembering that in naive patients with no cannabinoid tolerance, especially in the elderly, low doses might suffice.

CANNABIS THERAPY SUMMARY

It is beyond the scope of this book to delve into the challenges of treating opiate addiction, but therapeutics are inadequate and cannabis is not a panacea. For it to be a successful adjunct therapy, the patient needs to be committed and would benefit from supportive coaching or psychotherapy. Many patients will not be cooperative with opiate weaning, even when they say they'd like to achieve that result. For example, there was another elderly patient in her 80s who was truly addicted/attached to her opiates, about 60 mg/day of Norco, also with the aid of a caregiver. Every year she came to see me to be able to continue using cannabis, which she smoked, and every year we talked about using it therapeutically to decrease her opiate use. Yet, she gave her caregiver a very hard time, was verbally abusive, if she dared to lower the opiate dosage. The exact opposite of the elderly patient reported earlier. Don't be surprised when this kind of resistance happens, as it often does with addictive substances. Another case was the 60-year-old male patient who had been on opiates for 30 years. His dose was high, up to about 360 mg of Oxycontin per day. His doctor told him he could no longer prescribe those high doses so he needed to cut back. He and his wife came in to see if cannabis could help. She did most of the talking, as he seemed kind of dissociated, not too involved in the conversation. I could tell he had no interest in finding a solution here, but came at his wife's insistence. I didn't even waste my time reviewing his options, what cannabis to use, etc. I looked them both straight in the eye, and said "I don't think you're prepared to follow through on whatever I might suggest. You may need to go to an inpatient rehabilitation program, or at least be in a supportive counseling environment." I commented, "Sir, you have been numb, physically and emotionally for 30 years. Are you both ready for your feelings to come back, to feel not only your physical pain, but your life?" Needless to say, they left my office without a cannabis approval and never returned. At best, you can offer alternatives, but the patient has to want to take it.

As far as the dose range that has been successful is concerned, I've seen anywhere from 5 mg of a CBD/THC mix 3×/day be helpful, up to 50 mg of THC-rich cannabis 3×/day. The dose one might need is individualized, and depends on the patient's opiate dose, pain level and cannabis tolerance, but always should include some THC for its synergistic properties. Many patients do best on a CBD/THC 1:1 mix. The success of opiate reduction depends upon so many factors, not least of which are the underlying motivation, the level of pain, the type of opiate and its dosage, the duration of opiate dependence and emotional factors.

REFERENCES

1. Wiese B, Wilson-Poe AR. Emerging evidence for cannabis' role in opioid use disorder. *Cannabis Cannabinoid Res.* 2018;3.1.
2. Bachhuber MA, Saloner B, Cunningham CO, Barry CL. Medical cannabis laws and opioid analgesic overdose mortality in the United States, 1999–2010. *JAMA Intern Med.* 2014;174(10):1668–1673.
3. Hayes MJ, Brown MS. Legalization of medical marijuana and incidence of opioid mortality. *JAMA Intern Med.* 2014;174(10):1673–1674.
4. Bellnier T, Brown GW, Ortega TR. Preliminary evaluation of the efficacy, safety, and costs associated with the treatment of chronic pain with medical cannabis. *Ment Health Clin* [Internet]. 2018;8(3):110–115.
5. Lucas P. Rationale for cannabis-based interventions in the opioid overdose crisis. *Harm Reduct J.* 2017;14:58.
6. Nielsen S, Sabioni P, Trigo JM, et al. Opioid-sparing effect of cannabinoids: a systematic review and meta-analysis. *Neuropsychopharmacology.* 2017;42(9):1752–1765.
7. Sideris A, Khan F, Boltunova A, et al. New York physicians' perspectives and knowledge of the state medical marijuana program. *Cannabis Cannabinoid Res.* 2018;3:74–84.
8. Reiman A, Welty M, Solomon P. Cannabis as a substitute for opioid based pain medication: patient self-report. *Cannabis Cannabinoid Res.* 2017;2(1):160–166.
9. Lucas P, Walsh Z. Medical cannabis access, use, and substitution for prescription opioids and other substances: a survey of authorized medical cannabis patients. *Int J Drug Policy.* 2017;42:30–35.
10. Boehnke KF, Litinas E, Clauw DJ. Cannabis use is associated with decreased opiate medication use in a retrospective cross-sectional survey of patients with chronic pain. *J Pain.* 2016;17:739–744.
11. Haroutounian S, Ratz Y, Ginosar Y, et al. The effect of medicinal cannabis on pain and quality-of-life outcomes in chronic pain: a prospective open-label study. *Clin J Pain.* 2016;32:1036–1043.
12. Lucas P, Baron EP, Jikome N. Medical cannabis patterns of use and substitution for opioids & other pharmaceutical drugs, alcohol, tobacco, and illicit substances: results from a cross-sectional survey of authorized patients. *Harm Reduct J.* 2019;16:9.
13. Campbell G, Hall WD, Peacock A, et al. Effect of cannabis use in people with chronic non-cancer pain prescribed opioids: findings from a 4-year prospective cohort study. *Lancet Public Health.* 2018;3:e341–e350.
14. Cichewicz DL. 2004. Synergistic interactions between cannabinoid and opioid analgesics. *Life Sci.* 74(11):1317–1324.

15. Bushlin I, Rozenfeld R, Devi LA. Cannabinoid-opioid interactions during neuropathic pain and analgesia. *Curr Opin Pharmacol.* 2010;10(1):80.
16. Welch SP. Interaction of the cannabinoid and opioid systems in the modulation of nociception. *Int Rev Psychiatry.* 2009;21:143–151.
17. Abrams DI, Couey P, Shade SB, Kelly ME, Benowitz NL. Cannabinoid-opioid interaction in chronic pain. *Clin Pharmacol Ther.* 2011;90(6):844–851.
18. Roberts JD, Gennings C, Shih M. Synergistic affective analgesic interaction between delta-9-tetrahydrocannabinol and morphine. *European J Pharmacol.* 2006;530(1–2):54–58.
19. Johnson JR, Burnell-Nugent M, Lossignol D, et al. An open-label extension study to investigate the long-term safety and tolerability of THC/CBD oromucosal spray and oromucosal THC spray in patients with terminal cancer-related pain refractory to strong opioid analgesics. *J Pain Symptom Manag.* 2013;46:207–218.
20. Manini AF, Yiannoulos G, Bergamaschi MM, et al. Safety and pharmacokinetics of oral cannabidiol when administered concomitantly with intravenous fentanyl in humans. *J Addict Med.* 2015;9:204–210.
21. Prud'homme M, Cata R, Jutras-Aswad D. Cannabidiol as an intervention for addictive behaviors: a systematic review of the evidence. *Subst Abuse.* 2015;9:33–38.
22. Scavone JL, Sterling RC, Van Bockstaele EJ. Cannabinoid and opioid interactions: implications for opiate dependence and withdrawal. *Neuroscience.* 2013;248:637–654.

41 Osteoarthritis, Joint Pain

OSTEOARTHRITIS, JOINT PAIN AND CANNABIS

This section focuses on the commonly encountered arthritis of aging, most often felt in the joints. Osteoarthritis (OA) affecting the spine is often diagnosed as back pain and is also presented in another section (see Chapter 21). Autoimmune-mediated arthritis is presented elsewhere as well (see Chapter 16). Osteoarthritis is a common, frequently painful condition, especially in the elderly. Research suggests that cannabis-based therapies may be effective in the treatment of arthritis and the other and degenerative back and joint disorders.[1] Patients are able to reduce their usage of potentially harmful non-steroidal anti-inflammatory drugs (NSAIDs) and/or opiates when using cannabis for arthritis or joint pain. The use of cannabis as a treatment for joint pain both internally and topically has been handed down as a folk-remedy and used for centuries. In fact, the common Mexican practice of soaking cold cannabis leaves in alcohol and applying the mix to joints has had a great influence on the use of cannabis in topical form. The Arthritis Society of Canada states:

> Since 2001, medical cannabis (also known as marijuana) has been a legal treatment option in Canada for certain health conditions, including arthritis. An estimated two thirds of Canadians who use cannabis for medical purposes do so to help manage arthritis symptoms.[2]

Survey results presented at the 2019 Annual European Congress of Rheumatology (EULAR) meeting stated that of 1,059 arthritis patients (22% were diagnosed with OA), 37% have tried cannabis, and of those, 97% said it helped their symptoms.[3]

Osteoarthritis was at one time considered a "noninflammatory arthritis," but this is now known to be simplistic and inflammation is an important component of joint damage. Cannabis and its constituents are effective for joint pain due to their antinociceptive, analgesic and anti-inflammatory properties (see Chapters 25 and 39 for a review of analgesic action). In addition, cannabis helps to loosen stiff joints due to its muscle-relaxant properties. A review of the anti-inflammatory action of cannabinoids summarizes:

> Studies have shown that cannabinoids, for the most part, suppress the production of cytokines in innate and adaptive immune responses, both in animal models and in human cell cultures. . . . [T]hese drugs might have anti-inflammatory effects and could therefore be used for the treatment of chronic inflammatory diseases.[4]

Evidence now exists to support the anti-inflammatory and analgesic properties of both cannabis and its main cannabinoids, not only CBD and THC but also THCA and CBDA, the forms found in raw cannabis. Cannabinoids have been shown to inhibit cyclooxygenase (COX) enzymes and affect the potency of NSAIDs potentially via modulation

DOI: 10.1201/9781003098201-52

of the COX pathway. In vitro studies showed that THC, THCA and CBD inhibited prostaglandin production, but CBDA stimulated it.[5] Another report showed CBDA has a dual inhibitory effect on COX, through downregulation and enzyme inhibition.[6] The difference is likely concentration dependent. The anti-inflammatory actions of THC are attributed in great part to its action at CB2 receptors and modulation of the COX pathway as described earlier. The anti-inflammatory effects of CBD are mediated via multiple pathways, acting at multiple receptors, CB receptors, adenosine A2A receptors, TRPV1 receptors, GPR55 receptors and CB2/5HT(1A).[7] The TRPV1 receptor was found to mediate the anti-hyperalgesic effect of CBD in a rat model of acute inflammation.[8] Another study in mice found that CBD suppresses persistent inflammatory and neuropathic pain by targeting the alpha-3 glycine receptors.[9] A major terpene in cannabis, β-caryophyllene, is also anti-inflammatory, and has been found to act at CB2 receptors. In an animal model of arthritis, it was concluded that atypical cannabinoid receptors are involved in joint nociception that may be advantageous for the treatment of inflammatory pain.[10] A study of CB2 receptor agonists in rats concluded:

> Joint damage and spinal CB2 receptor expression are correlated. . . . Activation of CB2 receptors inhibits central sensitization and its contribution to the manifestation of chronic OA pain. These findings suggest that targeting CB2 receptors may have therapeutic potential for treating OA pain.[11]

A recent review of how cannabis may act concludes:

> There is a widely held view that natural cannabis may have advantages over pure THC in a number of cases owing to the "added value" of the beneficial effects produced by these other molecules (other phytocannabinoids). . . . Although it does appear that CBD can be of benefit for treating pain under some circumstances, the molecular/cellular basis for such effects are still far from clear.[1]

In OA experimentally induced in rats, a one-time dose of injected CBD dose-dependently decreased joint firing rate, and increased withdrawal threshold and weight bearing, and acute joint inflammation was reduced. Pretreatment with CBD prevented the development of joint pain and was found to be neuroprotective.[12] A review of cannabinoid action for joint pain concluded that "limited clinical evidence has been provided to support this therapeutic use of cannabinoids, despite the promising preclinical data."[13] It is unfortunate that no reports from human studies are available to date, especially because OA and joint pain are such prevalent complaints in the general population. A recent review of endocannabinoid involvement and how cannabinoids may be used for the treatment of OA pain relies mostly on animal models and still documents the need for human research.[14] A clinical trial is in progress to compare the effects of vaporized CBD/THC combinations of different ratios in patients with knee OA.[15]

PATIENT REPORTS

To move on to patient results from my practice, I saw patients with arthritis with ages in the 50–90s. In fact, there were few elderly patients I saw that did not show some signs of OA. Many of the elderly had multiple diagnoses and are described elsewhere in patient reports of their more debilitating conditions. Here are a few illustrative case reports.

Patient 1: This is a 77-year-old female who complained of hip and hand pain for many years. She preferred not to take pharmaceuticals and was on none. She was new to cannabis use. She lived in a senior community and ended up referring several friends to see me as she was so pleased with the effects of cannabis. I advised a CBD/THC 2:1 tincture, which she took at a dose of only 5 mg/day. Over the course of the next year, she required a pacemaker and was put on Metoprolol and Eliquis. She sometimes used topical cannabis if her pain level increased. In a recent communication from her, she wrote,

> Most of my friends who started using cannabis when I did, about 7 years ago [she is now 84], have long given up self-dosing and returned to using opioids. I used to think they were too lazy to self-medicate, but the majority do not have a primary physician who supports cannabis use, as mine does. But my doctor can't tell me what cannabis product and dosage might work best for me. Sales staff at the dispensary is knowledgeable but certainly not a substitute for your own doctor. I've tried the oils but have gladly returned to the alcohol-based tincture. My go-to medicine is 2:1, which is exactly what you recommended for me that many years ago. I'm continuing to stay away from opioids by altering doses, which is pretty much what you told me I would need to do, and it works. Unfortunately, my friends have returned to drugs and now worry that their own doctors won't refill their opioid prescriptions due to overuse and much needed scrutiny.

Pearls: You have to work with a patient's belief system. This patient was already interested in using an alternative therapy, making it easier for her to stick with cannabis. Without a supportive belief system, it's difficult to stay the course. Having a supportive primary care physician is not ensured, and is so valuable, especially in the elderly.

Patient 2: This is a 65-year-old female with OA in most joints. She was taking Celebrex daily, and rare ibuprofen. She had been using cannabis for 3 years. She had just relocated from another "medical marijuana" state. She recounted that she did edibles to get off opiates, now she is smoking more. It sounded like she had received some good advice. I counseled her to use cannabis daily as an anti-inflammatory, which she did in the form of a CBD/THC 1:1 tincture and an indica edible at night. She was then able to discontinue Celebrex. She also added topical to her regimen.

Pearls: Pain is not the only motivating factor to use cannabis. You need to counsel patients about daily use as an anti-inflammatory in chronic conditions. If not specifically advised, if they don't hurt, they won't use it.

Patient 3: This is a 61-year-old male with chronic knee pain. He had three surgeries on his knee due to injuries, with ongoing pain. He had been using cannabis for many years, both smoked and topical applied to the knee, not daily. He was taking no medications, and had it treated by a chiropractor. He still enjoyed playing tennis, for which he used a brace. I advised applying the topical before the activity rather than after.

Pearls: This case illustrates the preventive use of cannabis to alleviate inflammation, here as a topical. But it is worthwhile to point out that both internal and external use are methods that can be used to keep the inflammatory response subdued, either in a chronic condition or before exercise.

Patient 4: This is a 66-year-old female with joint pain and swelling in multiple joints, the hips, shoulders, hands and feet. Her diagnoses included OA, shoulder bursitis and tendonitis and partial rotator cuff tear. She was taking sulindac 150 mg 2×/day, and was already using cannabis, as a chocolate once/day, dosage unknown. Over the next year, she increased cannabis to a chocolate 2×/day plus topical for her shoulders 2×/day. This continued for several more years, while the sulindac was discontinued and the patient was awaiting shoulder surgery.

Pearls: This is not an uncommon result, that sufficient cannabis dosing can decrease or eliminate the need for anti-inflammatory medications. The dosage is critical. Just as sulindac was prescribed at twice/day, so did cannabis by edible require twice/day dosage.

Patient 5: This is a 75-year-old female with OA in multiple joints and her back. She also had lumbar disc disease and experienced episodic sciatic pain. She already had one hip replaced and it was likely she'd need to have the other done. She was already using 10 mg of a CBD-rich tincture 2×/day and some vaporized cannabis. Over the next few years, her dosage did not change, but with a new diagnosis of shoulder bursitis her pain increased and insomnia due to pain became an issue. We then added a CBD/THC 1:1 tincture at night. During the next year, she had the other hip replaced. Continued pain post-surgery resulted in the addition of tramadol 25 mg 2×/day and she added an additional 5 mg of an indica edible before bed.

Pearls: This is typical with the elderly that the incorporation of THC-rich cannabis, to aid pain and sleep, is a slow process due to the patient's fear of and/or dislike of its psychoactive effects. The transition from a CBD/THC 20:1 mix, to a 1:1 mix, to effectively a 1:2 mix before bed is typical of how best to manage this progression. It is especially important in cases of insomnia due to pain to increase the sedation provided by cannabis in the p.m. dose.

CANNABIS THERAPY SUMMARY

Many components of cannabis are useful for this condition. Preparations with a high CBD/THC ratio and/or with THCA or CBDA, all of which would not be psychoactive make it an ideal therapeutic intervention. A good product would be a CBD/THC/THCA 1:1:1 mix, which acts on multiple receptors and which actually can be found in some dispensaries. Typical dosing may be 5–10 mg of cannabinoids 3×/day. Very few of the elderly were comfortable with smoking cannabis and I did not see it useful for this population, but for younger patients with joint pain, such as from trauma, smoking a THC-rich cultivar will likely be the preferred delivery chosen by the patient. As regard terpenes, β-myrcene, D-limonene and β-caryophyllene enhance anti-inflammatory action. As compared to immune-mediated arthritis, topical is likely to be helpful here, in addition to or instead of internal use. Topical applications of cannabis are especially useful for localized pain, such as at joints, and can be applied to the affected area without causing psychoactive effects.[16] One elderly patient was adamant that she only wanted to use topical as she was fearful even of CBD internally. She ended up using a topical with CBD and THC every morning. On follow-up she had discontinued all cannabis as she said it didn't help much. This patient was typical of most of the elderly patients who have trepidation about taking "marijuana" in any form. The issue here is to educate the patients to use the topical at least 3×/day, because it won't last all day. Of course, if the arthritic pain is mild, and is only felt occasionally then prn use is fine. An important example of this is preventive application of topical or an internal dose pre-exercise if a flare-up is expected post-exercise. It's common that patients think of cannabis as an adjunct to bring added relief, while staying on their NSAID or opiate. Keep suggesting it. Sometimes it takes several visits to get these patients to change habits. Patients often find that they can accomplish more movement, more stretching and feel less pain with less side effects when using cannabis.

REFERENCES

1. Miller RJ, Miller RE. Is cannabis an effective treatment for joint pain? *Clin Exp Rheumatol.* 2017;35 (Suppl. 107):S59–S67.
2. Arthritis Society. Position Paper. Research Medical Cannabis. www.arthritis.ca/AS/media/pdf/Treatment/Medical-Cannabis-Position-Paper-EN-FINAL.pdf Accessed October 3, 2019.
3. Gelman L. 57% of arthritis patients have tried marijuana or CBD for medical reasons (and more than 90% say it helped). https://creakyjoints.org/eular-2019/medical-marijuana-cbd-usage-arthritis-patients-study/ Accessed March 5, 2020.
4. Klein TW. Cannabinoid-based drugs as anti-inflammatory therapeutics. *Nat Rev Immunol.* 2005;5(5):400–411.
5. Ruhaak LR, Felth J, Karlsson PC, et al. Evaluation of the cyclooxygenase inhibiting effects of six major cannabinoids isolated from cannabis sativa. *Biol Pharm Bull.* 2011;34(5):774–778.
6. Burstein S. 2015. Cannabidiol (CBD) and its analogs: a review of their effects on inflammation. *Bioorg Med Chem.* 2015;23(7):1377–1385.
7. Pellati F, Borgonetti V, Brighenti V, Biagi M, Benvenuti S, Corsi L. Cannabis sativa L. and nonpsychoactive cannabinoids: their chemistry and role against oxidative stress, inflammation, and cancer. *Biomed Res Int.* 2018;1–15:Article ID 1691428.
8. Costa B, Trovato AE, Comelli F, Giagnoni G, Colleoni M. The non-psychoactive cannabis constituent cannabidiol is an orally effective therapeutic agent in rat chronic inflammatory and neuropathic pain. *Eur J Pharmacol.* 2007;556(1–3):75–83.
9. Xiong W, Cui T, Cheng K, et al. Cannabinoids suppress inflammatory and neuropathic pain by targeting alpha 3 glycine receptors. *J Exp Med.* 2012;209(6):1121–1134.
10. Malfait AM, Gallily R, Sumariwalla PF, et al. The non-psychoactive cannabis constituent cannabidiol is an oral anti-arthritic therapeutic in murine collagen-induced arthritis. *Proc Nat Acad Sci.* 2000;97:9561–9566.
11. Burston JJ, Sagar DR, Shao P, et al. Cannabinoid CB2 receptors regulate central sensitization and pain responses associated with osteoarthritis of the knee joint. *PLoS One.* 2013;8(11):e80440.
12. Philpott HT, O'Brien M, McDougall JJ. Attenuation of early phase inflammation by cannabidiol prevents pain and nerve damage in rat osteoarthritis. *Pain.* 2017;158(12):2442–2451.

13. La Porta C, Bura SA, Negrete R, Maldonado R. Involvement of the endocannabinoid system in osteoarthritis pain. *Eur J Neurosci.* 2014;39(3):485–500.

14. O'Brien M, McDougall JJ. Cannabis and joints: scientific evidence for the alleviation of osteoarthritis pain by cannabinoids. *Curr Opin Pharmacol.* 2018;40:104–109.

15. McGill University Health Centre/Research Institute. A randomized double blind placebo controlled, proof-of-concept, crossover clinical trial of vapourized cannabis in adults with painful osteoarthritis of the knee. https://clinicaltrials.gov/ct2/show/NCT02324777 Accessed March 18, 2020.

16. Hammell DC, Zhang LP, Ma F, et al. Transdermal cannabidiol reduces inflammation and pain-related behaviours in a rat model of arthritis. *Eur J Pain.* 2016;20(6):936–948.

42 Parkinson's Disease

PARKINSON'S DISEASE AND CANNABIS

One of the primary treatments for Parkinson's disease (PD) is the supplementation of dopamine (DA) production by its precursor, L-dopa, but tolerance develops and increasing doses are required over time. Only 1–5% of supplemental administered L-dopa makes it into the target neurons where it is needed. After continued use of such medications, side effects such as dyskinesias often develop making this a less than satisfactory outcome. Treatments that slow the progression of cell death of DA-producing cells in the substantia nigra have yet to be developed. Often concurrent therapies for fatigue, depression, low appetite or a sleep disorder are also needed. Cannabis can be therapeutic for PD in several respects. Aside from treating symptoms of tremor, dyskinesias, fatigue, agitation, sleep, etc., it may also be therapeutic for the disease and augment traditional treatment.

It is well-documented that cannabis can provide neuroprotection, slow cell death of neurons, promote repair, reduce inflammation in the brain and thus potentially slow the progression of neurodegenerative disease.[1] Endocannabinoids are abundant in dopaminergic pathways, including the striatum where they act as a retrograde feedback system to modulate dopamine transmission.[2] This activity is affected by either the activation or the blockade of the endocannabinoid system (ECS).[3] A review of the effect of THC on DA expression concludes that acute THC causes increases in DA release and neuron activity, but long-term use causes reduced release. They point out that preclinical studies done with humans have shown variable results.[2] Endocannabinoid levels are altered in PD patients. One study investigating the endocannabinoid levels in PD patients found a doubled anandamide level in their cerebrospinal fluid.[4]

Most of the research concerning PD and cannabis use comes from animal models and anecdotal patient reports. There are a few human studies, but they are small and yield inconclusive results. Several reviews are helpful.[3,5,6] To recap the most instructive findings, we start with a survey of 85 PD patients who ate raw, chewed cannabis, about ½ teaspoon of fresh or dried leaves daily. Patients reported subjective improvements, especially with dyskinesias after 3 months of use.[7] This is unusual because raw cannabis really speaks to the effect of cannabinoid acids, in this case THCA, not commonly studied. Help with dyskinesias was also reported with nabilone at a dose of 0.3 mg/kg.[8] This contrasts with a 4-week trial using Cannador, a THC/CBD 2:1 cannabis extract, in which up to a 0.25 mg/kg dose failed to show any significant effect on dyskinesias, parkinsonian traits, motor symptoms or quality of life.[9] The authors suggest, "As the phenomenology of dyskinesia in PD is complex it is possible that cannabinoids differentially affect different types of dyskinesia."[9] Alternatively, because many study participants did not reach the target dose, the dose was too low. This is an ongoing challenge with

DOI: 10.1201/9781003098201-53

PD patients to reach clinically relevant levels of THC-containing medicine due to its disorienting effects. Yet, patients with PD who smoked cannabis showed immediate improvement (after smoking 0.5 gram) on the standard Unified Parkinson's Disease Rating Scale (UPDRS). It dropped from 33 before they smoked to 24 after inhalation. This study also documented decrease in parkinsonian tremor.[10] Investigation into a non-psychoactive cannabinoid therapy led to a study of the effect of THCV on parkinsonian symptoms in animals. It showed reduced motor inhibition in parkinsonian rats, via increased glutamergic transmission. They propose that THCV might be therapeutic for use in humans.[11]

There are several studies that indicate that CBD, at high doses of 300 mg/day, can help quality of life, although not significant for the total UPDRS.[12] At a lower concentration, CBD was anecdotally reported to help REM sleep behavior disorder, a problem some PD patients develop. The doses used here were still high, most were 75 mg at night.[13] This is as expected knowing that high doses of CBD are sedating, while low doses may be alerting. PD patients with psychosis also benefit from CBD.[14] The authors hypothesize:

> Because the psychotic symptoms of these patients were possibly associated with the use of the dopaminergic drugs, the observed antipsychotic effect of CBD may have occurred through the attenuation of dopaminergic activity in areas related to the production of psychotic symptoms.

In an older study of the effect of CBD on PD patients, they found:

> At 100 to 200 mg/day, there was a decrease in clinical fluctuations and in dyskinesia scores (by 30%) without a significant worsening of the parkinsonism. At 300 to 400 mg/d, there was no further improvement in the dyskinesia. But CBD withdrawal resulted in several weeks of increased sensitivity to Sinemet, suggestive of a drug holiday effect.[15]

This brings up the intriguing possibility that CBD or other cannabinoids may prove an avenue for the reduction of Sinemet.

Patients using cannabis commonly report other supportive benefits in the reduction of symptoms of PD.[16] These include improvement in depressed mood and fatigue, improvement in anxiety and improvement in neuromuscular symptoms such as tremors, dystonias and rigidity. The use of cannabis in PD should be used with caution, as it's psychoactive properties can be disorienting. The question of whether cannabis can help PD symptoms is still apparently an individualized answer, and may depend upon the stage of the disease the patient has reached, how long they have been on dopaminergic medicine.

PATIENT REPORTS

To move on to patient results from my practice, these patients were very hesitant about starting an alternative regimen. Of those who came in for consultation, less than half ever began cannabis therapy. All change was difficult. Dose modulation was generally slow, thereby taking years to come to a useful regimen, compounded by the progression of the disease. Patients were older, from the mid-50s to the 70s. Here are a few illustrative case reports.

Patient 1: This is a 53-year-old male with a 12-year history of PD. He had been using cannabis for 35 years, 1–2 puffs by smoking several times/day. He was on Sinemet up to 15 tabs/day, and trihexylphenidyl 4x/day. He was still experiencing much stiffness and shaking. He stated that cannabis reduced these symptoms. Over the next year, his cannabis usage did not change, but his symptoms improved due to deep brain stimulation. His medications did reduce significantly to ½ tab of Sinemet 3x/day. I advised increasing to a CBD-rich tincture, but was not successful in influencing his cannabis use over the 5 years we worked together. He continued to smoke cannabis 3–4x/day, which he said helped his mood and reduced stiffness.

Pearls: This is typical of PD patients, that change in habits are rare, and/or slow to happen. In this case, the patient used cannabis positively for mood and symptom control. It is of no small significance that he had a long history of cannabis use and was comfortable with it.

Patient 2: This is a 69-year-old male with PD for many years, and cannabis use for 35 years. He was relatively functional, still working, but was taking high doses of Sinemet, 5x/day, as well as seligeline, amantadine and Mirapex. He stated that cannabis helped with stiffness and creativity. Over the next year, his Sinemet usage increased to 10 tabs/day, then he had deep brain stimulation, after which his medication was reduced to 1/2 tab 4x/day. He continued to inhale cannabis, but now was vaporizing some of the time. He continued to use smoked and vaporized cannabis, preferring sativa during the day for stiffness and fatigue. His condition remained stable over the next few years. I again advised adding a CBD-rich tincture, but the patient declined to do this.

Pearls: As with the aforementioned patient, cannabis was successful for mood and stiffness. Again, deep brain stimulation was a successful intervention. This patient highlights the benefit of sativa strains for creativity and fatigue. We were not able to add a CBD regimen. Most experienced cannabis users do not find the expected mood alteration with CBD products, and especially with PD patients, it's hard to effect change without obvious reward.

Patient 3: This is a 66-year-old male with a 5-year history of PD, adult-onset diabetes, also complaining of low back pain, knee pain and depression. His medications included Azilect 1 mg/day, Sinemet 25/100 1.5 tabs 3x/day, oral diabetic medications and blood pressure medicine. He wasn't taking anything for pain or mood. He had been using a small amount of cannabis regularly for 25 years by smoking, not daily. I advised him to use a CBD/THC 1:1 tincture, about 5 mg 3x/day to start. At our next visit, he was using the tincture rarely, due to cost, he said. A new tremor had onset. I directed him to cannabis compassionate use discount programs at several dispensaries. At our next visit, he was still smoking and/or using tincture irregularly, still due to cost. I was unable to convince him to use cannabis regularly, therefore he did not reap maximal benefits from its use.

Pearls: This patient seemed to benefit from a low dose of smoked cannabis. One might be tempted to consider the effects of low usage of cannabis as a microdosing example, but erratic use is more often a result of a cost consideration and/or apprehension of becoming dependent on cannabis medicine.

Patient 4: This is a 65-year-old female who initially presented with complaints of muscle spasm, insomnia, foot and low back pain. She had used cannabis in the distant past. Her medications included Trazodone, Lunesta and Remeron, which helped her sleep. We focused on using cannabis to reduce some of her medications. Over the next year, she was able to stop Lunesta by using a CBD/THC 1:1 tincture at night. The muscle spasm had progressed to rigidity and she was newly diagnosed with PD. Over the next year, she began Sinemet 1-tab 3x/day, and switched to an indica tincture for sleep. I advised vaporizing and a CBD-rich tincture for daytime symptoms, but this did not happen. The next year brought new onset anxiety with increased dosage of Sinemet. The stiffness and muscle spasm progressed to more rigidity. I continued to recommend a CBD-rich tincture during the day. Her regimen remained the same for the next few years.

Pearls: The patient was comfortable using THC-rich cannabis at night for insomnia, yet daytime use remained a challenge. In this case, the patient was not comfortable with cannabis as it had not been a recent habit, and again, daytime use even of CBD was declined. There was a reluctance to try not only a CBD tincture but also another herbal tincture I recommended for muscle spasm. In my experience with PD patients, willingness to try an alternative medicine is slow to come by.

CANNABIS THERAPY SUMMARY

There is some evidence for the efficacy of cannabis to treat PD dyskinesias and tremor. Research seems to indicate that THC may be the most effective cannabinoid for this, by inference from positive results with nabilone, Surprisingly, unheated cannabis also gave positive results indicating some potential for cannabinoid acids. The use of THC-rich cannabis in PD patients is a double-edged sword due to its disorienting effects, but some PD patients finds it relieves fatigue and depression. In such cases it's best to use low doses and mix it with some CBD. A CBD/THC 1:1 mix either by ingestion or inhalation would be a good choice, although often one to two puffs of a sativa strain can be well-tolerated. Can cannabis reduce some of the amount of dopaminergic medicine required? We tried to evaluate this in one patient with a relatively new diagnosis of PD. He was already vaporizing cannabis to treat tremor and some dystonia. After titrating up to 150 mg/day of ingested THC-rich cannabis, an attempt to wean off Sinemet (10/100) mg 3x/day, resulted in depression, possibly as a result of dopamine depletion. Sinemet was immediately resumed. Clearly, there needs to be more research done to answer this question. As far as treatment of the underlying neurodegeneration is concerned, there have been no long-term studies to establish whether cannabinoids or cannabis can slow the progression of the disease. But often, neuroprotective effects take time to manifest, and results may not be discernible for weeks to months. The role of CBD in the treatment of PD manifests in several ways. It reduces the psychoactivity of coadministered THC, and it may be considered for neuroprotective function. Another anecdotal use of CBD is in treating REM sleep behavior disorder, which affects up to 30% of PD patients, ordinarily treated with Klonapin. In my patient population, those PD patients who smoked or vaporized THC-rich cannabis stayed with it, while those using CBD often did not follow-up, not finding any immediately discernable results. The ongoing challenge with PD patients, of initiating a new change in therapy, is a common theme in dealing with this condition. Repeat instructions, having frequent follow-ups, be patient with slow progress and work with a patient's support system to reinforce advice on cannabis therapy.

REFERENCES

1. Fernandez Ruiz J. The endocannabinoid system as a target for the-treatment of motor dysfunction. *Br J Pharmacol.* 2009;156:1029–1040.
2. Bloomfield MAP, Ashok AH, Volkow ND, et al. The effects of Δ9-tetrahydrocannabinol on the dopamine system. *Nature.* 2016;539:369–377.
3. Bassi MS, Sancesario A, Morace R, Centonze D, Iezzi E. Cannabinoids in Parkinson's disease. *Cannabis Cannabinoid Res.* 2017;2(1):21–29.
4. Pisani A, Fezza F, Galati S. High endogenous cannabinoid levels in the cerebrospinal fluid of untreated Parkinson's disease patients. *Ann Neurol.* 2005;57(5):777–779.
5. Lim K, See YM, Lee J. A systematic review of the effectiveness of medical cannabis for psychiatric, movement and neurodegenerative disorders. *Clin Psychopharmacol Neurosci.* 2017;15(4):301–312.
6. Gandor F, Ebersbach G. Cannabinoids in the treatment of Parkinson's disease. *Neurology Int Open.* 2017;1:E307–E311.
7. Venderová K, Rzicka E, Vorísek V, Visnovský P. Survey on cannabis use in Parkinson's disease: subjective improvement of motor symptoms. *Mov Disord.* 2004;19(9):1102–1106.
8. Sieradzan KA, Fox SH, Hill M, et al. Cannabinoids reduce levodopa-induced dyskinesia in Parkinson's disease: a pilot study. *Neurology.* 2001;57(11):2108–2111.
9. Carroll CB, Bain PG, Teare L, et al. Cannabis for dyskinesia in Parkinson disease: a randomized double-blind crossover study. *Neurology.* 2004;63(7):1245–1250.
10. Lotan I, Treves TA, Roditi Y, Djaldetti R. Cannabis (medical marijuana) treatment for motor and non-motor symptoms of Parkinson disease: an open-label observational study. *Clin Neuropharm.* 2014;37(2):41–44.
11. García C, Palomo-Garo C, García-Arencibia M, et al. Symptom-relieving and neuroprotective effects of the phytocannabinoid D9-THCV in animal models of Parkinson's disease. *Br J Pharmacol.* 2011;163:1495–1506.
12. Chagas MH, Zuardi AW, Tumas V, et al. Effects of cannabidiol in the treatment of patients with Parkinson's disease: an exploratory double-blind trial. *J Psychopharmacol.* 2014;28(11):1088–1098.
13. Chagas MH, et al. Cannabidiol can improve complex sleep-related behaviours associated with rapid eye movement sleep behaviour disorder in Parkinson's disease patients: a case series. *J Clin Pharm Ther.* 2014;39:564–566.
14. Zuardi AW, Crippa J, Hallak JE, et al. Cannabidiol for the treatment of psychosis in Parkinson's disease. *J Psychopharmacol.* 2009;23(8):979–983.
15. Snider SR, Consroe P. Beneficial and adverse effects of cannabidiol in a Parkinson patient with Sinemet-induced dystonic dyskinesia. *Neurology.* 1985;35(Suppl):201.
16. Finseth TA, Hedeman JL, Brown RP, et al. Self-reported efficacy of cannabis and other complementary medicine modalities by Parkinson's disease patients in Colorado. *Evid Based Complement Alternat Med.* 2015;2015:874849.

43   Post-Traumatic Stress Disorder

POST-TRAUMATIC STRESS DISORDER AND CANNABIS

The symptoms associated with post-traumatic stress disorder (PTSD) may include persistent re-experiencing of the traumatic event, avoidance of usual activities and symptoms of increased arousal, such as hypervigilance and irritability. This disorder involves dysregulation of neurotransmitter, hormonal and pain receptor metabolism as well as the hypothalamic-pituitary-adrenal (HPA) axis. The "fight or flight" response is under constant stimulation. The endocannabinoid system plays an important role in the regulation of hormonal and neurotransmitter regulation and is integral in processes that regulate learning and emotional responses, especially those related to traumatic experiences. The hyperconsolidation of traumatic memories in PTSD is potentiated by glucocorticoid activation of norepinephrine release regulated by CB1 receptors. Cannabinoid agonists, presumably including THC, impair memory retrieval while facilitating memory extinction, thereby diminishing the excessive retrieval of trauma experienced by PTSD patients.[1] Interestingly, CBD may also play a role in trauma relief. CBD at a dose of 32 mg by inhalation was found to facilitate the extinction of aversive conditioning, but only when administered immediately after, and not before the process.[2] In addition, CBD is effective in reducing both the cardiovascular responses and anxiogenic effects caused by stress.[3] Cannabis is also helpful for nightmares, anxiety, depression and emotional as well as physical pain that may be experienced by PTSD patients.

Evidence from multiple studies show reduced endocannabinoid (eCB) levels in PTSD. Patients with PTSD were found to have increased levels of CB receptors and reduced peripheral levels of anandamide (AEA). CB1 receptors have shown increased availability in chronic stress situations such as found in PTSD.[4] CB1 receptor upregulation may be a result of low receptor occupancy caused in turn by the deficiency AEA.[5] Serum 2-arachadonylglyderol (2-AG) was also found to be diminished in survivors of the World Trade Center attack.[6] This may represent a possible "clinical endocannabinoid deficiency syndrome," hypothesized for multiple conditions, and more recently extended to include PTSD.[7] In such cases, exogenous cannabinoids may be helpful in bringing homeostasis. Although PTSD has also been proposed to present an endocannabinoid deficiency syndrome, due to lower levels of AEA in some cases, the complexity of eCB regulation does not always correlate with measured levels. Because eCBs inhibit the HPA axis, higher levels of endocannabinoids may ultimately be induced in someone perpetually needing to amplify the HPA system to manage stress. This may explain the success of THCV as a therapy for PTSD, as it is a CB1 antagonist that would counteract CB1 upregulation. Homeostatic management of the HPA axis along with variable glucocorticoid levels makes anticipating the effects of cannabis also complex.

DOI: 10.1201/9781003098201-54

THC or its analogs may be helpful for sleep in PTSD patients. Nabilone, a synthetic form of THC, decreased treatment resistant nightmares in PTSD subjects. The majority of patients (72%) receiving nabilone experienced either cessation of nightmares or reduction in intensity. Male military personnel with PTSD and trauma-related nightmares who were given 0.5–3 mg of nabilone showed a reduction of nightmares of up to 50% as compared to 11% for placebo.[8] Patients taking 5 mg of THC sublingual twice a day showed significant improvement in global symptom severity, sleep quality, frequency of nightmares and PTSD hyperarousal symptoms.[9]

PTSD is a major condition for qualifying patients in the New Mexico medical cannabis program. Most of these patients are veterans. In a chart review of 80 such patients, the clinician administered PTSD scales (CAPS) were significantly reduced compared to non-cannabis users. Patients reported more than 75% reductions in all three areas of PTSD symptoms while using cannabis.[10] A survey of 588 medical cannabis patients with PTSD in Canada also reported improvement in quality of life, mood, sleep, concentration and a large number reported improvement in pain with cannabis use.[11] Similar results were found in a study of PTSD patients in Israel, in which 2–3 grams/day of cannabis sativa strain resulted in a significant improvement in quality of life and pain scores, with some positive changes in CAPS scores. Patients also reported lowering the dosage of pain killers and sedatives.[12]

Environmental and social issues are of significance regarding cannabis use in PTSD. Cross-sectional studies have found a direct correlation between severity of PTSD symptomatology and increased motivation to use cannabis especially among patients with difficulties in emotional regulation or stress tolerance.[13] Patients with PTSD, especially veterans, are often marginalized. Post-traumatic stress symptom severity was associated with greater marijuana use coping motives. Non-judgmental acceptance was found to partially mediate the association.[14] In comparing veterans' cannabis use, a survey found that relative to recreational users, medical cannabis users reported significantly greater motivation for using cannabis for sleep disturbance, reporting increased sleep quality and reduced nightmares. Medical cannabis patients with PTSD also reported a lower frequency of alcohol use.[15]

Nevertheless, in literature reviews of cannabis use for PTSD, it was concluded that "We found insufficient evidence regarding the benefits and harms of plant-based cannabis preparations for patients with PTSD."[16] "The studies with the highest quality ratings generally find an association between PTSD and marijuana use, but the study designs do not allow for determination if one causes or aggravates the other, or if both are associated with some unknown third factor."[17] And, "Current literature is suggestive of a potential decrease in PTSD symptomatology with medical marijuana, but also suggests a correlation with problematic cannabis use."[18] Confounding is a problem in the many studies that have correlated cannabis use with an increase in cannabis use disorder, especially in veterans with PTSD. Due to the large percentage of these patients who have been classified as substance abusers rather than medical patients, these conclusions reflect bias. At the start of my cannabis practice, veterans were denied prescription opiates if they tested positive for THC (indicating cannabis). Fortunately, the VA has recently issued a new policy, as of December 2017. It states that "Veterans must not be denied VHA [Veterans Health Administration] services solely because they are participating in State-approved marijuana programs."[19] It also encourages veterans to discuss medical cannabis use with their VA providers. I can attest to the great relief that has brought to medical cannabis patients, to not have to hide what they're doing from their providers. And, an important corollary is that their cannabis use should ordinarily no longer be considered as a disorder.

It is not surprising that a large percentage of patients with PTSD are drawn to use cannabis, whether medical or recreational. Cannabis can treat autonomic, physiological, psychiatric and sleep disturbances, all challenges encompassed in the PTSD diagnosis.

PATIENT REPORTS

To move on to patient results from my practice, patients presented from all ages, teens through the 60s. Emotional trauma was not reserved for any subset of patients, and even though I practiced in an area with a significant number of veterans, they did not make up the bulk of my PTSD patients. Depending upon which of the many aspects of PTSD the patient was experiencing, choice of the cannabis product(s) varied widely. This is a condition that truly requires individualized treatment. Further discussion of these aspects can be found in the appropriate sections (see Chapters 15, 26 and 33). Here are a few illustrative case reports.

Patient 1: This is a 15-year-old male who came in with his newly appointed guardian, having been removed from living with his parents due to an abusive situation. He had been diagnosed with bipolar disorder at age 8, which later was changed to PTSD. He had a history of childhood abuse from an early age. He had been on multiple medications in the past, all stopped 3 years ago. He had problems with sleep and was recently smoking an indica strain before bed. He also complained of depression. At our visit he was interactive and agreeable to what his guardian wanted regarding supervised cannabis medicine. I advised a CBD/THC 2:1 strain for daytime use and an indica before bed. He actually got these directions reversed and reported doing well on the indica during the day and the CBD-rich at night. He reported that his mood "escalated" on CBD and it was not helpful during the day. He also complained of lack of appetite and found the THC-rich strain better for appetite and mood management. He was doing counseling and felt more stabilized. I then advised a CBD/ THC 1:1 tincture for longer duration. At our last visit, he had been placed on a low dose of Lexapro, and was trying CBD honey by dabbing. I again advised a tincture, and to limit dabs to after school use, even with CBD-rich oil.

Pearls: The range of cannabinoids this young patient says helped him was instructive for me, noting that a THC-rich indica was most helpful for daytime use. Then after a year of stabilizing in his new supportive environment, and on an antidepressant, a CBD-rich product was more useful. To see a young person voluntarily switch from THC to CBD is rare, but reflective of the needs of his evolving mood. Also, the type of cannabis most effective is likely to change with new psychiatric medications.

Patient 2: This is a 59-year-old Vietnam veteran with PTSD as well as low back pain. He had been using cannabis for 12 years by smoking and vaporizing approximately 1 gram/day. He also had a 7-year history of opiate use for back pain, escalating over this time to 50 mg of hydrocodone/day. Over the past year, this was weaned off under VA supervision. He complained of chronic depression, but was on no anti-depressants. His new pain management protocol included ongoing exercise at a gym. He continued to smoke or vaporize a sativa strain for 2 years. He reported improvement in mood, but still nightmares at night. I advised an indica strain before bed. He found that a CBD-rich capsule was calming. He took 35 mg 3–4×/day and vaporized or smoked THC-rich cannabis as needed for mood management.

Pearls: Again, we see the evolving nature of cannabis efficacy as the patient's chemistry, pain level and mod transitions occur. Early on we were dealing not only with PTSD, but pain and a recent opiate discontinuance. THC was effective for depression, pain and sleep. As these improved, a high CBD dose was useful for mood management.

Patient 3: This is a 61-year-old female who initially presented with complaints of anxiety and insomnia. She reported crying a lot and routinely awake several times a night. She was seeing a psychotherapist, but was on no medications other than progesterone cream 2 weeks/month. She was smoking cannabis before bed and again in the middle of the night. She also felt she had environmental sensitivity. She was taking multiple supplements and homeopathic remedies. She reported a history of a previous marriage to a paranoid schizophrenic. I thought she might be exhibiting symptoms of PTSD, but this was as yet undiagnosed. I advised an indica tincture before bed for longer duration of action than smoking, with avoidance of alcohol as she was sensitive to it. I also advised using progesterone nightly. Her sleep improved on this regimen, she said, for the first time in 20 years. Over the next few years, she changed therapists and had started doing EMD/R (a rapid eye movement technique) for her new diagnosis of PTSD. Sleep was much improved and she no longer needed the tincture, now smoking indica before bed and sleeping through the night.

Pearls: One of the hallmarks of PTSD is interrupted sleep, and in this case, treating that with a longer acting form of cannabis before bed was of benefit. The EMD/R therapy was an important element of mood issue resolution as well. Often mood lability and insomnia during post-menopausal hormone alterations, treated with daily progesterone topical, are transitory, and further medication, that is, cannabis, can be adjusted as improvement happens.

Patient 4: This is a 65-year-old male, Vietnam veteran, with complaints of PTSD, insomnia with nightmares and leg pain due to a service-connected injury. His medications were extensive, including duloxetine 60 mg/day, aripiprazole 7.5 mg/day, valproic acid 500 mg twice a day and bupropion 200 mg twice a day, Trazodone 100–200 mg at night and Percocet 2–4/day among other cardiovascular medications. He was doing counseling at the VA regularly. He smoked about one joint/day for many years. He said of cannabis, "It's one of the best, possibly the best for PTSD and dreams." I advised him to try an edible or tincture of indica before bed, while he continued to smoke during the day. He tried this, but found he preferred smoking. I advised him again to use an edible for better sleep, yet over the 4 years we worked together, his usage nor his medications changed. He did say that some days he used more cannabis, up to 2 joints/day.

Pearls: PTSD as a result of military trauma is an ongoing issue for many years post-trauma. Many veterans of this age group turned to smoking cannabis long ago, before medical cannabis had been approved. In fact, smoking cannabis to help with nightmares is a practice that many older PTSD patients found out about before research on its efficacy was widely known.

Patient 5: This is a 63-year-old male, Vietnam veteran, with complaints of PTSD, and insomnia with nightmares. He had been using medical cannabis most nights for 4 years to help with sleep. He stated that smoking or using an edible before bed helps with the nightmares. He has previously taken an antidepressant and did counseling at the VA. I advised him to make sure he chose an indica strain and to see which gave better sleep, inhalation or ingestion. Over the next few years, his usage did not change. Even though he only got 5 hours of sleep with smoking cannabis, he preferred it to the edibles. He did not use cannabis during the day. He tried to resume counseling, but was unable to be accommodated at his local VA office.

Pearls: Many Vietnam veterans have used cannabis by smoking, although in this case it was a newly instituted practice, used only 4 years after decades of insomnia and nightmares. The patient was opposed to "inebriation of any kind" and felt it justified to use cannabis only after it was medically approved. Again, we see that THC-rich cannabis does help with nightmares and sleep. If we were successful in switching to a longer-acting form, a longer duration of sleep may have been possible.

CANNABIS THERAPY SUMMARY

The more we've learned about the effects of endocannabinoids and cannabis on the myriad of symptoms that PTSD encompasses, the more evidence there is that cannabis effects a multifactorial in a therapeutic manner. Not only does THC-rich cannabis promote extinction of aversive memories and reduce the stress response, but it affects REM sleep in a way that reduces nightmares. The dosage of THC is critical in determining its effects on REM sleep. At low doses it can reduce it, while at high doses it can prolong it, exhibiting a biphasic effect (see Chapter 33). The issue of tolerance has not been adequately studied in this regard. It is preferable to keep the THC dose in the low to moderate range as we know it is effective for nightmares in this range, that is, a few puffs before bed, or a 10 mg edible. During the day, there are other options, such as a CBD/THC mix, that would address anxiety, depression and mood stabilization. THCV as a therapy for PTSD also looks promising as a way of balancing an overstimulated endocannabinoid system, yet with limited psychoactivity and should be investigated further. Its clinical use has been hampered by the lack of availability of cultivars rich in this cannabinoid. There is scant information on the dosing of THCV, but a place to start would be 5–10 mg. Recently, THCV containing cultivars and products have become available at some dispensaries.

REFERENCES

1. Trezza V, Campolongo P. The endocannabinoid system as a possible target to treat both the cognitive and emotional features of post-traumatic stress disorder (PTSD). *Front Behav Neurosci.* 2013;7:100.
2. Das RK, Kamboj SK, Ramadas M, et al. Cannabidiol enhances consolidation of explicit fear extinction in humans. *Psychopharmacology.* 2013;226:781–792.

3. Bittencourt RM, Takahashi RN. Cannabidiol as a therapeutic alternative for post-traumatic stress disorder: from bench research to confirmation in human trials. *Front Neurosci.* 2018;12:502.

4. Neumeister A, Normandin MD, Pietrzak RH, et al. Elevated brain cannabinoid CB1 receptor availability in posttraumatic stress disorder: a positron emission tomography study. *Mol Psychiatry.* 2013;18(9):1034–1040.

5. Hill MN, Bierer LM, Makotkine I, et al. Reductions in circulating endocannabinoid levels in individuals with post-traumatic stress disorder following exposure to the World Trade Center attacks. *Psychoneuroendocrinology.* 2013;38:2952–2961.

6. Russo EB. 2016. Clinical endocannabinoid deficiency reconsidered: current research supports the theory in migraine, fibromyalgia, irritable bowel, and other treatment-resistant syndromes. *Cannabis Cannabinoid Res.* 2013;1(1):154–165.

7. Fraser G. The use of a synthetic cannabinoid in the management of treatment-resistant nightmares in posttraumatic stress disorder (PTSD). *CNS Neurosci Ther.* 2009;15(1): 84–88.

8. Jetly R, Heber A, Fraser G, Boisvert D. The efficacy of nabilone, a synthetic cannabinoid, in the treatment of PTSD-associated nightmares: a preliminary randomized, double-blind, placebo-controlled cross-over design study. *Psychoneuroendocrinology.* 2015;51:585–588.

9. Roitman P, Mechoulam R, Cooper-Kazaz R, Shalev A. Preliminary, open-label, pilot study of add-on oral Δ9-tetrahydrocannabinol in chronic post-traumatic stress disorder. *Clin Drug Investig.* 2014;34(8):587–591.

10. Greer GR, Grob CS, Halberstadt AL. PTSD symptom reports of patients evaluated for the New Mexico Medical Cannabis Program. *J Psychoactive Drugs.* 2014;46(1):73–77.

11. Chan S, Blake A, Wolt A, et al. Medical cannabis use for patients with post-traumatic stress disorder (PTSD). *J Pain Manage.* 2017;10(4):385–396.

12. Reznik I. 2011. Medical cannabis use in post-traumatic stress disorder: a naturalistic observational study. Abstract presented at the Cannabinoid Conference 2011, 8–10 September, Bonn, Germany. www.cannabismed.org/studies/ww_en_db_study_show.php?s_id=481 Accessed October 10, 2019.

13. Betthauser K, Pilz J, Vollmer LE. Use and effects of cannabinoids in military veterans with posttraumatic stress disorder. *Am J Health Syst Pharm.* 2015;72(15):1279–1284.

14. Bonn-Miller MO, Vujanovic AA, Twohig MP, et al. Posttraumatic stress symptom severity and marijuana use coping motives: a test of the mediating role of non-judgmental acceptance within a trauma-exposed community sample. *Mindfulness.* 2010;1:98–106.

15. Metrik J, Bassett SS, Aston ER, Jackson KM, Borsari B. Medicinal versus recreational cannabis use among returning veterans. *Transl Issues Psychol Sci.* 2018;4(1):6–20.

16. O'Neill ME, Nugent SM, Morasco BJ, et al. Benefits and harms of plant-based cannabis for posttraumatic stress disorder. *Ann Intern Med.* 2017;167(5):332–340.

17. Campos-Outcalt D, Hamilton P, Rosales C. Arizona Department of Health Services Medical Marijuana Advisory Committee Report. 2012. Medical marijuana for the treatment of post traumatic stress disorder: an evidence review. www.azdhs.gov/documents/licensing/medical-marijuana/debilitating/Debilitating-Conditions-PTSD.pdf Accessed October 3, 2019.

18. Yarnell S. The use of medicinal marijuana for posttraumatic stress disorder: a review of the current literature. *Prim Care Companion CNS Disord.* 2015;17(3):10.4088/PCC.15r01786.

19. US Department of Veteran's Affairs. VA and marijuana – what veterans need to know. www.publichealth.va.gov/marijuana.asp Accessed October 3, 2019.

44 Schizophrenia, Psychosis

SCHIZOPHRENIA, PSYCHOSIS AND CANNABIS

Cannabis has historically been considered to be harmful when taken by schizophrenics or those at risk for the condition. In fact, in the era of THC-rich cannabis as the primary type available (before 2010), this diagnosis was traditionally designated as one of the conditions for which a medical cannabis recommendation was contraindicated. The evidence supporting the basis for harm is contradictory and elicited from studies with poorly defined cannabinoid content. If you look at many of the studies done in the last half-century, the notion that there was an association between cannabis use and schizophrenia was prevalent. Studies were generated with the goal of proving this hypothesis. In fact, associations were found, but rarely proved to be causal, and minimized or found not significant when confounding factors were taken into account.

In a review of the literature up until 2006, which, by necessity included only THC-rich cannabis, they found:

> Associations between cannabis and psychotic symptoms or other psychopathology scores were more inconsistent. . . . Few studies adjusted for baseline illness severity, and most made no adjustment for alcohol, or other potentially important confounders. Cannabis use was consistently associated with increased relapse and non-adherence.[1]

A meta-analysis concluded:

> Continued cannabis use after onset of psychosis predicts adverse outcome, including higher relapse rates, longer hospital admissions, and more severe positive symptoms than for individuals who discontinue cannabis use and those who are non-users. These findings point to reductions in cannabis use as a crucial interventional target to improve outcome in patients with psychosis.[2]

Conversely, some studies actually showed cognitive improvement with cannabis use in schizophrenics.[3]

> The extent to which cannabis use might alter the clinical course of schizophrenia remains a point of contention within the literature. As a result, these patients have a better prognosis, exhibit fewer negative symptoms, have better social skills, and have an enhanced treatment response compared with nonusers.[4]

In addition, a recent meta-analysis the authors also referred to, one study showing increased cognitive performance in those with cannabis use disorders compared with

DOI: 10.1201/9781003098201-55

nonusers. The question of whether cannabis could cause psychosis in otherwise normal and/or predisposed individuals was also looked at extensively. Again, the poor exclusion of confounding factors clouds the results. A report of an adjusted odds ratio for any psychotic symptom associated with any cannabis use was found to be 0.72. "Neither of these estimates provides meaningful evidence that cannabis causes schizophrenia."[5] Another review concluded:

> Overall, cannabis does not, seem to represent a sufficient cause for the development of schizophrenia. However . . . there are consistent findings that cannabis use does indeed increase the risk for schizophrenia and other psychotic disorders in vulnerable people.[6]

So where does that leave us? Well, in light of the fact that all of these studies involved THC-rich cannabis, because that was what was commonly available, we know that THC might be contraindicated with schizophrenic patients. But that may be more problematic with sativa strains than indica strains, which hasn't been identified in studies. Evidence suggests that cannabis may somehow trigger schizophrenia in those who are already at risk of developing the disorder. Use of THC-rich cannabis especially in adolescents genetically or otherwise predisposed to developing schizophrenia "might" bring it on at a younger age (see "Psychosis Risks" in Chapter 6).[7]

As a result of the studies that have come out on the effects of CBD for psychosis and schizophrenia, we know that THC mixed with CBD is not harmful, and that CBD is helpful, possibly even a therapeutic medicine. The clinical studies reviewing the effects of CBD in psychosis or schizophrenia have been carried out since 1982 and are reviewed.[8,9] A review of the effect of CBD on cognition in schizophrenia concluded, "To date, there is one clinical investigation into the effects of CBD on cognition in schizophrenia patients, with negative results for the Stroop test. CBD attenuates Δ9-THC induced cognitive deficits."[10] The effect of smoked cannabis with varying CBD/THC ratios was studied by analysis of hair samples of subjects. Subjects with THC only showed higher levels of positive psychotic symptoms than the groups with THC+CBD or non-cannabinoids in hair.[11] Also, the ingestion of a combination of 0.5 mg/kg THC + 1 mg/kg CBD lozenges significantly reduced the anxiety and the psychotomimetic symptoms as compared to 0.5 mg/kg THC lozenges.[12] CBD (1,000 mg/day) or placebo was taken by subjects alongside their existing antipsychotic medication. The CBD group had lower levels of positive psychotic symptoms. It was concluded: "As CBD's effects do not appear to depend on dopamine receptor antagonism, this agent may represent a new class of treatment for the disorder."[13] In a trial of CBD (600–800 mg/day for 4 weeks) compared with amisulpride on psychosis in individuals with schizophrenia, CBD was as effective as the antipsychotic in treating psychotic symptoms and had fewer adverse effects, including fewer extra pyramidal symptoms and weight gain.[14]

The mechanism through which CBD exerts this antipsychotic effect is multifactorial. An explanation involving a purely biological genetic factors has not been fully elucidated.

> However, the significant association observed in cannabidiol-treated patients between improvement of clinical symptoms and serum anandamide levels suggests that the

ability of cannabidiol to inhibit the FAAH activity and enhance intrinsic anandamide signaling might be a functionally relevant component of its antipsychotic properties.[14]

An interesting and promising avenue of research is the potential that cannabis or rather the role a group of compounds found in cannabis might offer in treating schizophrenia. Cannabidiols have been shown to provide therapeutic value in the treatment of schizophrenia with a relatively low risk of adverse effects.[15]

We know that clinically CBD is antianxiety, antipsychotic and is a mood stabilizer in bipolar disorder (see Chapters 15 and 26). It should be no surprise that CBD-dominant cannabis may actually be useful for schizophrenia patients. The problem lies in ensuring that those are the strains that actually are used. It is also possible that low doses of an indica product could be calming and help with sedation and appetite.

There is also the element of harm reduction in using cannabis in this population. Many schizophrenics turn to alcohol, tobacco or recreational drugs, for which cannabis can be a less harmful substitute, especially if used correctly. These harmful habits are noted in clinical practice and confirmed by studies. In an analysis of this issue, it was found, "Problem use of drugs and alcohol by people with schizophrenia is greater than in the general population, but absolute numbers are small. Tobacco use is the greatest problem."[16] Another review found that more than 70% of patients with chronic schizophrenia are nicotine dependent. This same review did not consider cannabis as a harm reduction agent, rather as a substance of abuse.[6]

PATIENT REPORTS

To move on to patient results from my practice, they were in the younger adult range, from their 20s to 40s. The patients represented here were those that actually followed up multiple times and sought my advice. I have also seen many of another category of patient, those who wanted to smoke THC-rich cannabis because they liked the feeling it gave them, but did not return as I tried to dissuade them from that practice. Here are a few illustrative case reports.

Patient 1: This is a 46-year-old male with a long-term diagnosis of schizophrenia. He had a history of Thorazine prescribed, but was currently not on any medications, just cannabis. He reported that he's been using cannabis for 30 years, and has been a medical marijuana patient for 15 years. He also had a history of Hepatitis C, was under a physician's care, and was losing weight. His initial medical cannabis recommendation was for appetite stimulation. He consistently smoked an indica strain 4×/day to "keep his behavior in check," and it also helped his appetite. On exam he had an unkempt appearance, but is mental status showed no delusions, no hallucinations, normal speech and was able to follow our conversation with no difficulty. I saw this patient for 5 years, during which time he steadfastly remained on a smoked indica regimen without deviation.

Pearls: The big question, did cannabis serve as an antipsychotic all these years, was his schizophrenia atypical or was the diagnosis in error? We'll come back to this in concluding remarks. In this case it was useful for appetite stimulation to use a THC-rich strain.

Patient 2: This is a 36-year-old male with a diagnosis of schizophrenia and insomnia. He occasionally took Zyprexa to help with sleep. He identified as having been a Rastafarian, liked natural remedies and was on a vegetarian diet. On exam he was a kind, gentle fellow who liked gardening and was a handyman. He had no delusions, no hallucinations, normal speech and was able to follow our conversation with no difficulty. He has been using cannabis for 15 years, because as he said, "It's gentler on my consciousness, and just makes me feel more present. It also calms, relaxes and rejuvenates me." While he smoked THC-rich cannabis, some of the time he switched recently to CBD-rich tinctures to help him relax. He also utilized flower essences and essential oils. I saw this patient for 4 years, during which time he stopped Zyprexa entirely, and instead used an indica cookie on occasion to sleep. He said his mood became stabilized, and no longer considered himself schizophrenic. His ongoing cannabis regimen was smoking 2x/day, using a CBD-rich tincture rarely, and an indica edible rarely.

Pearls: Is this another atypical schizophrenic patient? Perhaps CBD helped to stabilize his mood. Significantly, here is a patient who was able to stay away from pharmaceuticals to a great extent. Did his herbal regimen result in success due to less exposure to antipsychotic medications and their side effects? It is likely that these compliant patients who returned to work with me represent milder forms of schizophrenia or misdiagnosed individuals.

Patient 3: This is a 29-year-old male who presented for shoulder pain, also carrying a diagnosis of schizophrenia. The patient was delusional 1 year ago, and started on antipsychotic medications while in jail. He reported a second delusional episode 5 years earlier, but took no medications before this time. He had a 15-year history of cannabis use, smoking about 1 gram/day, unspecified as to sativa, indica, or hybrid. He was happy with his use, and maintained that he was not schizophrenic. Currently, he was not incarcerated, but maintained his regimen of Haldol by injection every 2 weeks, and Zyprexa 10 mg twice/day as mandated by the court. As was the practice with possibly non-compliant patients, I issued a temporary 2-month recommendation with advice to vaporize or smoke a CBD-rich strain for symptoms of anxiety, stress or escalating mood. He was to return with a note from his psychiatrist stating he was informed of this therapy, and approval from his probation officer. Upon follow-up his condition was unchanged, with the addition of Trazodone 50 mg at night, and Zyprexa down to 5 mg. He reported trying a CBD/THC 2:1 strain but preferred the THC-rich indica that he was used to taking. I explained to the patient that this was not the recommended course and I couldn't extend the recommendation.

Pearls: What about this patient caused me to not extend his recommendation? This is the clinician's personal choice, and I had been coached that schizophrenia was one of those conditions where non-indica THC-rich strains may exacerbate the patient's condition, so promoting accessibility to cannabis if the wrong type was going to be used was not wise. In fact, now that cannabis is decriminalized in California, I'm sure that this patient is using whatever strain he chooses and may be worse off for it.

CANNABIS THERAPY SUMMARY

In the early days of my practice when CBD-rich cannabis was unavailable, all we could offer was a caution to use low-dose indica varieties and avoid sativas at all costs. Some patients saicannabis helped them, and others were exacerbated by its use, saying it increased paranoia. Cultivar specificity is imperative in making therapeutic recommendations for this condition.The most important aspect of cannabis therapy for schizophrenia or psychosis is to keep in mind that THC-rich cultivars that are stimulating or using high doses of THC is contraindicated, not only in young adults that have a predisposition for developing schizophrenia, but also in any individuals at risk for or who are experiencing psychotic symptoms. After having established that, we do see that some THC-rich varieties, such as the more sedating indicas, may have a place in helping with sleep and/or in inducing a shift in perspective. In some of these cases, an aspect of harm reduction may be a therapeutic response, as regards the reduction of other drugs of abuse, alcohol or tobacco. What is usually really helpful are products that provide CBD, even with as much THC as may be in a CBD/THC product with a 2:1 ratio. CBD has been documented as having antipsychotic properties and may be considered a useful therapeutic intervention in this condition. How much to use is dependent on the patient's severity of symptoms, but may begin as usual for CBD, at 10 mg/dose. That may not always be the case. Another patient I've seen diagnosed with schizoaffective disorder found that CBD acted as a mood stabilizer. Here the patient was taking several antipsychotic medications, hence a high dose of CBD up to 50 mg 2×/day was required to have an impact. It is important to note that individuals with mild forms of schizophrenia presented as patients, the more severe cases may not choose to participate in medical cannabis consultations. Having patients agree to try CBD-rich cannabis is not always easy, as they often prefer the psychoactive effects of THC. Poor compliance is a hallmark of treatment of schizophrenia patients, an ongoing challenge. If recommendation for specific cannabis products were regulated for medical cannabis patients, it would serve this population well.

REFERENCES

1. Zammit S. Effects of cannabis use on outcomes of psychotic disorders: systematic review. *Br J Psychiatry.* 2008;193:357–363.
2. Schoeler T, Monk A, Sami MB, et al. Continued versus discontinued cannabis use in patients with psychosis: a systematic review and meta-analysis. *The Lancet Psychiatry.* 2016;3(3):215–225.
3. Løbegr E, Hugdahl K. Cannabis use and cognition in schizophrenia. *Front Hum Neurosci.* 2009;3:53.
4. LynchMJ,RabinRA,GeorgeTP.Thecannabispsychosislink.*PsychiatricTimes.*January 12, 2012. www.psychiatrictimes.com/schizophrenia/cannabis-psychosis-link#sthash.en52 agT0.dpuf Accessed October 3, 2019.
5. Macleod J, Davey Smith G, Hickman M, Egger M. Cannabis and psychosis. *The Lancet.* 2007;370(9598):1539.
6. Winklbaur B, Ebner N, Sachs G, et al. Substance abuse in patients with schizophrenia. *Dialogues Clin Neurosci.* 2006;8(1):37–43.
7. Rodrigo C, Rajapakse S. Cannabis and schizophrenia spectrum disorders: a review of clinical studies. *Indian J Psychol Med.* 2009;31(2):62–70.
8. Zuardi AW, Crippa JA, Hallak JE, et al. A critical review of the antipsychotic effects of cannabidiol: 30 years of a translational investigation. *Curr Pharm.* 2012;18:5131–5140.

9. Rohleder C, Müller JK, Lange B, Leweke FM. Cannabidiol as a potential new type of an antipsychotic. A critical review of the evidence. *Front Pharmacol.* 2016;7:422.

10. Osborne AL, Solowij N, Weston-Green K. A systematic review of the effect of cannabidiol on cognitive function: relevance to schizophrenia. *Neurosci Biobehav Rev.* 2017;72:310–324.

11. Morgan CJA, Curran V. Effects of cannabidiol on schizophrenia-like symptoms in people who use cannabis. *Br J Psychiatry.* 2008;192:306–307.

12. Zuardi AW, Crippa JA, Hallak JE, Moreira FA, Guimarães FS. Cannabidiol, a cannabis sativa constituent, as an antipsychotic drug. Braz *J Med Biol Res.* 2006;39:421–429.

13. McGuire P, Robson P, Cubala WJ, et al. Cannabidiol (CBD) as an adjunctive therapy in schizophrenia: a multicenter randomized controlled trial. *Am J Psychiatry.* 2018;175(3):225–231.

14. Leweke FM, Piomelli D, Pahlisch F, et al. Cannabidiol enhances anandamide signaling and alleviates psychotic symptoms of schizophrenia. *Transl Psychiatry.* 2012;2:e94.

15. Hamilton I, Monaghan M. Cannabis and psychosis: are we any closer to understanding the relationship? *Curr Psychiatry Rep.* 2019;21(7):48.

16. McCreadie RG. Scottish Comorbidity Study Group. Use of drugs, alcohol and tobacco by people with schizophrenia: case-control study. *Br J Psychiatry.* 2002;181:321–325.

45 Seizure Disorder, Epilepsy

SEIZURE DISORDER, EPILEPSY AND CANNABIS

Cannabis has historically been used to treat seizures, as far back as in early Ayurvedic and Islamic medicine. In fact, 50 years ago, studies in the 1970s showed promise for cannabinoids, including THC and CBD to treat seizures. More recently, CBD has attracted the most interest as a therapy for epilepsy, especially in refractory pediatric cases. The first FDA drug derived from a cannabis extract was approved in 2018 as a Schedule V drug, Epidiolex (99% pure oil-based CBD extract of constant composition, GW Pharmaceuticals) for two types of refractory childhood epilepsy: Dravet syndrome and Lennox-Gastaut syndrome. The US legal classification of CBD has been unclear until the Farm Bill of 2018 decriminalized the use of CBD derived from hemp (less than 0.3% THC content).[1]

The endocannabinoid system (ECS) is involved in seizure regulation affecting the initiation, propagation and spread of seizures. In animal studies, 2-arachadonoylglycerol increased within the hippocampus, suggesting that endocannabinoids modulate seizure termination and duration through activation of the CB1 receptor. The ECS is strongly activated by seizures, and the upregulation of CB1 receptor activity has been found to have anti-seizure effects.[2] Reduced levels of anandamide, downregulation of CB1 receptors, as well as sprouting of GABAergic axons with CB1 receptors have been found in cerebrospinal fluid and tissue biopsy derived from patients with epilepsy.[3]

In the case of THC, anti-seizure activity seems to be mediated to an important extent by its partial agonist action on the CB1 receptor.[4] Additionally THC is associated with a serotonin-mediated anticonvulsant effect.[5] However, THC, as other CB1 agonists exhibit contradictory pro- and anticonvulsant effects. "Evidence from 34 studies from 6 animal species demonstrate that Δ9-THC is anticonvulsant in 61.8% (21/34), proconvulsant in 2.9% (1/34), mixed in 2.9% (1/34), and shows no significant effect in 32.4% (11/34) of seizure models."[6] Because the effects of dosage of THC are contradictory and due to its psychoactivity, THC has not been favored as an agent to treat seizures. This has led to increased interest in the application of other cannabinoids, CBD being the most studied, but it is not the only effective agent.

Multiple other cannabinoids have anti-seizure activity. In animal studies, anticonvulsant effects were found for the following cannabinoids in order of approximate effective dose (ED50): 11-OH-Δ9-THC (14 mg/kg), Δ8-THC (80 mg/kg), Δ9-THC (100 mg/kg), CBD (120 mg/kg), Δ9-THCA (200–400 mg/kg), cannabinol (CBN) (230 mg/kg).[7] Note the very high concentrations used in this experiment, well above what is clinically applicable. It is interesting that the strongest cannabinoid is the metabolic product of THC, 11-OH-Δ9-THC, opening the possibility that the

DOI: 10.1201/9781003098201-56

success of using THC may be more potent by ingestion where an increased amount of 11-OH-THC is circulated. Other anticonvulsant cannabinoids of interest include THCV and CBDV.[6,8,9] THCA has been found to possess anticonvulsant activity in preclinical investigations.[3] In one case, THCA-rich therapy proved effective when treatment with CBD and THC failed to deliver satisfactory results.[10] Combinations of cannabinoids as well as cannabis extracts with terpenes show more promise than single agents. A test of the anticonvulsant properties of several CBD-rich cultivars was investigated. These results suggest that not all CBD-rich extracts have the same anticonvulsant properties, and that comprehensive phytocannabinoid profiling can enable to evaluate the potential anticonvulsant properties of cannabis extracts.[11]

The mechanism of action of CBD to treat seizures has not been fully elucidated and is considered partially to be mediated by CB1 and CB2, receptors as well as by several other non-CB receptors. Other mechanisms include agonism or antagonism at multiple 7-transmembrane receptors, ion channels and neurotransmitter transporters. Effects on adenosine reuptake and antagonism of G protein-coupled receptor 55 (GPR55) have been suggested.[3] The effect of CBD in epilepsy has been the subject of several reviews.[3,7,12,13]

Specific reports of CBD use to treat epilepsy include several studies of note. In a trial of Epidiolex to treat patients with severe, intractable, childhood-onset, treatment-resistant epilepsy, CBD at 2–5 mg/kg/day, up-titrated to a maximum dose of 25–50 mg/kg/day for 12 weeks, seizures were reduced by 36.5%.[14] In a recent study, 74 patients with refractory epilepsy were treated with sublingual cannabis oil extract containing a CBD/THC ratio of 20:1, given three times daily. Daily dose ranged from 2 to 27 mg/kg/day. A reduction in seizure frequency was found in 89% of the subjects.[15] A retrospective study of patients with epilepsy using CBD cannabis extracts found generally similar results as compared with clobazam therapy. The dose of CBD oil used showed wide variability from 0.02 to 50 mg/kg/day. Twenty two percent of patients were able to decrease anti-seizure medication levels with CBD.[16] One comprehensive review, reviewing clinical data from 670 patients, treated with CBD-rich cannabis extracts or purified CBD, with average daily doses between 1 and 50 mg/kg, and duration of treatment from 3 to 12 months. They found, "The results of efficacy in the studied population suggest that treatment with CBD-based products significantly reduces seizure frequency, even for this otherwise treatment resistant population."[13] An average of 64% of the patients had a reduction in seizure frequency with rates ranging from 37% to 89%. Improvement after using CBD-rich cannabis extracts was greater (71%) than those treated with purified CBD (36%). The average daily dose reported for purified CBD was 27.1 mg/kg/day, while the average daily dose reported for CBD-rich cannabis extract was 6.1 mg/kg/day. Adverse effects were more frequent in the purified CBD studies at the higher doses than in CBD-rich extracts. The most common adverse events reported were appetite alteration, sleepiness, gastrointestinal disturbances/diarrhea, weight changes, fatigue and nausea. They conclude:

> This data suggests that CBD is 4 times "more potent" when administered in herbal form, probably because other minor compounds present in the extract may contribute to its therapeutic effect. Apparently, CBD-rich Cannabis extracts are more potent and have a better safety profile (but not higher efficacy) than products with purified CBD.[13]

It's important to consider possible side effects of taking such a high dose of CBD. A recent dosing trial for patients with Dravet syndrome compared safety and tolerability of 5, 10 and 20 mg/kg/day of purified CBD. There were some adverse effects, including pyrexia, somnolence, decreased appetite, sedation, vomiting, ataxia and abnormal behavior, all of which were well tolerated. Some patients developed elevated liver enzymes, which normalized after the study.[17] High doses of CBD may be expected to cause adverse drug interactions (DDIs), via its inhibition of CYP 450 enzymes potentially causing significant medication interactions with anticonvulsants (AEDs) (see "Drug Interactions" in Chapter 6). Phenytoin and carbamazepine may decrease CBD concentrations, while CBD is known to increase concentrations of clobazam to >60%.[18]

The dose of CBD needed when provided in a cannabis extract is much lower than when provided by Epidiolex. In an observational study of 272 patients using cannabis in various forms, all CBD-rich, but some with the inclusion of THC or THCA, seizure reduction was noted in 86% of cases. One of the authors observed anticonvulsive effects in patients at doses as low as 0.02 mg cannabinoids/kg/day. They point out that the effect of terpenes in the extract, especially D-linalool or D-limonene that are anticonvulsant, may confer an advantage. In some of these patients, small doses (0.1–1 mg/kg/day) of THCA were used, corresponding to 0.01–0.1% of the patient's body weight in THCA.[10]

PATIENT REPORTS

To move on to patient results from my practice, seizure disorder occurred across all ages, child, youth and adult, but the preponderance of cases was in the pediatric category. Here the parents were mostly concerned with the effects of anti-seizure medications, or the cases were medically refractory, or simply had heard about CBD and wanted to try it. Often there were multiple diagnoses, including developmental delay, autism and/or behavioral disorders. Here are a few illustrative case reports. There are several represented here, both adults and children, as their protocols are generally different.

Patient 1: This is a 42-year-old female with multiple conditions, including generalized convulsive epilepsy, migraine headaches, fibromyalgia and anxiety. Her seizures appeared at age 13, then diminished until age 28. At the time of her visit, her seizures disorder was described as stable on Lamictal and Klonapin, but she reported two breakthrough seizures per month, lasting less than a minute. She had been using cannabis for 25 years by pipe or edible once/day. She had not correlated seizure events to any particular trigger or if they occurred on edible days versus pipe days, that is, relative to cannabis intake. Her anxiety had been severe, for which she was taking 6 mg of Klonapin per day. She was relatively well-functioning, a mother of three children, and was doing counseling. She wanted to use cannabis more wisely to reduce seizures and other medications. She began a regular dose of an indica edible overnight, and reported seizure reduction from 2×/month to 2× in the past year. She used a CBD mouth spray for those occasions which helped the seizures. Ongoing, the seizures stayed reduced at 3 episodes/year. She had switched to using concentrated CBD oil to ward off seizures when she felt an aura. She continued cannabis by mostly smoking due to a lesser cost.

Pearls: This is a complex case, with multiple conditions. The patient's cannabis use was inconsistent, but her seizure frequency did decrease. It is unclear if she was taking enough to prevent seizure episodes per se, but she did find the cannabis useful for stress relief and was comfortable with it. The addition of concentrated CBD, by oil or by mouth spray, seemed to provide benefit for "stopping" a seizure, and is a strategy used by several patients.

Patient 2: This is a 20-year-old female with a genetic abnormality, resulting in autism, intellectual delay, seizure disorder, osteopetrosis, small stature and difficulty chewing and swallowing. Her weight was 85 lb. The seizure disorder was described as medically refractive symptomatic epilepsy. Seizures were occurring approximately 3x/month, primarily while asleep, on a regimen of Keppra and Lamictal, having been unable to tolerate higher doses of various other anticonvulsants. She began a tincture of CBD-rich 20:1 cannabis, about 7 mg 2x/day. Her mother did not advance her up to the recommended dose of 10 mg 3x/day. She reported that seizure frequency had decreased to 1x/month. The next year we increased the dose to 10 mg 2x/day and 10 mg before bed with 30% THC content to help with sleep. This did not eliminate seizures, which continued at 1–2x/month, but sleep was improved, and the seizures were no longer nocturnal, but pre-menstrual. Her seizure medications then were reduced at mom's request. Keppra ultimately was reduced from 3,000 mg/day to 1,500 mg/day, and Lamictal decreased from 400 mg/day to 300 mg/day. No increase in seizures occurred.

Pearls: This is a case where cannabis may be considered an adjunct to pharmaceutical seizure management, in fact allowing a decrease in medications, and better sleep. Mom asked if she should reduce the medications further, which began a detailed discussion of using cannabis as a primary seizure control medication. In fact, this patient was eligible for Epidiolex treatment by her neurologist. She decided to defer changing the protocol just now and focus on improving her daughter's diet, which was high in gluten, and not maximally nutritious.

Patient 3: This is a 10-year-old male with a mild form of epilepsy, having absence seizures daily. The seizures had been occurring for the past 5 years, about 20 times/day. Anti-seizure medications were of no help and had been discontinued 2 years earlier. He was new to cannabis use. I advised a CBD/THC 20:1 tincture at a relatively low dose, 10 mg 3x/day, which provided a dose of about 2.3 mg/kg/day. The seizures decreased to about 3 per day on this regimen. We then tried a somewhat higher dose, of 15 mg 3x/day. After another year, we went to 20 mg 3x/day but the seizures remained at 3–5/day. Sleep was an issue, so we added some THC at night, utilizing a CBD/THC 4:1 oil for the nighttime dose, on which sleep improved. After 4 more years, the patient continued to have 3 absence seizures/day. At this point, the patient was taking 28 mg of cannabis oil by capsule 2x/day containing 62% CBD, 2% THC and 36% cannabinoid acids, as well as 28 mg of the 4:1 mix at night, which provided 1.3 mg/kg/day of cannabinoids. We agreed to increase the dose back up to the 2 mg/kg range to adjust for his increase in weight. The family was pleased with this protocol, reporting good cognition and school performance, decreased stress and still on no medications.

Pearls: This is another case of treatment-resistant seizures that responded well to cannabinoid treatment. In this case, the inclusion of cannabinoid acids (THCA and

CBDA) seems to have brought similar results at a lower dose than a CBD/THC 20:1 extract. The use of cannabinoid acids for seizure control is a rarely used strategy, as the medicine is not easy to obtain. It's important to consider a combination of CBD and cannabinoid acids for seizures.

Patient 4: This is a 2-year-old male with medically refractive symptomatic epilepsy, developmental delay and a brain malformation since birth. He was having about one seizure/hour on a ketogenic diet, twice that when off. His medication included Keppra and Diastat. He started on a CBD-rich tincture that was made from a 20:1 strain at home, concentration not determined. The dose was titrated based upon symptoms, determined for each batch. His seizures remarkably reduced 0–3/day, and over the next 5 years, stayed steady at that level. We attempted to estimate the dose as he was taking 2 dropperfuls twice/day with a relatively weak tincture, perhaps 5 mg of cannabinoids/ml, providing a dose of 300 mg/20 kg weight = 1.5 mg/kg/dose. All fluids and nutrition were delivered by nasogastric tube. Antiseizure medications were discontinued on this regimen, with the addition of baclofen recommended by his pediatric neurologist who supported his cannabis use. Around this time, Epidiolex became available for medically refractive epilepsy and the patient was switched off cannabis onto this medication and care continued through the neurologist. He was still on a ketogenic diet. On follow-up a few years later, the parents reported that the Epidiolex dose was currently 1.9 ml of a 100 mg/ml solution providing a dose of 190 mg/25 kg = 7.6 mg/kg, a fivefold increase over the previous cannabis dose. Seizures occurred now only a few times/week. The dad said he's done so much better on cannabis or Epidiolex, as not only did AEDs not work, but they were "dimming him."

Pearls: This is a case where CBD-rich cannabis made a remarkable difference to seizure control in a brain malformation, medication-resistant condition. The use of homegrown cannabis to provide an otherwise potentially expensive medicine is full of challenges. In this case, the correct strain was successfully grown, extracted and dosed! It is of note that the transition to Epidiolex went smoothly, albeit at a much higher dose.

Patient 5: This is a 7-year-old male with focal partial epilepsy for 3 years. On the current medications, he was having only 2 seizures/month on sleep to wake. His medications included divalproex, Trileptal and Onfi. Mom wanted to try and replace some of these medications with CBD. We began at a dose of a CBD extract providing 0.5 mg/kg/day by tincture, titrated up to 1 mg/kg/day, divided into two doses. We then increased the dose to 3 mg/kg/day in preparation for medication reduction. He was mostly seizure-free for several years, was doing well at school and sleeping well. Mom was still interested in weaning the anticonvulsants but was hesitant to begin this process.

Pearls: This is a case where cannabis was used at a high-enough dosage to actually potentially replace an anticonvulsant, yet this did not ensue. It is always challenging for parents to go against the advice of their child's neurologist, especially with a protocol that is successful. I question whether this patient needs to stay on the CBD at all, because his seizures prior to this considerable dose were mild and only occurred 2×/month. Hopefully, as more pediatric neurologists become familiar with cannabis for seizures, a combination protocol could be supported.

CANNABIS THERAPY SUMMARY

Research indicates that several cannabinoids can be effective for seizure control, including 11-OH-THC, THC, CBD, THCA, CBDA and potentially THCV and CBDV. In practice, the focus of clinical attention has been on CBD culminating in the approval of Epidiolex for certain pediatric seizure disorders. Not all cases of intractable epilepsy respond with much success to cannabis therapy, yet often they respond as well as AEDs and may be able to replace one or more of them. The use of THC when delivered by ingestion would provide the strongest of these resulting in 11-OH-THC that has largely not been pursued due to its psychoactive consequences. However, one of my 16-year-old patients with juvenile myoclonic epilepsy reported a reduction in seizures on smoked THC-rich cannabis from one episode/month to none.

It has been shown in several studies that CBD provided in a cannabis extract is more efficacious at a lower dose than pure CBD. This is what we found in several patients that a four- to fivefold reduced dose is required with the extract as compared to purified Epidiolex. As far as CBD-rich cannabis is concerned, the accepted practice is to titrate up to 2–5 mg/kg/day of a cannabis extract. The potency of the CBD, whether from a cannabis extract, a purified isolate, a hemp-derived product, with or without terpenes, all can and will affect the dosage required. Another practice, acute use of a concentrated CBD extract, either in alcohol or mid-chain triglyceride oil by spray, to mitigate the effects of an ongoing seizure, is one that has shown efficacy. We know that several terpenes have anticonvulsant action. Cultivars with higher levels of these terpenes, β-myrcene, D-limonene and to a lesser extent D-linalool, would make the most effective cannabis product for use with seizures. As the cannabinoid dose is high in these cases, there is a potential for adverse reactions, the most likely of which are excessive somnolence and diarrhea. Nevertheless, at the lower doses of cannabis extracts as compared to pure CBD, there are fewer documented cases of the need to adjust for DDIs with AEDs (see "Drug Interactions" in Chapter 6).

The inclusion of cannabinoid acids has recently been gaining in favor, a useful therapeutic intervention as these would not be expected to provide the same level of sedation as CBD. We know that THCA can be effective, possibly at <1 mg/kg/day, and it may be that CBDA can be used as well. Another pediatric patient I treated showed a 50% seizure reduction while using a CBDA cannabis extract, at a dose of approximately 4 mg/kg/day. Sparse research data indicates a much lower dose can be effective when cannabinoid acids are provided in conjunction with other cannabinoids, such as CBD. The untapped potential of propyl analogues such as THCV or CBDV has not been adequately tested. It is important to remember that while CBD-rich cannabis extracts are favored, notably in pediatric cases, we cannot forget that other cannabinoids have value, and should not be ignored, especially in adult patients. Often the cost of the medicine is an issue, especially with the high doses required leading to possible discontinuance of the cannabis medicine. The need for continual medication management, especially while titrating the dose of CBD up to higher levels, and/or AED reduction requires careful coordination with the patient's neurologist, which has been a challenge.

REFERENCES

1. Mead A. Legal and regulatory issues governing cannabis and cannabis-derived products in the United States. *Front Plant Sci.* 2019;10:697.
2. Maroon J, Bost J. Review of the neurological benefits of phytocannabinoids. *Surg Neurol Int.* 2018;9:91.
3. Perucca E. Cannabinoids in the treatment of epilepsy: hard evidence at last? *J Epilepsy Res.* 2017;7(2):61–76.
4. Wallace MJ, Blair RE, Falenski KW, Martin BR, DeLorenzo RJ. The endogenous cannabinoid system regulates seizure frequency and duration in a model of temporal lobe epilepsy. *J Pharmacol Exp Ther.* 2003;307(1):129–137.
5. Ladino LD, Hernández-Ronquillo L, Téllez-Zenteno JF. Medicinal marijuana for epilepsy: a case series study. *Can J Neurol Sci.* 2014;41(6):753–758.
6. Rosenberg EC, Tsien RW, Whalley BJ, Devinsky O. Cannabinoids and epilepsy. *Neurotherapeutics.* 2015;12(4):747–768.
7. Devinsky O, Cilio MR, Cross H, et al. Cannabidiol: pharmacology and potential therapeutic role in epilepsy and other neuropsychiatric disorders. *Epilepsia.* 2014;55(6):791–802.
8. Hill A, Weston SE, Jones NA, et al. Δ^9-Tetrahydrocannabivarin suppresses in vitro epileptiform and in vivo seizure activity in adult rats. *Epilepsia.* 2010;51(8):1522–1532.
9. Hill AJ, Williams CM, Whalley BJ, Stephens GJ. Phytocannabinoids as novel therapeutic agents in CNS disorders. *Pharmacol Ther.* 2012;133(1):79–97.
10. Sulak D, Sanneto R, Goldstein B. The current status of artisanal cannabis for the treatment of epilepsy in the United States. *Epilepsy Behav.* 2017;70(Pt B):328–333.
11. Berman P, Futoran K, Lewitus GM, et al. A new ESI-LC/MS approach for comprehensive metabolic profiling of phytocannabinoids. *Cannabis Sci Rep.* 2018;8:14280.
12. Gloss D, Vickrey B. Cannabinoids for epilepsy. *Cochrane Database Syst Rev.* 2014 Mar 5;3:CD009270.
13. Pamplona FA, da Silva LR, Coan AC. Potential clinical benefits of CBD-rich cannabis extracts over purified CBD in treatment-resistant epilepsy: observational data meta-analysis. *Front Neurol.* 2018;9:759.
14. Devinsky O, Marsh E, Friedman D, et al. Cannabidiol in patients with treatment resistant epilepsy: an open-label interventional trial. *Lancet Neurol.* 2016;15(3):270–278.
15. Hausman-Kedem M, Kramer U. Efficacy of medical cannabis for treatment of refractory epilepsy in children and adolescents with emphasis on the Israeli experience. *Isr Med Assoc J.* 2017;19:76–78.
16. Porcari GS, Fu C, Doll ED, Carter EG, Carson RP. Efficacy of artisanal preparations of cannabidiol for the treatment of epilepsy: practical experiences in a tertiary medical center. *Epilepsy Behav.* 2018;80:240–246.
17. Devinsky O, Patel AD, Thiele EA, et al. Randomized, dose-ranging safety trial of cannabidiol in Dravet syndrome. *Neurology.* 2018;90:e1204–e1211.
18. Campbell CT, Phillips MS, Manasco K. Cannabinoids in pediatrics. *J Pediatr Pharmacol Ther.* 2017;22(3):176–185.

46 Skin Conditions

SKIN CONDITIONS AND CANNABIS

Psoriasis, eczema and multiple other skin conditions are regulated by the endocannabinoid system (ECS), as is the case for any other organ system. The ECS is involved in the regulation of skin cell proliferation, differentiation and survival, all required for cutaneous homeostasis. It influences skin health in multiple ways, from modulating allergic response to mediating skin-derived sensory signaling. This includes central and peripheral sensory effects such as pain and itch. The mechanism involves activation of CB1 and CB2 receptors, and by stimulating receptors such as TRPV1 at sensory nerve terminals and inflammatory cells.[1] It has long been shown that cannabinoids can reduce inflammation and hyperalgesia by interaction with peripheral CB receptors.[2] Endocannabinoids also enhance lipid synthesis and induce apoptosis in sebocytes. It was shown in cell studies that, "Endocannabinoids (AEA, 2-AG) are produced by sebocytes, and that these endocannabinoids (at physiologically relevant concentration) stimulate sebocyte lipid synthesis and apoptosis in a CB2-mediated manner."[3] Administration of AEA and 2-AG dramatically increased lipid production via sebocytes, an intervention of particular interest in dry skin conditions.[4] These results implicate cannabinoids as possible therapeutic agents for dry skin as well as acne, among others.[5]

Immune dysfunction plays a major role in pathologies of the skin such as acne, allergic contact dermatitis, eczema, psoriasis and rosacea. Psoriasis is an inflammatory disease also characterized by epidermal keratinocyte hyper-proliferation. The exact pathophysiology of psoriasis is not entirely understood, but the immune system and its interaction with nervous system has been investigated as the underlying mechanism.[6] It has been found that multiple cannabinoids (THC, CBD, CBN, CBG) all inhibited keratinocyte proliferation in a non-CB receptor concentration-dependent manner.[7] This inhibition of proliferation is applicable to the effect of cannabinoids on skin tumors as well.

The results of several studies have contributed to our understanding of cannabinoid action on skin conditions, yet sparse information has been gathered about the effect of full plant formulations. Topical (subcutaneous) application of THC (5 mg/kg), reduced allergic inflammation in mice, and helped them heal faster from skin allergies.[8] THC application effectively decreased contact allergic ear swelling and myeloid immune cell infiltration not only in wild-type but also in CB1/2 receptor-deficient mice. Notably, THC was also shown to be able to bypass cannabinoid receptors entirely and directly stimulate keratinocytes to decrease inflammation. In a mouse model of allergic contact dermatitis, topical THC administration showed decreases in myeloid immune cell infiltration, with these beneficial effects existing even in mice with deficient CB1 and CB2 receptors.[9] These results support a potentially wide anti-inflammatory activity of topical THC. THC also reduces pruritis. In

DOI: 10.1201/9781003098201-57

mice, systemic THC reduced the scratching response. Additional mice were treated with an inhibitor of fatty acid amide hydrolase (FAAH). The authors concluded that neuronal FAAH suppression reduces pruritus via CB1 activation, establishing the therapeutic role of cannabinoids in pruritus.[10]

A report of patients with prurigo, lichen simplex and pruritus who applied an emollient cream with a cannabinoid agonist stated an average reduction in itch of 86.4%. In an observational, prospective cohort study of 2,456 patients with atopic dermatitis (AD), the average itch was reduced from 4.89 to 1.97 after 39 days of treatment with a cannabinoid agonist cream – PEACE. PEACE not only reduced pruritus but improved dryness, excoriation, lichenification, scaling and erythema in 70% of patients with AD. Globally, AD symptoms improved substantially in 56% of participants and reduced weekly topical steroid use by 62%. A complete resolution of pruritus was noted in 38% and significant improvement in further 41%.[11] "Topical cannabinoid agonists represent a new effective and well-tolerated therapy for refractory itching of various origins. Creams with a higher concentration may be even more effective with broader indications."[12]

CBD is anti-inflammatory and may be useful for skin conditions as well, although human studies are lacking. In cell studies it was shown that "CBD also exerted complex antiinflammatory actions that were coupled to A2a adenosine receptor-dependent lipostatic, antiproliferative, and antiinflammatory effects, CBD has potential as a promising therapeutic agent for the treatment of acne vulgaris."[13] Mechanisms of CBD inhibition of sebum secretion and sebocyte proliferation include TRPV1, 3 and 4 activation.[14] A retrospective study of 20 patients with psoriasis, atopic dermatitis, or outcome scars showed that topical treatment with CBD-enriched ointment significantly improved spymptoms.[14]

The effect of cannabis and cannabinoids on skin cancer conditions that are systemic such as melanoma is reviewed in a recent publication and discussed in general elsewhere (see Chapter 23).[15] Internal administration of synthetic and phytocannabinoids has been shown to be effective in inducing apoptosis and tumor growth inhibition in vitro and in vivo in multiple skin tumor models.[14] Local application of cannabinoids may be effective in localized skin cancers such as basal cell carcinoma, with many anecdotal reports of success with a concentrated cannabis oil with high THC content. To date, no clinical trials of such a therapy have been reported.

Cannabinoids not only possess anti-inflammatory, immunomodulating, anti-itch qualities, they also are antimicrobial and antifungal. In concert with similar qualities in various terpenes, a cannabis formulation, both internal and topical, provides a potent therapy for many skin conditions. Of the major terpenes found in cannabis terpenes, we recall that β-caryophyllene has antibacterial, antifungal, anti-inflammatory and analgesic effects. α-Pinene is also anti-inflammatory, antibacterial, antifungal, D-linalool is antibacterial, α-humulene is anti-inflammatory and antibacterial, and perhaps most useful of all for skin formulations, D-limonene is antibacterial, antifungal and also assists in the absorption of other terpenoids and cannabinoids through the skin. In general, topical cannabis is the preferred delivery method for skin conditions. The use of topical cannabis for skin disorders ranging from itching, to scaling, swelling and redness has been gaining popularity among medical cannabis patients, and often can substitute for steroid creams or other medications. Transdermal penetration of pure highly lipophilic phytocannabinoids is usually low, they tend to accumulate in the most superficial layers of the epidermis. Balms and salves that have less water content are preferred for eczema treatment.

PATIENT REPORTS

To move on to patient results from my practice, simple skin disorders such as eczema can present in all ages, but those with psoriasis were adults in their 30–60s. Some elderly patients reported pruritis, perhaps as a consequence of their medications or an underlying metabolic condition. Most of the patients represented here had a major skin condition disorder, psoriasis. Other patients seen with skin conditions include dermatitis, pruritis and an account of successful treatment of skin cancer with a cannabis formulation is reported in a subject I followed for 3 years, my cat (see Chapter 12). Here are a few illustrative case reports.

Patient 1: This is a 58-year-old male presenting for "skin spots" and low back pain. He had been using cannabis rarely by vaporizing for low back pain. His history included scarring of his legs from a bout of severe poison ivy as a child. He had multiple actinic keratoses on his legs. On presentation he was not using cannabis for dermatitis issues. I advised applying a topical to his keratotic lesions. At our next visit, he had developed dermatitis on his thorax and arm after a bout of shingles. He was now using an edible daily, and applying topical to his legs but had not applied topical to the post-herpetic lesions, which I then advised. At our last visit, most of the post-herpetic lesions had resolved and he was on a maintenance level of cannabis, applied topically as needed, with rare internal use.

Pearls: The topical benefits of cannabis for skin conditions are not as widely disseminated as its psychoactive or pain-relieving effects. As is the case with many patients, appropriate education about these functions may be left to the professional consultant, even with massive online promotions, especially for CBD-rich topicals. Even with a patient who became aware of topical benefits, he didn't automatically extend this use to additional skin dermatitis issues.

Patient 2: This is a 42-year-old female returning patient with multiple medical conditions including psoriasis, insomnia and fibromyalgia. She had a 28-year history of occasional cannabis use. She had been using cannabis topically for psoriasis plaques, and edibles occasionally for sleep. She was getting acupuncture for her conditions, but was on no medications. She made her own salve and said it "is like magic." She used the topical daily but still had psoriatic rashes on her extremities. Over the next few years, she continued on this regimen and added fresh raw juiced cannabis when available, which helped.

Pearls: Topical cannabis routinely helps to reduce psoriatic plaques. The addition of juiced cannabis is likely to add internal anti-inflammatory benefit. This was a very health-conscious patient, who followed a strict anti-inflammatory diet, exercised and preferred non-psychoactive forms of cannabis, hence daily topical and juiced forms. The effect of cannabinoid acids on autoimmune conditions has been well-documented. It would be interesting to see its effect on psoriasis in topical form, but this has not been reported.

Patient 3: This is 37-year-old male with psoriatic arthritis and psoriasis. He was taking leflunomide daily but still had rashes. He was new to cannabis use. He used topical THC-rich cannabis on his plaques, and he reported that they resolved within 6 weeks. We discussed adding internal use by tincture, which he tried for a while, but stopped, seeing no appreciable change. He did not use enough tincture, nor for a long enough period to make this assessment with finality, but he was satisfied sticking with the topical.

Pearls: This is another case of THC-rich topical being effective for psoriasis. Here, used in conjunction with an immunosuppressive drug, complete remission was achieved. The comorbidity of psoriatic arthritis and psoriasis is common, the former requiring internal cannabis therapy, while often the latter is treated sufficiently with topical.

Patient 4: This is a 65-year-old male who presented with psoriasis, low back pain, hypertension, gout and insomnia. He was new to cannabis use, and on blood pressure medications. He had psoriatic plaques on his arms and legs. We began with a tincture for sleep and topical for psoriasis. He later began a prescription medication for gout. He was erratic in cannabis use, using it only as needed, for pain, psoriasis and sleep. The plaques continued with episodic use of a CBD-rich topical. I advised regular use of a THC-rich topical, which seemed to be more effective.

Pearls: We are often asked which topical is better, CBD or THC? The answer depends on the condition, and, of course, to concentration of the topical. Not all topicals are equivalent, but it may be that THC-rich topicals work better for psoriasis compared to CBD at the same dosage. Although they have both been proven to be effective.[16]

CANNABIS THERAPY SUMMARY

The primary condition for which my patients sought cannabis therapy was psoriasis, in which case both CBD- and THC-containing cannabis creams have been effective. As this is an autoimmune disorder, the addition of internal cannabis and/or THCA-containing topicals would add benefit. In general, it is wise to continue a maintenance dose of once/day of topical with chronic psoriatic plaques even when they are reduced. For more severe cases, 3x/day dosing is preferred. For dermatitis, topical cannabis, especially salves, is also helpful. Salves have the added benefit of forming a water impermeable barrier on the skin, which helps eczema and prolongs action at the epidermal level. For neuropathy such as in pruritis or shingles, a more permeable carrier is recommended for topical use (see discussion of topicals in Chapter 7). Of interest here is the permeation enhancing effect of n-limonene in particular, so products containing this terpene would pass through the dermal layer more effectively than preparations without it. There are currently many formulations over the counter containing CBD that are now being promoted for antiaging and regenerative purposes for skin. Studies are lacking as the efficacy of such a therapy, and should be done. We can anticipate that anti-inflammatory, antioxidative and lipostatic functions as well as the hydrating effects of an appropriate carrier might yield good results.

REFERENCES

1. Bíró T, Tóth B I, Haskó G, Paus R, Pacher P. The endocannabinoid system of the skin in health and disease: novel perspectives and therapeutic opportunities. *Trends Pharmacol Sci.* 2009;30(8):411–420.
2. Richardson J, Kilo S, Hargreaves K. Cannabinoids reduce hyperalgesia and inflammation via interaction with peripheral CB1 receptors. *Pain.* 1998;75(1):111–119.
3. Dubrosi N, Toth BI, Nagy G, et al. Endocannabinoids enhance lipid synthesis and apoptosis of human sebocytes via cannabinoidreceptor-2-mediated signaling. *FASEB J.* 2008;22(10):3685–3695.
4. Zákány N, Oláh A, Markovics A, et al. Endocannabinoid tone regulates human sebocyte biology. *J Investigative Dermatol.* 2018;138:1699–1706.
5. Tóth KF, Ádám D, Bíró T, Oláh A. Cannabinoid signaling in the skin: therapeutic potential of the "c(ut)annabinoid" system. *Molecules.* 2019;24(5):918.
6. Derakhshan N, Kazema M. Cannabis for refractory psoriasis-high hopes for a novel treatment and a literature review. *Curr Clin Pharmacol.* 2016;11(2):146–147.
7. Wilkinson JD, Williamson EM. Cannabinoids inhibit human keratinocyte proliferation through a non-CB1/CB2 mechanism and have a potential therapeutic value in the treatment of psoriasis. *J Dermatol Sci.* 2007;45(2):87–92.
8. Karsak M, Gaffal E, Date R, et al. Attenuation of allergic contact dermatitis through the endocannabinoid system. *Science.* 2007;316:1494.
9. Gaffal E, Cron M, Glodde N, Tüting T. Anti-inflammatory activity of topical THC in DNFB-mediated mouse allergic contact dermatitis independent of CB1 and CB2 receptors. *Allergy.* 2013;68(8):994–1000.
10. Marks DII, Friedman A. The therapeutic potential of cannabinoids in dermatology. *Skin Ther Lett.* 2018;23(6):1–5.
11. Eberlein B, Eicke C, Reinhardt HW, Ring J. Adjuvant treatment of atopic eczema: assessment of an emollient containing N-palmitoylethanolamine (ATOPA study). *J Eur Acad Dermatol Venereol.* 2008;22(1):73–82.
12. Stander S, Reinhardt HW, Luger TA. Topical application of a cream with N-palmitoyl ethanolamine had a good antipruritic effect in most patients. *Hautarzt.* 2006;57:801–807.
13. Olah A, Tóth BI, Borbíró I, et al. Cannabidiol exerts sebostatic and antiinflammatory effects on human sebocytes. *J Clin Invest.* 2014;124(9):3713–3724.
14. Scheau C, Badarau IA, Mihai LG, et al. Cannabinoids in the pathophysiology of skin inflammation. *Molecules.* 2020;25(3):652.
15. Bachari A, Piva TJ, Salami SA, Jamshidi N, Mantri N. Roles of cannabinoids in melanoma: evidence from in vivo studies. *Int J Mol Sci.* 2020;21(17):6040.
16. Palmieri B, Laurino C, Vadalà M. A therapeutic effect of CBD-enriched ointment in inflammatory skin diseases and cutaneous scars. *Clin Ter.* 2019;170(2):e93–e99.

47 Women's Health

WOMEN'S HEALTH AND CANNABIS

Cannabis use for gynecological issues has been documented throughout history.[1] Many of the conditions that might be classified under women's health have multi-factorial components, including mood, pain, poor sleep and/or dysregulation of hormonal balance. Because cannabis can influence all of these regulatory systems, it is an effective choice for women's health complaints. The capacity of cannabis to act as an anti-inflammatory agent, a muscle relaxant, and a pain reliever, all at the same time, make it ideal for pelvic pain conditions, as well as its ability to elevate mood in cases of premenstrual syndrome (PMS), common in younger female patients, or perimenopausal syndrome, common in older female patients.

The endocannabinoid system (ECS) is implicated in all aspects of reproductive physiology and affects hormonal regulation. Female pelvic organs have a high density of cannabinoid receptors. CB1 receptors are highly expressed in the uterus and other non-reproductive organs such as the bladder.[2] Elevated levels of endocannabinoids have been documented in patients with dysmenorrhea and dyspareunia, implying that levels may increase in response to pain. Increased anandamide (AEA) and 2-arachidnylglycerol (2-AG levels) correlate with decreased local CB1 expression in endometriosis, suggesting a negative feedback loop regulation.[3] CB1 receptor agonists decrease, whereas CB1 receptor antagonists increase, endometriosis-associated pain, implying a role for THC in pain reduction.[4] Studies have shown that AEA levels are correlated with serum luteinizing hormone (LH), follicle-stimulating hormone (FSH) and estradiol, but not progesterone levels, throughout the menstrual cycle. Cannabinoids bind not only to CB1 and CB2 receptors but also to G protein-coupled receptors, transient receptor potential ion channels and nuclear peroxisome proliferator-activated receptors in pelvic tissue.[5] Monkey studies showed that high doses of THC given IM or IP through several menstrual cycles transiently disrupt the hypothalamic-pituitary-ovarian (HPO) axis function. THC (2.5 mg/kg) suppressed serum estradiol, progesterone, LH and prolactin, and inhibited ovulation and menses, but the monkeys developed tolerance to these effects.[6] These results have not yet corroborated in humans.

Patients with pelvic pain disorders use cannabis regularly to alleviate pain and uterine cramping. The most common syndrome of pelvic pain in women is associated with PMS and dysmenorrhea, including premenstrual cramping. PMS is a hormonal disorder with a wide range of physical and emotional symptoms that affects about 50% of menstruating women. There is often pelvic/abdominal cramping and bloating, craving for sweets or chocolate, fatigue, breast tenderness and/or mood swings. Cannabis has long been known to alleviate menstrual cramps, one of the most common women's health complaints, affecting up to 80% of younger female patients. As a matter of fact, female patients often list menstrual cramps as a reason for wanting

DOI: 10.1201/9781003098201-58

to use medical cannabis. A 2017 survey of women with PMS or PMDD (premenstrual dysphoric disorder) achieved relief with cannabis.[7] Contrary to expectations however, many patients listing menstrual cramps as a reason for medicinal cannabis use, do use it throughout the month, indicating that they are using it for more than just episodic monthly symptoms. Older female patients also benefit from cannabis, especially in perimenopausal years. A survey-based study conducted in 2016 found that cannabis alleviates certain menopause symptoms, such as sleep problems, irritability, depression and joint pain.[8] A particularly trying symptom is hot flashes, ordinarily responsive to hormone therapy. The fact that CBD-rich cannabis also offers relief is an alternative intervention. This may explain why menopausal sleep disorder is often more responsive to CBD than other forms of insomnia. Other pelvic pain syndromes include endometriosis and uterine fibroids. The effect of the ECS on endometriosis pain has been studied. The long-term consequences of endometriosis result in chronic inflammation, not only pain. Both inflammatory and neuropathic mechanisms contribute to endometriosis-associated pains. Women with endometriosis have lower levels of CB1 receptors in their uterine tissue, and decreased activation of these receptors may lead to worsening pain. As mentioned earlier, CB1 agonists decrease pain, implying a strong role for THC in pain management. The anti-inflammatory action of CBD would be of benefit as well. Cannabinoids may also have antiproliferative effects on endometriosis, in a biphasic, dose-dependent manner.[2] An interview with a researcher at the National Institute of Complementary Medicine (NCIM) Health Research Institute at Western Sydney University revealed the results of a survey done on patients with endometriosis.

> Over 50 per cent of women who were utilising cannabis for their symptoms in the survey, which was about one in 10, had a reduction of 50 per cent of their pharmaceutical usage. . . . They also showed fairly significant improvements across the domains of things like anxiety, depression, sleep, nausea, vomiting and gastro-intestinal upsets.[9]

A recent survey found that patients who used cannabis to address their chronic pelvic pain had a 5.9-point reduction in pain score, as compared to 2.9 points in the control group.[10] In a survey of gynecological cancer patients, 30% were using cannabis regularly, primarily for pain, but as with other cancers, also for appetite, nausea, sleep and mood. Of the women using cannabis, almost half decreased prescription opiates.[11] A group in Canada treating urologic chronic pelvic pain (UCPPS) comment on the frustrations of working with cannabis with their patients for this disorder, applicable to all clinical work with cannabis. They say:

> We have been prescribing medical marijuana for a number of years and are slowly figuring out how to do this properly. We had no textbook, no manual, and no instructions. The literature did not help us. It was really trial and error, with our patients teaching us the optimal strategies for the use of marijuana in UCPPS.[12]

A hot topic currently is cannabis and women's sexual health, some proponents claiming aphrodisiac like effects. Cannabinoids and endocannabinoids interact with the hormones and neurotransmitters that affect sexual behavior. Increases in both physiological and subjective indices of sexual arousal have been significantly associated with decreases in AEA and 2-AG.[13] Early studies on sexuality with cannabis were poorly designed, and did not take into effect tolerance, strain or covariant factors. The influence of cannabis intake on sexual behavior and arousability is thought to be dose-dependent in both men and women. Investigations also reveal a suppression of gonadotropin release by cannabinoids in a dose-dependent fashion.[14] A survey of 373 women found that the use of cannabis products before sexual activity increased sex drive and decreased pain.[15] The challenge here, as with all mood-related issues, is that the causative factors are often multifactorial, may or may not require psychotherapeutic intervention and may or may not require actual hormonal intervention. The actions of cannabis as an aphrodisiac for both women and men is not an area that is easily generalized, nor should it be. Again, we return to the caveat, that cannabis prescription is intimately tied to one's own endocannabinoid and broader physiology.

PATIENT REPORTS

To move on to patient results from my practice, several conditions are represented here for which cannabis has been helpful that specifically happen in females. These include PMS, perimenopausal syndrome, endometriosis and pelvic pain. The age range of patients here is mostly younger and mid-aged adults, up to perimenopause. Here are a few illustrative case reports.

Patient 1: This is a 44-year-old female with perimenopausal symptoms, including mood swings, insomnia and tension headaches. She had a non-total hysterectomy 4 years earlier due to severe menstrual cramping. Her diagnosis was actually PMD, premenstrual disorder, due to her low mood. She had been using a small amount of cannabis for 24 years, about ½ gram/week, now mostly by vaporizing. She said "it removes problems instantly, and I feel capable of doing daily duties." She was on no medications. I suggested she try a small dose of an indica edible before bed for longer sleep, and try a CBD/THC mix for vaporizing. This helped her sleep. Over the next few years, she switched to CBD-rich edibles, 10 mg each day, and vaped indica at night. The mood disorder continued, feeling more like anxiety than depression.

Pearls: This age range from mid-40s to mid-50s in females often brings much endocrine instability, sometimes referred to as premenopausal syndrome. It is not uncommon to have patients who previously complained of PMS now move right into perimenopausal complaints, including insomnia, anxiety and hot flashes. Here we see how the medicine of choice has changed from a THC-rich variety, more helpful for depression, to a CBD-rich cannabis, more helpful for anxiety.

Patient 2: This is a 34-year-old female with endometriosis and anxiety. She had been using cannabis for 15 years, now mostly by 5–10 mg of an edible daily. She was also taking birth control pills, Zoloft and Klonapin, as needed. She preferred the cannabis to Klonapin. I suggested she try a CBD-rich edible, which did help anxiety such that she was able to lower the Zoloft from 100 mg to 50 mg after 10 years on this drug. She also continued an indica edible as needed for sleep. Over the next few years, she was able to find cannabis vaginal suppositories, which were THC-rich, effective for endometriosis pain. She continued to wean Zoloft to 25 mg. The dose of edible she used for sleep increased to 25 mg, so we discussed a tolerance break of

1 night/week. We also discussed how to make her own suppositories, as they were hard to find and costly.

Pearls: Vaginal suppositories are an excellent delivery method to treat any kind of pelvic pain. They are delivered and absorbed primarily locally, so the psychoactive effects are much reduced, allowing for a higher dose of THC acting in the target area. An added benefit was the reduction of Zoloft from 100 mg to 25 mg, facilitated here by a CBD-rich product.

Patient 3: This is a 41-year-old female with menstrual cramps and insomnia. She had been using indica cannabis occasionally by vaporizer. She was on no medications. She reported that it worked immediately for cramps and sleep. As she got older, sleep got worse and she switched to an edible as needed before bed. Cramps worsened as well. I suggested a CBD-rich edible or tincture for daytime use. This helped with cramps and nausea associated with menses. She reported pure CBD was no help, but a CBD/THC mix was helpful.

Pearls: We recall that CBD in pure isolate or distillate form requires a much higher dose that cannabis extracted full-spectrum CBD products. It is no surprise that pure CBD was not effective. Nevertheless, it's usually smart to use a cannabinoid mix for cramps as well as nausea, because both CBD, THC and some terpenes address these issues.

Patient 4: This is a 25-year-old female who presented with post-partum depression and anxiety. She was on Zoloft 50 mg/day. Cannabis use was intermittent for the past 8 years. She was currently off cannabis since the birth of her second child 6 weeks prior. She was concerned about using THC as she was nursing. I advised CBD-rich cannabis. She did find mood improvement with CBD edibles daily, plus rare sativa smoked for relief of depression and fatigue. Hip pain had developed since the delivery, and when she stopped nursing, she increased her THC dose to treat the pain. The post-partum depression was now improved, but her cannabis use increased. She settled upon a regimen of THC-rich edibles, 25 mg, 2×/day, plus CBD capsules. She was advised about tolerance and reducing her dose.

Pearls: The use of cannabis during breastfeeding is a much-disputed issue (see "Pregnancy Risks" in Chapter 6). This patient was able to manage post-partum depression with a CBD-rich product. Products that help depression without THC might be those containing the terpene D-limonene, which acts as a mood elevator, or α-pinene, which helps with fatigue. I don't know the terpene profile of the edible she was using; it was likely not specified. In the case of smoked cannabis while nursing, I always tell my patients to use only 1–2 puffs and do it right after breastfeeding, as its peak effect will occur in 2 hours and will wane before the next feeding. The key here is to not build up an excess that is stored in the milk.

Patient 5: This is a 64-year-old female with chronic pelvic floor pain. This onset after anal fissure repair 15 years earlier. She has not found a useful pain management program, although Paxil helped for a few years, then it stopped being helpful. Currently, she was using a small, 0.25 mg dose of Klonapin prn for pain. Her pain was accompanied by vulvodynia and vaginal spasm, as well as spasm of multiple pelvic perianal, abdominal and low back muscles. She was doing physical therapy and yoga. Her previous cannabis use was erratic. She has tried a CBD/THC 20:1 tincture, and smokes one puff 2–3×/day. This was clearly a case where suppositories would be useful, but they were hard to find in dispensaries. I coached her in how to make them herself and advised 2x/day use. On a 2-month follow-up, she was feeling better, using a low-dose homemade CBD-rich suppository 2x/day. The dose was unclear, but it may have been 10–15 mg. I advised a higher dose suppository, up to 50 mg, used overnight by rectal or vaginal insertion, or rotated between these two. This patient was then lost to follow-up.

Pearls: This case illustrates two important points. Advise suppositories for pelvic, rectal, vaginal or anal pain. It usually works well. And, chronic pelvic pain often has an emotional component, possibly some previous trauma. Cannabis helps the trauma as well as the pain and spasm.

CANNABIS THERAPY SUMMARY

There are a great range of conditions for which cannabis is beneficial in women's health. As far as knowing what, and how much to use, it is best to refer to the relevant chapters on individual conditions, such as anxiety, depression insomnia, muscle spasm or chronic pain. What is unique here is the effect of cannabinoids on hormonal regulation, an area that has yet to be fully explored, let alone understood. As with all endocannabinoid regulation, a small amount of an exogenous cannabinoid, especially THC, goes a long way. An endocannabinoid agonist such as THC can boost a deficient endocannabinoid tone, something that can easily happen during times of hormonal transitions, that is, menstruation, pregnancy, childbirth, post-partum and perimenopause. For this reason, I do encourage the inclusion of some amount of THC-containing cannabis in these conditions. CBD/THC mixed products will likely be the most successful in hormonal regulation, with the least psychoactivity.

The fact that the vagina has a mucous membrane that can readily absorb medicinal products makes vaginal suppositories uniquely suited to treating conditions affecting the women's reproductive system, especially for pelvic pain. Topicals come in handy for menstrual cramps, applied to the uterine area as well as the low back. Topicals can also be applied vaginally, for pain, spasm or for relief of genital herpes. One of my patients reported that vaginal topical use did not help her lichen sclerosis, but did help the itch. Unfortunately, often suppositories are hard to find, but the internet does offer recipes for home production. The inclusion of indica products is especially useful for muscle spasm complaints, either vaginally, topically or internally, because β-myrcene is also a muscle relaxant.

REFERENCES

1. Russo E. Cannabis treatments in obstetrics and gynecology: a historical review. *J Cannabis Ther.* 2002;2(3–4):5–35.
2. Bouaziz J, Bar On A, Seidman DS, Soriano D. The clinical significance of endocannabinoids in endometriosis pain management. *Cannabis Cannabinoid Res.* 2017;2(1):72–80.
3. Sanchez AM, Cioffi R, Viganò P, et al. Elevated systemic levels of endocannabinoids and related mediators across the menstrual cycle in women with endometriosis. *Reprod Sci.* 2016;23:1–9.

4. Dmitreiva N, Nagabukuro H, Resuehr D, et al. Endocannabinoid involvement in endometriosis. *Pain*. 2010;151(3):703–710.
5. Luschnig P, Schicho R. Cannabinoids in gynecological diseases. *Med Cannabis Cannabinoids*. 2019;2:1.
6. Brents LK. Marijuana, the endocannabinoid system and the female reproductive system. *Yale J Biol Med*. 2016;89(2):175–191.
7. Slavin M, Barach E, Farmer S, Luba R, Earleywine M. Cannabis and symptoms of PMD and PMDD. *Addict Res Theory*. 2017;25(5):383–389.
8. Slavin M, Farmer S, Earleywine M. Expectancy mediated effects of marijuana on menopause symptoms. *Addict Res Theory*. 2016;24(4):322–329.
9. Medhora S. Could medicinal cannabis be the new frontier in treating period pain? 2020. www.abc.net.au/triplej/programs/hack/can-medicinal-cannabis-cure-symptoms-period-pain-endometriosis/11873296 Accessed March 10, 2020.
10. Johns C, Lachiewicz M. Cannabis for treatment of chronic pelvic pain: a survey of prevalence and effectiveness. *Obstet Gynecol*. 2019;133:90S.
11. Blake EA, Ross M, Ihenachoc U, et al. Nonprescription cannabis use for symptom management amongst women with gynecologic malignancies. *Gynecol Oncol Rep*. 2019;30:100497.
12. Nickel JC. Medical marijuana for urologic chronic pelvic pain. *Can Urol Assoc J*. 2018;12(6 Suppl 3):S181–S183.
13. Klein C, Hill MN, Chang SC, Hillard CJ, Gorzalka BB. Circulating endocannabinoid concentrations and sexual arousal in women. *J Sex Med*. 2012;9(6):1588–1601.
14. Gorzalka BB, Hill MN, Chang SCH. Male-female differences in the effects of cannabinoids on sexual behavior and gonadal hormone function. *Horm Behav*. 2010;58(1):91–99.
15. Lynn BK, López JD, Miller C, Thompson J, Campian EC. The relationship between marijuana use prior to sex and sexual function in women. *Sex Med*. 2019;7:192–197.

Appendix
Acknowledgment of Disclosure

I _____ (Patient Name), understand that cannabis is a medicine used in treating the suffering caused by serious and debilitating medical conditions. I understand that under the Controlled Substance Act of 1970 cannabis is categorized as Schedule I, defining it as having no proven medical value, with potential for abuse. I understand that the use of cannabis could impair my ability to drive or operate heavy machinery. I have been advised that cannabis smoke may cause a cough and contains chemicals that may be harmful to my health. I understand that side effects may occur while I am medicated with cannabis.

Side effects of cannabis use, specific to THC, can include, but are not limited to:

- Change in mood/sensation
- Nervousness
- Dizziness
- Problem with memory/confusion
- Palpitations/fast heart beat
- Dry mouth
- Impairment of motor skills, reaction time and physical coordination
- Difficulty in completing complex tasks
- Hunger

Side effects of cannabis use, specific to CBD, can include, but are not limited to:

- Change in mood/sensation
- Dry mouth
- Difficulty with sleep
- Loose stools

Cannabis varies in potency. The effects of cannabis can also vary with the delivery system. Estimating the proper cannabis dosage is very important. Overdosage is more likely to occur with ingestion and/or the use of concentrates. I understand that some patients can become dependent on cannabis and may experience withdrawal symptoms when they stop using marijuana. Signs of withdrawal can include feelings of depression, irritability, restlessness or mild agitation, sleep disturbance, unusual tiredness, trouble concentrating and loss of appetite. I understand that the cannabis plant is not regulated by the United States Food and Drug Administration and therefore may contain unknown quantities of active ingredients, impurities or contaminants.

Appendix: Patient History Questionnaire

Name _____ Male ❑/Female ❑ Date_____

Age _____ Date of Birth _____ Birthplace _____

Current Address_____
                        (street address)   (city)   (state)   (zip)

Phone _____ Cell phone _____ e-mail _____

Occupation _____ Unemployed ___ Retired ___ Disabled___Student/

Where? _____

Chief Complaint:
List the medical problems for which you use or would like to use cannabis (i.e. nausea, pain, sleep, etc.)

_____

Medical History: (✓ check box if you now have, or have ever had any of the problems listed)

❑ Arthritis (OA, RA, other)
❑ Back or neck pain
❑ Blood disorders (anemia, abn. clotting)
❑ Brain disorders (epilepsy, trauma, etc.)
❑ Bladder (cystitis, neurogenic)
❑ Cancer, specify:
❑ Chronic pain, specify:
❑ Circulation (stroke, phlebitis, etc.)
❑ Diabetes
❑ Dystonia (spasms, tremors, Parkinsons)
❑ Ear (tinnitus, hearing loss)
❑ Eating disorder (anorexia, bulimia)
❑ Endocrine (thyroid, adrenal, hormones)
❑ Eye (glaucoma, cataracts, macular deg)
❑ Genital/GYN problems
❑ Headache/Migraine headache
❑ Heart disease

❑ Herpes/Herpes zoster (shingles)
❑ High blood pressure
❑ HIV/AIDS
❑ Intestinal disorders (ulcers, colitis, IBS, reflux)
❑ Kidney disease (stones, renal failure)
❑ Liver disease (cirrhosis, hepatitis)
❑ Lung disease (asthma, emphysema, COPD)
❑ Mental health disorders (see below)
❑ Multiple sclerosis (neurodegenerative disease)
❑ Prostate disease
❑ Rheumatic disease (Lupus, other autoimmune disease)
❑ Skin disorders (psoriasis, eczema, pruritis)
❑ Sleep disorders (insomnia, sleep apnea, restless legs)
❑ Substance abuse (see below)
❑ Weight loss/gain
❑ Other_____

Appendix: Patient History Questionnaire

Mental Health History:
Have you ever been diagnosed with any of the following? (enter approximate age or date)

ADD or ADHD_____ Anger_____ Anxiety_____ Bipolar disorder_____

Brain trauma_____ Dementia_____ Depression_____ Mood disorder_____

PTSD_____ Schizophrenia_____

Reproductive History (females):
# of pregnancies _____ # of children _____ Currently pregnant? Yes/No
Breastfeeding? Yes/No

Surgical History: Please list any surgeries and approximate dates

_____   _____

_____   _____

Health Care Information:
Name, location, phone of your health care professional (physician, chiropractor, therapist, etc.)

_____

Time of last visit?_____ Have you talked to your doctor about cannabis?
Yes/No

Current prescription medications (Or supplements, herbal medications, etc.):
Please list below
1. _____ Dosage _____ Frequency _____ Duration _____
2. _____ Dosage _____ Frequency _____ Duration _____
3. _____ Dosage _____ Frequency _____ Duration _____
4. _____ Dosage _____ Frequency _____ Duration _____

Lifestyle and Habits
Substance Use – Do you currently use?
Tobacco Yes/ No # cigarettes/day____, for how long____, Prior use? Yes/ No, Quit date? _____
Alcohol Yes/ No # of drinks/ week___, for how long____, Prior use? Yes/ No, Quit date? _____
Cocaine / Methamphetamine / Opiates / Heroin / Other Yes (circle which ones)
Are you on probation or parole? Yes/No   Do you have a pending cannabis case? Yes/No
Diet: Which do you eat on a daily basis? (circle all that apply)
Meat / Dairy / Processed foods / Fast food / Soda / Vegetables / Fruits / Sweets / White flour
How much coffee/or caffeine drinks do you drink in a day? _____
How much water do you drink in a day? _____

Appendix: Patient History Questionnaire

Exercise: What do you do for exercise? (circle all that apply)
Walk / Run / Bike / Sports / Dance / Swim / Martial arts / Other _____
Times/week? _____

Cannabis Use Pattern:
Are you new to cannabis use? Yes/No   How long have you been using cannabis?
_____
Have you ever been issued a cannabis recommendation? Yes/No
Preferred method of medicating: Circle all that apply
Pipe Bong Joint Vaporizer Concentrate (oil, keif) Edibles Tincture Topical Other
If you ingest, describe in what form _____
I use cannabis for my medical problem:
__every day or almost every day __more than once a week __more than once a
month.
On the days I use cannabis, I use it __1–2 times __ 2–3 times __more than 3 times
How much do you use per day/week/month? (i.e. #g/day, #oz/month) _____
My medicine comes from __grow my own __a dispensary __a delivery service __
other source
How does cannabis compare with your usual prescribed medicines in relieving your
symptoms?
_____
Do you take breaks from using cannabis? If so, for how long? _____ How often? _____
Reason for cannabis abstinence – check all that apply
___tolerance break ___financial – can't afford it ___access/can't find preferred form
of medicine ___health condition has improved ___other_____

All of the above is true to the best of my knowledge _____
                                                            (patient signature)

Appendix: Physician's Statement

Regarding California Health and Safety Code 11362.5

This statement certifies that

_____ DOB: _____

Is a patient under my consultative care and treatment for a serious medical condition.

The following is true:
1. I am a licensed physician in good standing in California and I have provided medical consultation services to the above patient.
2. I have examined this patient on the date specified below as "Examination Date."
3. I am identifying this patient as being qualified to use cannabis therapeutically due to his/her serious medical condition as defined by the California Health and Safety Code 11326.7 (h), and approve the medical use of cannabis by this patient.
4. I have discussed the medical benefits and risks of cannabis use with this patient as a treatment for this medical condition.
5. The patient has been advised to seek further medical consultation as appropriate for the duration of this recommendation.
6. The patient has authorized me to discuss the contents of this letter for purposes of verification.
7. This statement is a part of this patient's permanent medical record.

_____
MD Name
License #

Examination Date

_____

Expiration Date

_____

*TO VERIFY: Call _____

Patient Signature:

_____

Appendix: Elderly Patient Survey

1. Name/Date of birth/Date of interview

   _____

2. List of your medical conditions

   _____

3. Condition(s) for which cannabis is being used

   _____

4. Date cannabis begun/Discontinued? If so, why?

   _____

5. Dosage, delivery of cannabis, and product(s) used

   _____

6. List of medicines you're taking

   _____

7. Any change in medicines since using cannabis

   _____

8. Any change in symptoms since cannabis begun

   _____

9. How you feel about using cannabis

   _____

10. Any other comments?

    _____

Index

Printed in the United States
by Baker & Taylor Publisher Services